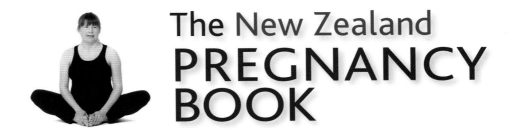

The New Zealand
PREGNANCY
BOOK

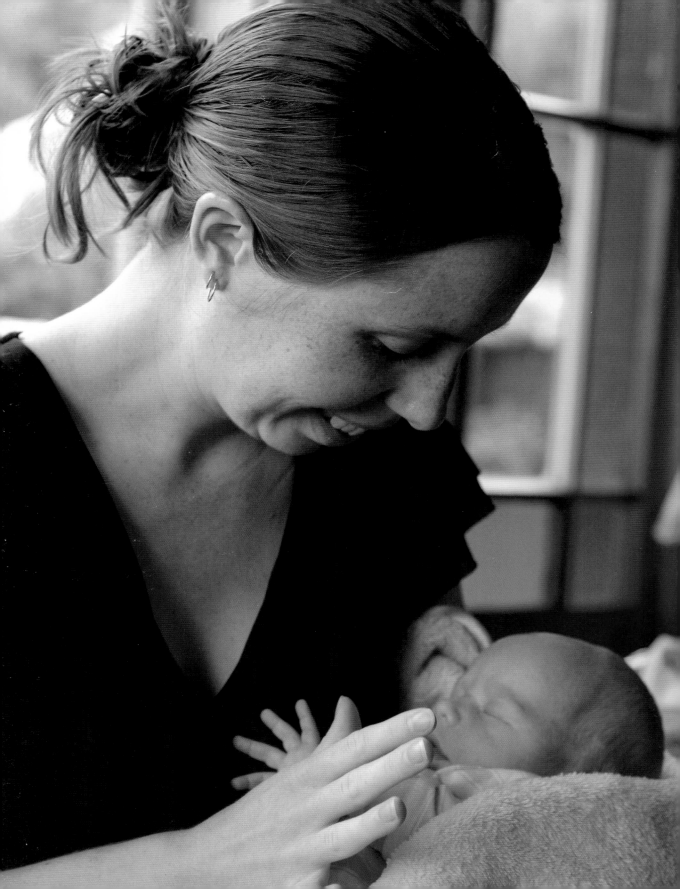

The New Zealand
PREGNANCY
BOOK

A guide to pregnancy, birth
and a baby's first three months

Third edition

Sue Pullon and Cheryl Benn

Photographer: Daniel Allen
Editor: Margot Schwass

 BRIDGET WILLIAMS BOOKS

Third edition published in 2008 by Bridget Williams Limited, P O Box 12 474, Thorndon, Wellington 6144.
Reprinted 2009, 2011.

The New Zealand Pregnancy Book was first published in 1991, with text written by Sue Pullon, illustrations provided by Becky Bliss and photographs by Louise Goossens. A second edition was produced, by the same team, in 1999. The third edition has been produced with the support of the BWB Publishing Trust.

National Library of New Zealand Cataloguing-in-Publication Data

Pullon, Sue.
The New Zealand pregnancy book: a guide to pregnancy, birth
and a baby's first three months / Sue Pullon and Cheryl Benn;
photographer Daniel Allen; editor Margot Schwass. 3rd ed.
Previous ed.: The New Zealand pregnancy book: conception,
pregnancy, birth and life with a new baby / Sue Pullon;
illustrations by Becky Bliss; photographs by Louise Goossens.
1999.
Includes index.
ISBN 978-1-877242-40-3
1. Pregnancy—New Zealand. 2. Childbirth—New Zealand.
3. Newborn infants—Care. I. Benn, Cheryl. II. Schwass, Margot.
III. Allen, Daniel. IV. Title.
618.200993—dc 22

Disclaimer Although every effort has been made to ensure that the information and advice given in the book is as accurate as possible, it is not intended to be a substitute for individual care and advice from a health professional. Information in a book such as this is necessarily of a general nature, and it may not apply to the particular circumstances of individual women. The authors can take no clinical responsibility for readers of this book. All women who are pregnant, contemplating pregnancy, or who have recently been pregnant are strongly advised to seek appropriate professional health care. Similarly, all parents and caregivers of babies and small children are urged to enrol with a Well Child and primary care provider, for both regular and emergency health care.

Photographs The photographs included fall into two groups. Many are included (without captions) to offer a general illustration of the experience of pregancy, birth or life with a new baby; these photographs are not specifically connected to the text or pages where they occur. Another group of photographs documents particular aspects of the experience: as their captions indicate, these photographs are related to the subject covered in the pages where they occur.

Edited by Margot Schwass, Susi Bailey and Ali Carew
Indexed by Diane Lowther
Photography by Daniel Allen (except as indicated above)
Illustrations by Adam Errington
Design and layout by Mission Hall Creative
Printed in Singapore by South Wind Production

Contents

Preface

This book first came into existence nearly 20 years ago, written when I was at home with my third baby, born in 1988. At the time, there was a dearth of good-quality, detailed pregnancy-related information for New Zealand women; I wanted to produce a resource that women in this country could use when contemplating pregnancy and first becoming mothers. Becky Bliss was a dedicated colleague, undertaking all the illustrations. Bridget Williams, then managing director of Allen & Unwin New Zealand, enthusiastically agreed to publish the book. Resources to produce that first edition were non-existent, but we harnessed enormous goodwill from many quarters and saw the book successfully launched in 1991. One of the outstanding contributions was made by photographer Louise Goossens, who did all the original photography for nothing more than the cost of the film she used. In 1999, the book was revised as a popular second edition.

For the third edition some ten years later, it was clear that a range of expertise would be required to create a contemporary resource for the next generations of parents. In particular, a significant midwifery component was essential, and I was delighted when Cheryl Benn agreed to co-author this new edition. Working with Cheryl on a large collaborative project previously, I had been impressed with her research integrity and international midwifery experience. It has been a privilege to welcome Cheryl onto the NZPB team.

For *The New Zealand Pregnancy Book* has become, after 18 years, a professional team effort. With Bridget Williams still as publisher, we have been joined by a photographer, Daniel Allen, writer Margot Schwass and physiotherapist Yvonne Ferguson, with Māori reviewers Hope Tupara and Donna Cormack. Many New Zealanders have shared with us their stories of pregnancy and birth; many more have shared their experiences through an amazing series of photographs. Experts in several fields have read, commented and written. The process of planning together and negotiating text, viewpoints, stories, comments, photography, illustrations and design in a way that serves modern families, and reflects societal and legislative change, has been an amazing team journey for everyone involved. It has been as much a challenge in its own way as writing the original manuscript on the end of the kitchen table, pen in one hand and baby-feeding spoon in the other.

These contributions enrich the book immeasurably, and we hope they will help to make it accessible to all kinds of people throughout New Zealand. As authors and coordinators for the project, Cheryl and I have also sought to present what we know about pregnancy, birth and baby care as clearly and fully as possible. Our views are of course our own, and we acknowledge that not all would share them: what we offer here is simply part of the range of views in this country about life in general, and pregnancy and parenting in particular. We hope that these pages, in various ways, will help women, their partners and their families with pregnancy, birth and the first months with a new baby.

Sue Pullon
July 2008

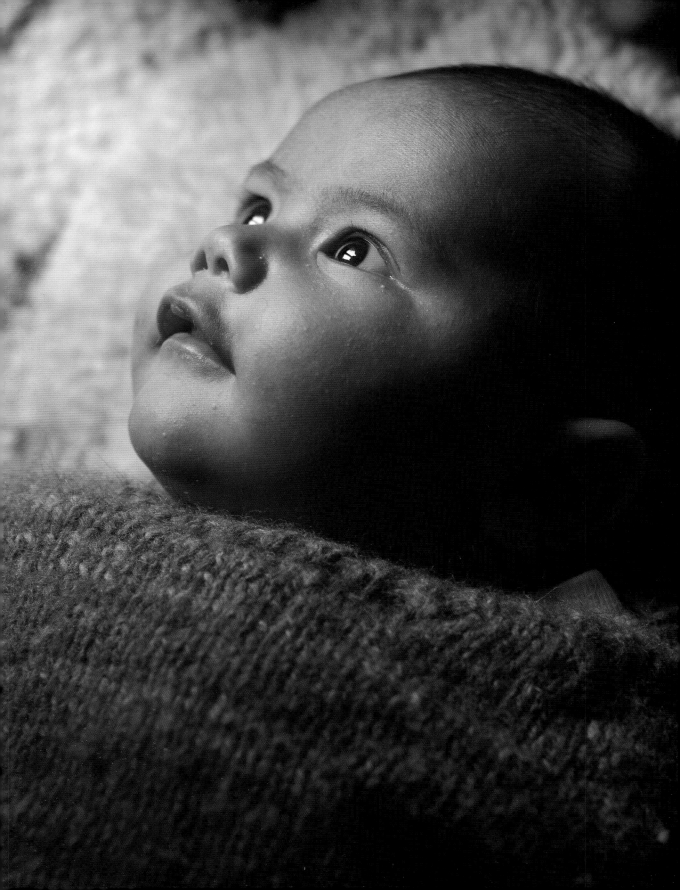

Introduction

The New Zealand Pregnancy Book has been a valued resource for New Zealand parents since it was first published in 1991. Many thousands of copies have found their way into New Zealand homes, midwifery and medical practices, antenatal groups and hospitals. Its popularity has reflected the ongoing demand for such a reference book, written expressly for and by New Zealanders. This completely revised and updated third edition now offers the next generation of parents the latest information about pregnancy, childbirth and life with a new baby.

In both health care and family life, there has been enormous change in New Zealand over recent decades – changes in the health system, in pregnancy care, and in women's and men's expectations about having children. The median age at which women bear children has climbed steadily to 30 years in 2008, from 25 years in 1968;[1] increasingly, too, women are remaining in paid work during their child-bearing years. Families tend to be smaller, with one or two children. Family groups are far more diverse than they used to be; single-parent families, same-sex parent families, blended families and extended families are common. Paid parental leave, reusable nappies, properly engineered buggies and backpacks, prenatal diagnostic testing, sophisticated infertility treatments, the routine offering of HIV testing in pregnancy, universal newborn hearing testing and many other new options have all become available in the last few years.

The care of women during pregnancy has also undergone considerable transformation. Since 1991, midwives have been able to practise independently to provide maternity care; and with the introduction of the Lead Maternity Care funding system in 1996, shared care between midwives and doctors largely disappeared. A small number of GPs still work with midwives to deliver babies, mainly in rural areas, but this arrangement is very unusual. Midwives now care completely for about 80 per cent of pregnant women in New Zealand, with the other 20 per cent choosing combined midwife and specialist obstetrician care.

Across the range of options for care, there has been a stronger commitment to providing services that meet the needs of Māori – services that acknowledge the role of whānau, for example, or that draw on traditional Māori tikanga and practices around childbirth and pregnancy. Health services have also developed in response to New Zealand's growing Pacific and new migrant communities.

One of the biggest shifts in the last decade has been the explosion of information on health, pregnancy and childbirth available online via the Internet. By world standards, New Zealanders are avid and expert Internet users. Many parents who read this book will no doubt supplement the information it provides by referring to the Internet, including the many useful websites listed in the Appendix.

The third edition of *The New Zealand Pregnancy Book* responds to all these developments, offering the next generation of parents a comprehensive guide to help them navigate this new landscape. Each step of pregnancy, childbirth and the baby's first months is set out with detailed information and clear diagrams. A remarkable set of photographs brings the journey to life, expressing the feelings that are so vividly present throughout. Personal stories amplify the text, offering readers insight into the joys and delights of this profound experience, and also the risks and difficulties.

The book draws on many years of experience in midwifery and maternal health care by the two expert authors, GP Sue Pullon and midwife Cheryl Benn. A wide range of evidence-based reference material has been consulted and incorporated, with specific references given where new or controversial information is included. Sources are listed at the end of the book. The book encompasses not only modern midwifery care and obstetric practice, but also primary health care, pre- and post-pregnancy care, and current welfare and health care legislation. While no single resource can provide the full range of perspectives or a complete range of information, *The New Zealand Pregnancy Book* will help prepare the pregnant reader, her partner and her family for what lies ahead, and provide an insight into what pregnancy and childbirth in New Zealand look like in the twenty-first century.

Using this book

The text is arranged chronologically, from pre-pregnancy to the end of the first three months with a new baby. In both the first and the last chapters, we have included information about general health and well-being for women (and their families), as this is so important in setting the scene for healthy pregnancy and good parenting. We describe women's health, pregnancy, birth and early parenting as part of a continuous life process, in which basic elements such as a good diet and regular exercise can have far-reaching benefits.

The book is designed to be read chapter by chapter as pregnancy progresses, but specific sections can equally well be dipped into as questions arise. Many chapters start with a section on 'What's happening?', explaining the remarkable physical changes that take place in a woman's body during pregnancy, birth and beyond; they also cover 'Feelings' and common problems such as tiredness, nausea and backache, and offer useful advice on 'Helping yourself'. Sections on 'Complications' and 'Continuing health care' are also part of most chapters. In addition, there are regular sections addressed to partners and support people, suggesting how best they can help a woman during pregnancy, birth and beyond. Throughout the book, the chapters are interwoven with extended life stories, in which New Zealand women and men share their own experiences of pregnancy and birth and as new parents. (In the interests of balance, the baby is referred to as 'he' in some chapters and 'she' in others: this is a book for all parents, regardless of whether they have a boy or a girl.)

We have avoided undue duplication by cross-referencing to different sections in the text; the glossary, index and contents list should help readers find their way around easily. Addresses for relevant websites and contact details for useful organisations are listed in the Appendix. Inevitably, new information will come to hand that may alter the current advice provided here. If in doubt, check alternative sources and ask health professionals for the most up-to-date information.

The people who made the book

The New Zealand Pregnancy Book was created by a team with a wide range of complementary knowledge and skills. To create such a rich resource, many people have given time and expertise to the project. Their contributions are outlined below. A particular debt is owed to those who shared, in photographs and stories, some of life's most intensely private and deeply felt experiences. Through their generosity, this book has gained a rare energy and immediacy.

Sue Pullon, the principal author, trained as a doctor and then as a GP in the 1970s and early 1980s. She has worked as a GP ever since, continuing part-time while her own three children were small. She has postgraduate qualifications in obstetrics, general practice and primary health care. Since 1994, she has been a Senior Lecturer in the Department of Primary Health Care and General Practice at the University of Otago, Wellington, where she teaches undergraduate medical students, supervises and teaches postgraduate studies for primary health care professionals, and researches women's health, health promotion and inter-professional learning.

Cheryl Benn, principal co-author, trained as a nurse and midwife in South Africa in the mid-1970s, and has practised as a midwife from that time on. After the birth of her two children, she moved to New Zealand in the early 1990s and worked as a lecturer in midwifery at Massey University. Since 2000 she has practised as a lead maternity carer while continuing her teaching and research into breastfeeding, midwifery practice and the health needs of women in New Zealand. Cheryl has been an International Board Certified Lactation Consultant since 1992, and is Midwifery Adviser to the MidCentral District Health Board.

Yvonne Ferguson, physiotherapist adviser and contributor, has post-graduate qualifications in women's health physiotherapy, and has provided expert physiotherapy care for pregnant women in the Nelson area for many years. She is passionate and knowledgeable about the role of exercise and movement in daily life, especially as part of the active enjoyment and management of pregnancy.

Margot Schwass worked with Sue Pullon and Cheryl Benn on the text, providing expert editorial advice for the book as a whole. Margot also worked with all the pregnant women and new parents who shared their stories for this new edition – some by writing, some by being interviewed. Margot has many years experience as a writer and editor, including working with people from different cultures and faiths to produce *Last words: Approaches to death in New Zealand's different cultures and faiths* (BWB). She works regularly with organisations such as the Bioethics Council, the Health and Disability Commissioner, and the Institute of Judicial Studies.

Hope Tupara and **Donna Cormack** reviewed the book from a Māori perspective, making a range of contributions. Hope Tupara (Ngāi Tamanuhiri, Ngāi Te Rangihouhiri, Kāi Tahu) is an experienced midwife with a background as a midwifery lecturer. She also served on the Midwifery Council of New Zealand and as a national committee member for the New Zealand College of Midwives. Donna Cormack (Waitaha, Kāti Mamoe, Kāi Tahu) is a health researcher at the Eru Pomare Research Unit at the Wellington School of Medicine and Health Sciences, University of Otago. Her research interests are Māori health, ethnic disparities in health, access to health services, and racism. Donna participated in this project as a new mother, her first child having been born as the book was being written.

Janice Wenn and **Lani Wills** provided Māori and Pacific Island perspectives. Janice Wenn (Ngāti Kahungungu ki Wairarapa) and Lani Wills from Tonga both have extensive nursing backgrounds. They have shared wise and special reflections from their experience.

Adam Errington has been illustrating for a wide variety of media since 1990, with clients in New Zealand and the UK. His work ranges from advertising storyboards to corporate logos, from diagrams to woodcuts. The diagram style used in this book was developed to convey information in the clearest way for a general audience.

Daniel Allen is an independent professional photographer whose work includes commissions for publishers in many fields. He was brought into the project by Robbie Burton, whose expertise in photographic publishing at Craig Potton Publishing is warmly acknowledged here. Dan and his wife, Sarah, have three young children and are based in Nelson, part of a large and vibrant community of parents and their children. Dan has been privileged to meet and get to know the many parents and prospective parents who agreed to be photographed for the book.

Jeanette Ware worked tirelessly with Dan and all the families involved to organise the photography, respecting what worked for people and what didn't, making sure people had all the information they needed, keeping the paperwork in order, and establishing and strengthening family and community networks.

Acknowledgements

The third edition of *The New Zealand Pregnancy Book* draws on the work of many people, some named above, some below, and others who wished to remain anonymous. Many in the community have also contributed in less identifiable ways. The publishers and authors offer here their heartfelt thanks to all who have participated.

Expert reviewers/contributors

Sharron Cole (Midwifery Council); Heidi Cooke (neuro-developmental therapist); Donna Cormack (as above); Joanne Dixon (cytogeneticist); Yvonne Ferguson (as above); Claude Preitner (medical advisor – aviation); Martin Sowter (obstetrician); Hope Tupara (as above); Jenny Visser (medical adviser – travel); Janice Wenn (as above); Lani Wills (as above).

Personal stories and other contributions

Natalie Anderson; Ngawari Carr; Donna Cormack; Charles Dawson; Victoria Feltham; Yuliya Gultekin; Ivy Liang; Anna Macey; Erena Powell; Chrissy Severinsen; Elinor Thomas; Michelle Wilson. Names and other identifying details in the personal stories and comments have been altered where requested.

Photography

The support of midwives, doctors and antenatal groups in establishing and strengthening connections in the Nelson area, where the photographer was principally located, was invaluable to this aspect of the book. The assistance of the Nelson-Marlborough District Health Board, Nelson Hospital, and the managers and clinical staff of Nelson Hospital Obstetric and Neonatal Units, where several of the birth sequences were photographed, and women and their babies cared for, is warmly acknowledged. The publishers are grateful also to photographers Shaun Barnett (pp.19, 123 and 404), Paul McCredie (pp.35 and 88) and Phil Press (p.122) for the contribution made by their work.

The following people all gave assistance with photography in different ways.
Midwives: Midwives in the Nelson region (especially Cat Allan; Anna Bannister; Paula Bethwaite; Ruth Brodbeck; Celia Butler; Vicky Chamberlayne; Wendy de Groot; Bridie Fahey; Gillian Gallacher; Janice Hayes; Suzi Hume; Aunouska Myer; Celia Rodley; Ellie Rudd). *Obstetricians:* Flora Gastrell; Kevin Hill; David Leadbetter. *Radiologist:* Chris Leaper. *Nurses and nurse managers:* Margaret Derry; Maureen Higgs; Lois Mctaggart; Katherine Rock; Jean Werry. *Other groups:* Aquanatal Group at Riverside Pool; Atawhai Playcentre; Birth Wise Wellington (especially Caroline McGlinchy); BodyPower Prenatal Yoga; Family Start; Nelson Multi-Ethnic Council; Nelson Parents Centre; Nelson/Tasman Settlement Support (especially Sonny Alesana); Te Korowai Trust (especially Carol Hunter); Whakatu Marae Health and Social Services (especially Carolina Hippolite); Aynsley and Derek Wilkinson, Baby on the Move.

The photographs reproduced here were selected from a wide-ranging collection, almost all taken especially for this book. Many people participated in the photography – pregnant women, couples, their families, friends, young women and men. Those who wish to be named are listed here.
Sarah Allen; Simon Beardsley; Jana Benbow; Keith Berrington and Noriko Matsumoto; Arko and Smita Biswas; Debbie Cole; Amy Danks and Marcus Roebuck; Karen and Hamish Darling; Julia de Weck; Carol Edmonds; Jason Elliot and Emily Street; Deborah and Peter England; Tineke Fancourt; Jonathan and Alana Hawke; Jenny and Niall Heeran; Katja Huibers; Clare Jones; Janine Kerr and Mark Neal; Nicola Kidson; Alarni Knowles; Karen Lewis; Hayley Lukies; Chris and Darlene Mahoney; Isabella Mason; Marcia and Brendyn Montgomery; Vera Moore; Sarah and Mathew Newton; Jessica Nicholas; Rochelle and Ray Nicholls-Clapp; Tania Norfolk and Matt Lawrey; Kereana Norton and her family; Rania Paul and her family; Andrea Pearson; Louise Percy; Katie Poole and Cameron West; Tanya Price; Ceridwyn Roberts and Carla Morris; Jasmine Robins and Doug Roberts; Jackie and David Sampson; River Seligman and Kainga Ropiha; Saskia Sheehan and Gavin Priest; Holly Joy Simpson; Fira and Jeff Smith; Annie Spurdle and Monica Manning; Tania Stanton; Kirsty Stark; Kim Stark; Yvonne Stirrup; Casey Thomas and Thomas Paton; Heidi and Chris Thompson; Louise Thornley; Tania Toa; Susan Todd; Liz Tui Morris; Rohan Wakefield and Annie Boanas; Lee-Anne Weenink; Roger and Anna Wilde; Anna Wills.

The babies and children whose photographs appear in this book are not named. Their place is acknowledged here: the book is for them and their generation.

Editorial and production team
Susi Bailey; Alison Carew; Diane Lowther; Mission Hall Creative (especially Eion Abernethy, Norris Childs, Chris Mahoney, Grant Sutherland); Margot Schwass; Jo Scully; Bridget Williams.

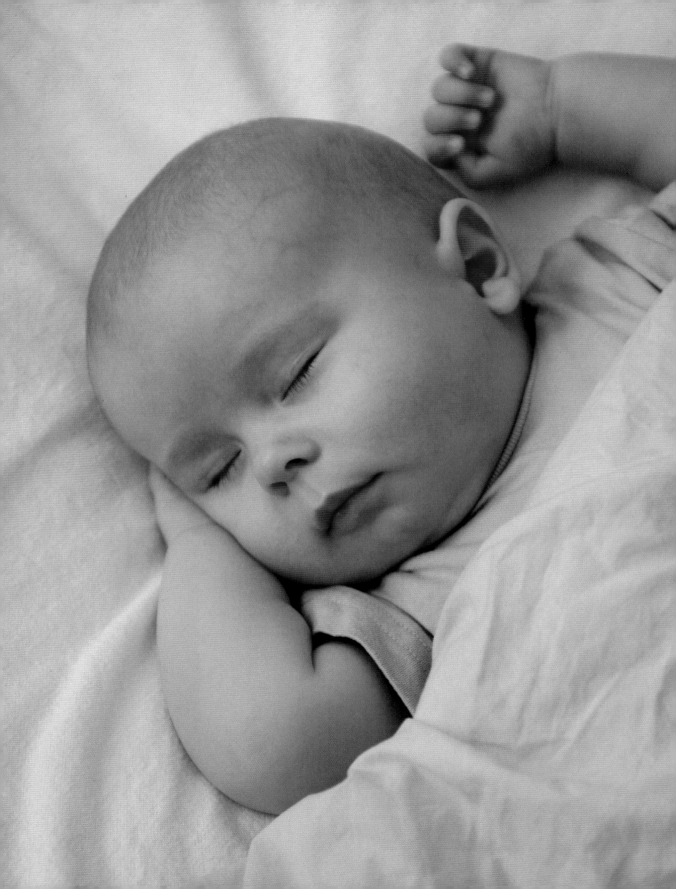

CHAPTER 1

Planning for pregnancy

1. Being in good health

So you're thinking about having a baby. The first step is to make sure you're in good health. But what's so good about being healthy? Aren't most younger New Zealanders reasonably healthy anyway? Yes – but only if they are physically active, eat good food in moderation, don't smoke or drink too much alcohol, don't take other recreational drugs, and feel reasonably good about themselves most of the time. Prevention and/or early treatment of common health problems like infections also help.

The pressures of modern life can easily compromise these basic elements of good health. Yet being in good physical, mental and emotional health is the best possible preparation for pregnancy.

For both women and men, conception, pregnancy and having children are all part of a continuum of social and reproductive life, and no single aspect occurs in isolation. A woman's pre-existing health greatly influences her pregnancy, and probably starts as early as the environment she herself experienced in the womb.[1] In turn, a healthy pregnancy may well be important for her child's own future reproductive health.

In countries like New Zealand, many of us tend to take good health for granted and forget that, at least in part, we owe our health to good nutrition, good sanitation and adequate housing. Those in developing countries often do not enjoy these privileges, let alone adequate health care. On a world scale, New Zealanders are generally privileged people, although it is still hard for some to find suitable housing or good food. But, as individuals, how good are we at taking responsibility for our own health?

Nutrition for all women

We can all choose what we eat. In New Zealand, our problem is generally not a lack of food but the ready availability of foods, especially those with a high fat content. The National Nutrition Survey 1997 showed that the average weight of New Zealanders increased by about 3kg between 1989 and 1997. In the future, it is likely that poor nutrition will lead to even more people becoming obese.

To choose the food that's best, it's good to know more about it. Much of the following information is based on Ministry of Health guidelines that draw on a wide range of nutritional evidence and take into account New Zealand lifestyles, eating habits, and preferred foods.[2]

Every food item contains one or more of the three main food types: proteins, carbohydrates (sugars and starches) and fats. In general, the food we eat should be mostly complex carbohydrates (starches), but also include a moderate amount of protein, a little fat, and a very small amount of simple carbohydrates (sugars).

Food also needs to contain a certain amount of indigestible matter (fibre), which is usually tough cellulose material from plants, although meat contains some fibre too. Fibre stays in the intestines while other substances are absorbed for the body to use. Fibre assists the passage of waste products through the small intestine, then the large intestine, and out of the body as faeces.

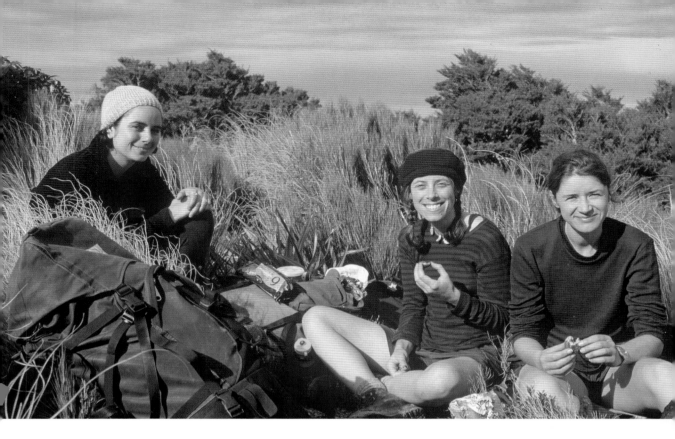

Vitamins and minerals are present in tiny amounts in various foods. These substances are required by the body to allow essential biochemical reactions to take place. For healthy people, all the minerals and vitamins they need are available in food – provided they eat a good variety, in approximately the right proportions.

Everyone needs a little salt to maintain correctly concentrated body fluid. But we need only tiny amounts, and our food usually contains enough natural salt to meet all our requirements. There is generally no need to add extra salt; if used at all, keep it to a minimal amount.

It's what we eat most of the time that counts, not what we eat occasionally. No one food is essential; variety minimises the chances of becoming deficient in any one area. Exactly how much we should eat, and of which foods, varies according to our individual energy requirements. A woman who is working hard physically or who is breastfeeding will need a lot more food than one who is sitting at a computer for much of the day. Some conditions – for example, diabetes or kidney problems – require particular foods to be precisely measured.

It's better to eat several times a day than all at once, so that the energy supply to the body is reasonably constant. It's also better to eat more food in the morning and early afternoon, and less towards the evening, as our energy requirements are generally higher during the day than at night.

Select from four main food groups each day:

- vegetables and fruit
- bread and cereals

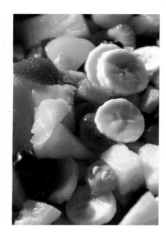

- milk and milk products
- lean meat, seafood, eggs, legumes, nuts and seeds.

Try to eat plenty of foods from the first two groups, and moderate or small amounts from the second two groups, keeping the fats to a minimum. This means using food-preparation methods that avoid adding fats, salt and sugar as much as possible. A suggested meal pattern using the above food groups is given opposite.

What should I eat?

Plenty of:

- *Raw fruits and vegetables* – e.g. apples, oranges, bananas, lettuce, raw carrots, tomatoes, capsicums, raw cabbage, watercress. These contain some sugars and starches, a little protein, vitamins A and C, a little iron, a little potassium, a little magnesium, and a generous amount of fibre.

- *Vegetables that can be boiled, steamed or microwaved* – e.g. potatoes, carrots, pūhā, watercress, broccoli, courgettes, peas, beans (all types), yams, taro. These all contain some fibre, and may contain starch (potatoes, carrots, peas, beans, yams, taro), protein (potatoes, beans, peas), vitamin A (carrots, broccoli) and vitamin C (carrots, potatoes, peas).

- *Unprocessed cereals* – e.g. bran, rolled oats, brown rice, barley. These contain a lot of starch and B vitamins (there are several), and are very high in fibre.

- *Wholemeal and wholegrain breads* – these contain starch, B vitamins and iron; they are also high in fibre.

A moderate amount of:

- *Dairy products* – e.g. milk, cheese, yogurt. These contain a lot of protein, calcium and some fat (depending on the particular food). Choose low-fat options where possible.

- *Other animal products* – e.g. meat, fish, chicken, eggs. These contain a lot of protein and some fat, and all contain iron. Red meat has the most concentrated iron.

- *Whole nuts and seeds (raw, not roasted)* – e.g. peanuts, almonds, brazil nuts, sesame seeds. These contain protein, some iron and some fats.

- *Dried fruits* – e.g. dried apricots, figs, prunes. These contain some starches, some magnesium, potassium and other minerals; however, they are high in sugar.

- *White bread* – this contains starches and B vitamins, but is low in fibre.

- *Processed cereals* – e.g. cornflakes, Weet-Bix. These contain starch, some fibre, and a variable amount of simple sugar.

A little of:

- *Rich dairy products* – e.g. butter and cream. These contain a lot of fat.

- *Highly processed foods* – e.g. tinned and packet soups, sauces. These contain some starches, but a lot of simple sugars and salt.

- *Sweetened foods* – e.g. sugared breakfast cereals, cakes and sweets. These contain little fibre and a lot of simple sugars.

- *Take-aways and deep-fried foods* – e.g. fish and chips, fried chicken, hamburgers. These contain some protein, some starch, and a lot of fat.

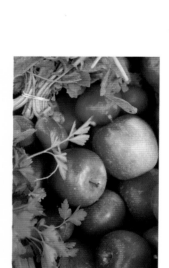

Breakfast

Wholegrain cereal and milk, fruit or juice, wholemeal toast and butter (or margarine or peanut butter). Very active people could add an egg, cheese or savoury dish. Unsweetened beverage.

Lunch or tea

Bread or rolls with various protein fillings and salad vegetables, or thick legume/vegetable soup with wholemeal bread. Include fresh fruit and an unsweetened beverage.

What should I drink?

- *Water*. Drink plenty every day – the equivalent of six to eight glasses (nine glasses when pregnant and ten when breastfeeding).
- *Milk*. Drink low-fat milk or milk drinks sometimes.
- *Other drinks*. Limit fruit juice, cordial and soft drinks – all are high in sugar. Limit coffee to no more than three to five cups per day. Avoid sugar in tea and coffee.

When you are pregnant, or planning to become pregnant, avoid energy drinks and smart (caffeinated) drinks. Limit herbal teas to everyday flavours such as mint, peppermint, orange, lemon and blackcurrant; have no more than two cups a day and use filtered teabags. Avoid coffee altogether, or have no more than 300mg caffeine per day (300mg caffeine is the equivalent of one long black coffee, or three cappuccinos, or four cups of plunger coffee, or six cups of instant coffee, or six cups of regular tea, or 400g plain chocolate).[3]

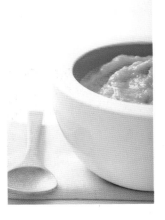

Dinner

Lean meat, fish, chicken, legumes or lentils. Potato, rice, pasta, taro or green banana. At least two other vegetables (one green), lightly cooked or raw. Dessert such as fruit, yogurt, ice-cream, milk pudding, or biscuits and cheese.

Snacks between meals

Avoid sweet food. Instead, choose from the following foods according to your energy needs: fruit, or raw vegetables; crackers, crispbreads, sandwiches, muffins; yogurt or milk drinks; water for thirst. (See also pp.134 and 402.)

Exercise

Our bodies are built to move, and we function best when we are active. Until the mid-twentieth century, most people exercised vigorously in the course of their daily lives. But thanks to mechanisation and technology, we are now in a highly unnatural situation where it is common to sit for long periods – for work, travel and leisure.

We need to redress this situation if our bodies are to work well: there's also good evidence to suggest that physical exercise directly benefits our minds. Mild or moderate exercise is generally good for everyone.[4] As well as making you feel better in yourself, exercise can help you:

- maintain an ideal weight
- improve asthma and related chest conditions
- get over coughs and colds more quickly
- cope with painful periods and premenstrual symptoms
- keep bones strong and muscles firm
- reduce depression and improve mood.

Sustained, strenuous exercise is for a select few. Women in this group are capable of achieving to a high standard in competitive sports, and seem to do particularly well in events calling for endurance. There are, however, potential health problems with this degree of exercise, and training programmes should take the special needs of women into account. Sustained, strenuous exercise may lead to:

- women being extremely underweight
- digestive problems
- lack of menstrual periods
- premature thinning of the bones (osteoporosis)
- overuse injuries to tendons, ligaments, muscles and bones.

Some of these conditions can adversely affect women's ability to have children, certainly in the short term and possibly in the longer term. Women who are competitive athletes need to keep in mind the possibility that they might want to become pregnant at some stage.

Even if you do no exercise at all, you may still get pregnant with no trouble, as long as you are not overweight. But it will be easier to get pregnant if you exercise moderately and keep your weight within, or near, the normal range for your height (see p.44). And pregnancy will certainly be easier for your body to cope with if you can do a little regular exercise before and during your pregnancy.

How much exercise?

Whether you are pregnant or not, it is well worth assessing your current exercise pattern and considering whether it is keeping you healthy.

Mild exercise

- Do you walk, run, swim, cycle or do other exercise for 30 minutes or more on most days?
- Do you do exercise that makes you puffed each week?
- Do you have a regular commitment to exercise, e.g. organised sport or a class?
- Do you enjoy some form of exercise?

If you answer 'yes' to most of these, then you're probably maintaining a basic level of fitness that's sufficient to keep your body in good working order.

Moderate exercise

- Do you exercise for more than one hour a day?
- Are you exercising as part of your daily work, e.g. constantly walking or cycling?

- Could you manage a hard game of netball, or a day's walking up and down hills?

If you answer 'yes' to one or more of these, then you're probably keeping yourself moderately fit and encouraging your body to function really well.

Strenuous exercise

- Do you exercise to your limit for two or more hours a day, five to seven days a week?
- Are you able to maintain a training programme for competitive sport for a good part of the year?

If you answer 'yes' to one or both of these, then you're probably very fit and your body is likely to be fully adapted to sustained, vigorous exercise.

Smoking affects your health

Cigarettes contain a variety of tar compounds and the drug nicotine. They give a feeling of well-being and relaxation when smoked, although this feeling is often short-lived and creates the desire 'for another one'.

Nicotine circulates quickly in the blood and is taken to all parts of the body. It affects the way all cells function, especially those in the blood vessels, making it more difficult for the cells to 'breathe'. They recover, but will become permanently damaged if they are given nicotine again and again. Nicotine is one of the most addictive substances known.

Compared to non-smokers, smokers are more likely to have higher blood pressure, more heart attacks, more strokes, more painful periods, more trouble with premenstrual symptoms, and a higher rate of pre-cancerous cell changes on the cervix.

The cells in the lungs and throat also have to cope with the tar compounds that get left in the tissues after each cigarette. This makes the lungs and throat less able to deal with coughs, colds, bronchitis and pneumonia, and more likely to suffer long-term damage from chronic bronchitis (also known as chronic obstructive pulmonary disease, or COPD) and cancers of the lungs, throat and mouth.

Women who are smokers are more likely to have:

- trouble getting pregnant
- a miscarriage
- high blood pressure or pre-eclampsia (toxaemia) in pregnancy (see p.139)
- intra-uterine growth restriction (IUGR), where the foetus is slow to grow (see p.142)
- premature birth or stillbirth
- trouble with breastfeeding
- babies with more colds, ear infections and asthma
- babies at greater risk of cot death (SIDS; see p.381).

If you are a smoker, you will really help your health in all ways if you stop smoking completely. If you're thinking about getting pregnant, or are already pregnant, you and your baby will be much healthier if you stop smoking now – and don't start again once your baby is born.

'Every time I thought about a cigarette I'd go and get in the shower. For the first weekend I was in the bathroom half the day. I was so incredibly clean ... I felt like a hospital ... But then after a while just the thought of yet another shower was often enough to put me off that smoke ...'

Giving up smoking – some suggestions[5]

- It's not easy giving up. Think hard about your reasons for giving up. Get mentally prepared for a real battle.
- Cut down gradually. Even cutting down will help your health, and your baby's health, straight away. Each morning, count out the number of cigarettes you're going to allow yourself that day and then ration yourself. Only smoke outside; keep your house and your car smoke-free.
- Some people do better by setting a definite date for quitting. On the chosen day, get rid of all your cigarettes, and then stop completely.
- If your partner or someone else in your household smokes, try to persuade them to give up with you.
- Have things to do with your hands, e.g. knitting, sewing or gardening.
- Identify activities normally associated with smoking and change them, e.g. drinking coffee after a meal.
- Prepare some snacks to have instead of a cigarette.
- For women who smoke more than about ten cigarettes a day, nicotine replacement therapy (NRT – nicotine-containing patches or gum) can help, especially if combined with a support programme.
- Try to keep out of smoky places, and keep away from others who smoke.
- If you can't manage it by yourself, ask for help. Increasingly, practice nurses and midwives are fully trained to assist. Quitline (0800 778778) is a national telephone support service that is effective for many people. (See Appendix: Quitline.)

Alcohol

'Because I knew that I might get pregnant at any time, I didn't ever drink – not a single glass of wine throughout the nine months and I'm not drinking now. I was a social smoker but I never smoked during the pregnancy. It just wasn't an issue. I am positive I will never smoke again.'

Most New Zealand women drink alcohol at some stage in their lives. Many, but not all, people can tolerate a modest amount well. However, women process alcohol more slowly than men, even if their body weights are the same. This means that the recommended safe limit for non-pregnant women (no more than 14 standard drinks a week) is lower than for men (no more than 21 standard drinks a week). A standard drink is approximately one can of beer, or one small glass of wine, or one nip of spirits. Both men and women should also have at least two or three alcohol-free days each week.[6]

Alcohol and your baby's health

During pregnancy, any form of alcohol can be a problem for the developing baby. Alcohol passes into the baby's bloodstream directly through the placenta, and also circulates in the amniotic fluid.

Exposure to alcohol during pregnancy increases the risk of a range of conditions known as foetal alcohol spectrum disorder (FASD). In the first 12 weeks of development, alcohol can affect the baby's brain, face, heart and kidneys, and can cause limb and joint deformities. Later in pregnancy, alcohol can cause miscarriage and intra-uterine growth restriction (IUGR; see p.142), and also increase the risk of the baby dying in the first few days after birth.

It used to be thought that only large amounts of alcohol would cause these problems. However, even quite a low alcohol intake in pregnancy can have permanent effects, although not every baby is affected, nor in the same way.[7]

Alcohol in pregnancy – current recommendations[8]

It's best to abstain from drinking alcohol completely if you are planning to become pregnant, and during pregnancy, for the following reasons:

- There is no established safe lower limit for drinking alcohol during pregnancy.
- Even one or two drinks can affect your baby's learning ability. Drinking more than that increases the risk of greater damage.
- It does not matter whether you drink beer, wine, spirits or RTDs (ready-to-drink pre-mixes) – all contain alcohol.
- Although the foetus is not always damaged when a pregnant woman drinks (which explains why some women have had the odd drink without apparent harm to their baby), it is impossible to know when harm will occur.
- Therefore, if you don't drink any alcohol, you can be certain your baby will not have FASD. (See Appendix: Alcohol.)

The reproductive/menstrual/ovulatory cycle

Most women have the potential to become pregnant from the time of their first period (menarche) to the time of their last period (menopause). A menstrual period is the shedding of the lining of the uterus, noticeable as bleeding from the vagina for a few days each month.

Each month there are a few days when a woman may become pregnant if, and only if, she has sexual intercourse with a man, or receives a man's semen into her vagina through artificial insemination.

Organs that change under the influence of the menstrual cycle

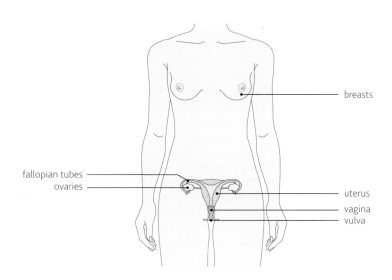

breasts

fallopian tubes
ovaries

uterus
vagina
vulva

The reproductive (or menstrual) cycle is said to extend from the first day of one period to the first day of the next. About half of all women have a 28-day cycle, while the rest vary from 21 to 35 days, or occasionally up to 42 days. This variation is normal, and the cycle may also vary from month to month. When women are taking the contraceptive pill they will usually have very regular cycles, and when they stop, their periods revert to a more variable, and fertile, pattern. Fertility usually returns rapidly. (See p.47.)

The menstrual cycle is under the control of four main hormones: follicle stimulating hormone (FSH), luteinising hormone (LH), oestrogen and progesterone. FSH and LH are produced in the pituitary gland at the base of the brain, and oestrogen and progesterone are produced in the ovaries. These hormones work together to coordinate all the changes during the reproductive cycle.

If the hormone sequence becomes muddled, the menstrual cycle may become irregular and ovulation may not take place. This is common during the first few years after menarche and the last few years before the menopause. Being underweight or overweight, undertaking regular strenuous exercise or being emotionally upset can also profoundly influence the hormones that control the reproductive cycle. Periods may stop completely in very stressful situations, while the cessation of periods in underweight women may be a sign of an eating disorder such as anorexia nervosa or bulimia.

The sequence of changes in a typical menstrual cycle

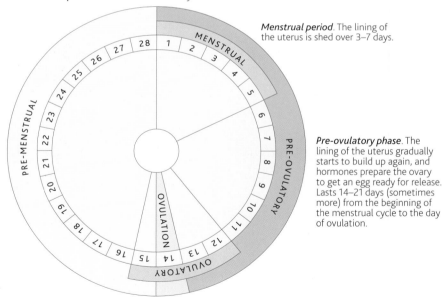

The next menstrual period. The start of another cycle.

Menstrual period. The lining of the uterus is shed over 3–7 days.

Premenstrual phase. The egg (smaller than a pinhead) moves into the end of the fallopian tube and then down the tube into the uterus. It will become fertilised if it meets sperm from a man; if not, it will pass through the uterus and out through the vagina. The mucous from the cervix becomes thick and white. Usually lasts 12–16 days from the day of ovulation.

Pre-ovulatory phase. The lining of the uterus gradually starts to build up again, and hormones prepare the ovary to get an egg ready for release. Lasts 14–21 days (sometimes more) from the beginning of the menstrual cycle to the day of ovulation.

Ovulatory phase. The mucous of the cervix becomes thin, copious and clear, and the egg is released from the ovary, leaving behind a little sac of fluid in the ovary called the corpus luteum. Lasts 4–6 days around the time of ovulation.

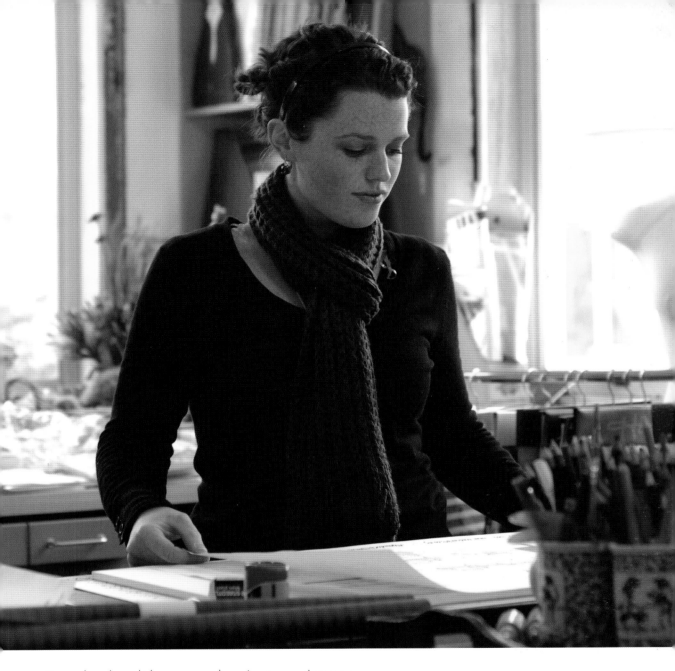

Regular health care – having a primary care provider

There are many benefits to enrolling with a regular primary care service, even if you are normally fit and well. Primary care services offer comprehensive health care from GPs (general practitioners, or family doctors), practice nurses and other health professionals. Once you enrol with a primary care service, you will nearly always become part of the population served by a primary health organisation (PHO), a larger grouping of health providers in a particular area. PHOs disburse government funding for primary care services, carry out quality checks on health services, and provide additional services that your local community might need. As a regular enrolled patient with a PHO, not only are you entitled to a wide range of benefits and services, but costs to you are also much lower than if you just visit on a casual basis.

Often, your local primary care service will be a health centre or general practice run by GPs and other health professionals. Comprehensive health services are also run by iwi and by community or commercial trusts. Māori health service providers aim to offer culturally appropriate services, but are by no means exclusive to Māori clients. These health services employ practice nurses, GPs and sometimes nurse practitioners to provide quality clinical services.

The primary care service you choose will depend on where you live, the services you require (including after-hours services) and your personal preferences. Try to find a practice you like and respect, and a regular doctor and nurse you feel you can talk to easily. Remember, you are free to change providers if you wish.

As part of their service to regular patients, primary care providers will recommend some periodic well-person checks, and it is their routine practice to remind you (as an enrolled person) when these are due. For well women, there are currently two recommended cancer-screening programmes: regular cervical smears to help prevent cervical cancer, and (for older women) regular mammograms to aid early detection of breast cancer.

Training for nurses and doctors in primary care

Regardless of the type of service they provide, all practice nurses, GPs and nurse practitioners must be fully trained to work in primary care, and they must be regularly recertified to continue to do so.

- *Practice nurses*. These are fully trained nurses with extra training in primary care delivery, including such skills as wound care, vaccination procedures and cervical smear-taking.

- *General practitioners (GPs)*. These are fully trained doctors, with additional postgraduate training (another five years minimum) to become vocationally registered in the speciality of general practice (FRNZCGP – Fellow of the Royal New Zealand College of General Practitioners).

- *Nurse practitioners*. In primary care these are fully trained nurses with postgraduate qualifications (a clinical masters degree with primary care scope – another two years minimum). They are able to undertake a wider range of health care than practice nurses, often including managing common illnesses and prescribing some medicines. This is a relatively new qualification, so numbers are still small.

Cervical smears

Why is it important to have a smear?

The place where the cells lining the vagina meet the cells lining the cervix is a vulnerable area. Every year, approximately 200 women in New Zealand develop cancer of the cervix, and about 70 women die from it.[9] These statistics are especially tragic because pre-cancerous changes in the cells of the cervix can nearly always be detected with regular smear tests before invasive cancer develops, allowing enough time for curative treatment. For this reason, regular cervical smears are recommended for nearly all women. (See Appendix: Cervical smears/testing.)

All women, young and not so young, are at risk of developing cervical cancer if they are, or ever have been, sexually active. Lesbians can develop changes in the cells on the cervix and are currently advised to have regular smear tests.

Cervical cancer, and pre-cancerous changes on the cervix, are known to be associated with sexual activity because of the easy and undetectable transmission of a family of common wart viruses known as human papilloma virus (HPV). Only some, not all, of the subtypes in the HPV family are known to be linked to the development of cervical cancer. These wart viruses may sometimes survive outside the body – on the skin, on condoms, or on sex aids. Sexual transmission may not be the only way of passing wart viruses from one person to another, but it is by far the most common.

Recently, a vaccine against a limited number of the HPV subtypes has been developed. This is a promising advance in the prevention of cervical cancer, and is now available in New Zealand, and due to be introduced as part of the funded vaccination schedule in 2008. However, the vaccine is active only against the wart subtypes most commonly implicated in the development of cervical cancer. Even if most people in the population are eventually vaccinated, it would be many years before any effects of the new vaccine are likely to be seen. To be most effective, the vaccine needs to be given to girls before they become sexually active and are exposed to HPV.[10]

What is a smear?

Your cervix is at the top end of your vagina and is the entrance to your uterus. It is normally firmly closed, leaving a tiny channel no bigger than a pin. Menstrual blood can pass down through the cervix, and semen from a man can pass up through it during sexual intercourse. A tampon cannot pass through the cervix.

You can feel your own cervix if you squat down and insert a clean finger gently into the vagina. Feel as far up and back as you can, and 'bear down' slightly. The cervix feels smooth and firm (compared to the softer, more spongy vaginal lining), and has a small dimple or groove in the middle. It is not recommended that you do this if you are already pregnant, although if you are gentle you are very unlikely to cause a problem.

A cervical smear is a sample of cells taken from the cervix during an internal vaginal examination ('VE', also sometimes referred to as a 'PV', or 'per vaginum'). Taking a smear is a highly skilled task done by a trained doctor or nurse. They will ask you to take off your lower clothing (usually just your trousers, underwear and shoes) and lie down on your back or side. You will often be given a sheet to put over yourself if you wish.

The nurse or doctor will then put on surgical gloves, gently insert a speculum into your vagina, and open it just enough to see the cervix. The speculum may be metal or plastic, and should be a comfortable temperature. It may have a light attached to it. The speculum may give you a rather odd, stretchy, uncomfortable feeling, but should not be painful. The more relaxed you are, the more comfortable it is – so help yourself by being as relaxed and 'floppy' as possible.

Cell junction at cervix

Different types of cells line the vagina and the uterus. A cervical smear samples cells from the junction.

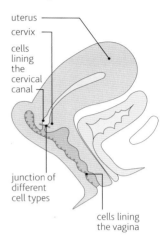

uterus
cervix
cells lining the cervical canal
junction of different cell types
cells lining the vagina

Feeling the cervix

cervix

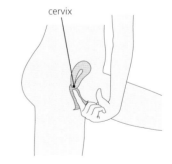

Vaginal examination (VE)

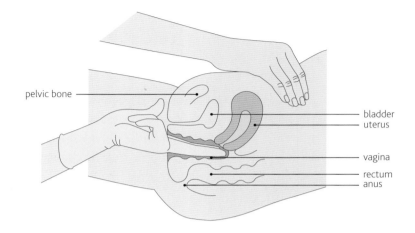

pelvic bone

bladder
uterus

vagina

rectum
anus

Once the doctor or nurse can see the cervix clearly, they will use a spatula or brush to wipe the surface of the cervix gently, which you will hardly feel. Sometimes swabs will be taken at the same time to check for infection: a small cotton-tipped stick is wiped on or near the cervix, then placed in a narrow transport tube and sent off to the laboratory.

The speculum will then be removed. Next, the doctor or nurse may check the uterus, tubes and ovaries by gently placing one hand on your tummy and two fingers in the vagina. The whole examination takes no longer than three or four minutes.

Cervical smears – current recommendations for New Zealand women[11]

- First smear from age 20 if sexually active.
- A second smear within one year.
- A smear every three years from then on.
- Stop smears at age 70 if all have been normal and there have been two smears within the last five years.
- If it has been more than five years since the last smear, have two smears a year apart and then one every three years.
- If any smear has ever been abnormal, they need to be done more frequently. Just how frequently depends on the nature of the abnormality.
- Women who have never been sexually active do not need regular smear tests.
- If the time for a routine smear test falls during the first few weeks of pregnancy, it can be done safely. Otherwise, it is better left until at least six weeks after the birth.

Taking a cervical smear

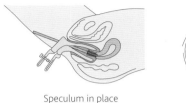

cervix

Speculum in place

'Cytobrush' being used
to take cell sample

The sample itself is either smeared onto a glass slide or immersed in a small jar of solution, and is then sent to the laboratory for examination under the microscope. The most common method involves smearing the cells directly onto a glass slide. Liquid-based cytology (for example, Thin Prep or Sure Path), where the cells are placed into a jar of solution, has not been shown to be any better than the direct smear method for most women.[12] However, it is better suited to digital technology analysis and will become more common in the future.

Sexually transmitted infections (STIs or STDs)

As well as the HPV subtypes that are linked to cervical cancer, a number of other infections can be passed on through sexual activity. Genital warts are also caused by some of the subtypes of HPV. Other viral infections include herpes (herpes simplex virus, or HSV), hepatitis B and HIV (human immunodeficiency virus, the cause of acquired immunodeficiency syndrome, or AIDS). Bacterial infections that are sexually transmitted include chlamydia, gonorrhoea and syphilis. (See Appendix: Sexually transmitted infections.)

All these infections can easily be passed on during unprotected sex. STIs may not cause any symptoms in the early stages, but can still cause problems later on. In women, untreated STIs can cause chronic, offensive vaginal discharge, infection in the fallopian tubes and surrounding tissue (pelvic inflammatory disease, or PID), chronic pelvic or abdominal pain, ectopic pregnancy and/or infertility. STIs such as hepatitis B, syphilis and HIV have other complications and can ultimately cause death.

Mutually faithful sexual relationships greatly reduce the chance of being exposed to STIs. Condoms also reduce the risk of getting STIs, but they do not eliminate it.

STIs can easily be checked for in women and men, even if there are no symptoms. If you think you may be at risk, or have had a new sexual contact, visit a GP, practice nurse, sexual health clinic or family planning clinic for an STI check.

For women, an STI check involves the same procedure as having a smear, but swabs will be taken instead of (or as well as) the smear sample. Sometimes, a urine test and a blood test will also be needed. For men, the genital area is examined, swabs are usually taken from the opening in the penis, and urine and blood tests are collected.

Results are usually available in a few days, and many infections can be treated with antibiotics. All recent sexual partners also need treatment at the same time, to avoid passing the infection on to others, or back and forth between current partners.

Chlamydia[13]

- Chlamydia is one of the most common STIs in New Zealand.
- In women, chlamydia may produce no symptoms, or cause a vaginal discharge, bleeding in between periods, pelvic inflammatory disease and/or abdominal pain.
- Repeated infection in women can cause permanent infertility.
- If chlamydia is present during pregnancy, it can cause miscarriage.
- If chlamydia is present during labour, the infection may be passed to the baby during birth and cause serious chest and eye infections. In the worst case scenario, this can lead to death or blindness.
- In men, chlamydia may produce no symptoms, or cause a discharge from the penis, pain with urination, or occasionally pain in the scrotum.
- Chlamydia can be detected with special urine and swab tests before and during pregnancy.
- Chlamydia is easily treatable with antibiotics (most commonly azithromycin or doxycycline), and as long as treatment is started promptly, it can be cured and complications avoided.

HIV-AIDS[14]

Human immunodeficiency virus (HIV) causes a breakdown in the body's normal immune response. This initially causes a transient flu-like illness, but then leaves the body increasingly prone to recurrent infections, as many of the cells that normally fight infection become fragile.

HIV infection may take months or years to cause the syndrome known as acquired immunodeficiency syndrome (AIDS). In people with AIDS, the body is unable to make essential types of new white blood cells. Infections become chronic and there is weakness, weight loss, the development of certain types of cancer and, ultimately, death.

- HIV is most often passed on during unprotected sex, but can also be passed on through intravenous drug use, and transfusion of unsafe blood products.
- It can be passed on through heterosexual and/or homosexual sex.
- It is not passed on by skin-to-skin touch, and is very rarely passed on through saliva.
- It has been more commonly acquired in New Zealand by men who have sex with men, but more women are now being diagnosed with HIV, acquired through heterosexual contact.[15]
- It can be passed from mother to baby during pregnancy and/or during breastfeeding (see p.315).
- It can easily be detected through a blood test, which is now routinely suggested early in pregnancy.
- It can be treated to greatly improve quality and length of life, although a total cure is not yet possible.

Breast examination

Like cervical cancer, breast cancer is common in this country. A New Zealand woman has a 10 per cent risk of getting breast cancer throughout her lifetime. The incidence increases with age, and three-quarters of women who get breast cancer are over 50.[16] Breast cancer is less common in younger women and is unusual in pregnancy, but it can occur. For all women, early detection and diagnosis make treatment and cure more likely.

The causes of breast cancer are not clear, and many women who get breast cancer have none of the known risk factors apart from increasing age. However, women have a somewhat higher risk of getting breast cancer if:

- they have already had cancer in either breast
- they have had treatment for some other cancers
- they have a sister, mother or daughter who has had breast cancer, especially at a younger age.

Early detection of breast cancer is not as easy as it is for cervical cancer. Breast cancers can be found by women noticing a new lump in their breast, although only a small proportion of all lumps found turn out to be caused by cancer.

If you do discover what you think might be a new lump, get it checked promptly by a nurse or doctor. As well as undertaking a breast examination, they may well arrange for you to have further tests, such as ultrasound, detailed mammography or a small biopsy known as a fine needle aspiration (FNA). In younger women, breast lumps are more likely to be caused by cysts or a condition called fibroadenoma, than by cancer. In pregnancy, many breast changes are normal (see p.119), but unusual lumps still need checking out. Breast pain and/or nipple discharge that are not associated with breastfeeding are uncommon signs of breast cancer, but if they persist they should be checked as well.

Mammography[17]

- Mammography is a soft-tissue X-ray of the breast, and is currently used as a screening test in New Zealand for well women aged between 45 and 69 years. This national screening programme is for non-pregnant women who have no symptoms of possible breast cancer.

- It can often detect breast cancer before any lump is noticeable, but it has variable reliability and is less reliable in younger women. As women get older, the breast tissue becomes less dense, making detection by mammography of possible breast cancers easier.

- It involves pressing the breast tissue between two clear plastic plates to get the best view. A few women find this painful, but most find it just uncomfortable. A very low level of radiation is used, and there is no evidence to suggest that the recommended screening procedure is harmful to breast tissue.

- It detects breast cancer earlier, and reduces (but does not eliminate) deaths from breast cancer when it is undertaken regularly by women over 50 years.

- It detects breast cancer earlier when it is undertaken regularly by women aged between 40 and 50 years, but to a lesser extent than for older women.

2. Sexuality and contraception

Most adults in New Zealand are sexually active, and many find sex satisfying and enjoyable. Some are sexually active only occasionally, while others enjoy an ongoing relationship and may have intercourse several times a week. There is a very wide range of what is considered normal. There is no evidence to suggest that long periods of celibacy are physically harmful, nor is there evidence to suggest that frequent intercourse is detrimental.

Desire for sexual activity has much to do with how successful or satisfying it is. Forcing someone – physically or emotionally – into sexual activity is likely to cause them physical and/or mental harm.

Comparing different methods of contraception and their reliability

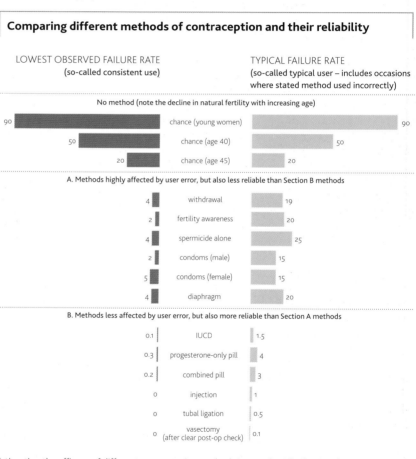

LOWEST OBSERVED FAILURE RATE
(so-called consistent use)

TYPICAL FAILURE RATE
(so-called typical user – includes occasions where stated method used incorrectly)

No method (note the decline in natural fertility with increasing age)

90	chance (young women)	90
50	chance (age 40)	50
20	chance (age 45)	20

A. Methods highly affected by user error, but also less reliable than Section B methods

4	withdrawal	19
2	fertility awareness	20
4	spermicide alone	25
2	condoms (male)	15
5	condoms (female)	15
4	diaphragm	20

B. Methods less affected by user error, but also more reliable than Section A methods

0.1	IUCD	1.5
0.3	progesterone-only pill	4
0.2	combined pill	3
0	injection	1
0	tubal ligation	0.5
0	vasectomy (after clear post-op check)	0.1

Estimating the efficacy of different contraceptive methods is complex. The figures above are expressed as approximations of user-failure rates per 100 women in the first year of use. The figures shown only approximate a percentage failure rate; nevertheless this is often a useful way of understanding the different reliability of different methods. For example, it is reasonable to say: 'Condoms can have a 15% failure rate for typical users, whereas the injection has only a 1% failure rate for typical users'. Information adapted from J. Guillebaud, *Contraception: Your Questions Answered*, 4th edn, Churchill Livingstone, Edinburgh, 2004, pp.14–15.

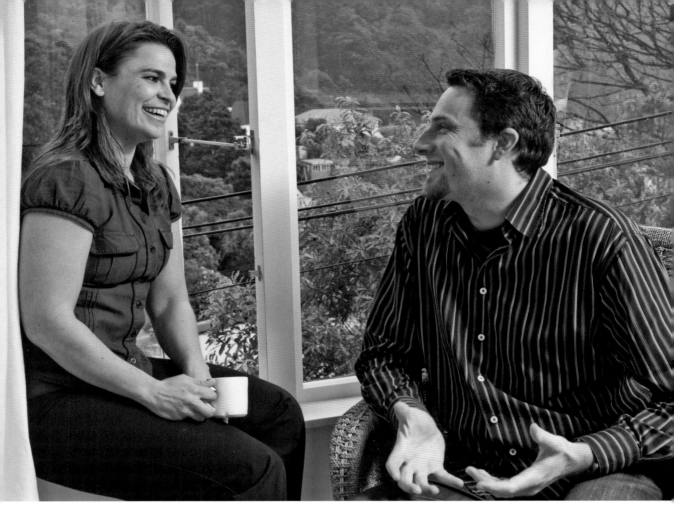

At any one time, only a small number of women who are sexually active want to become pregnant – hence the need for contraception. The term 'contraception' describes anything that attempts to prevent pregnancy (conception) in a woman who is sexually active with a man.

The idea of contraception is not new. Withdrawal (coitus interruptus), various calendar methods and types of sheath for the penis have been used for centuries by couples wishing to avoid pregnancy. Diaphragms and douches have also been around for a long time. But it is only in the last 50–60 years that more reliable methods of contraception have become readily available throughout the developed world, triggering a tremendous change in attitudes towards sexuality in general and pregnancy in particular.

Women are now able to control their fertility, whether or not they are sexually active. This is reflected in the trend towards smaller families, as well as the ever-widening role of women in the paid workforce.

The choice of whether to use contraception is a personal one that follows personal decisions about sex and sexuality. Pregnancy is likely to be a natural consequence of sexual intercourse unless you use some form of contraception. Choosing a method of contraception involves weighing up the potential risks against the potential benefits. Not all methods suit all people, and your needs may change as your circumstances and lifestyle change.

It is important to remember, too, that the risks of contraception need to be weighed up against the risks of repeated pregnancy for any particular woman. Our great-grandmothers, with their 12 or 14 children each, suffered high rates of maternal and infant mortality, as well as uncomfortably slack abdominal muscles, urinary incontinence and uterine prolapse.

Commonly used methods of contraception[18]

Fertility awareness (natural family planning)

See Chapter 1, p.48.

Coitus interruptus (withdrawal)

During intercourse, the man's semen is normally ejaculated at the top of the woman's vagina, around her cervix. If the man withdraws his penis from the woman's vagina just before he 'comes', then the sperm in the semen cannot make their way into the cervix.

For some couples, this method of contraception works. But for most people it is unreliable because it requires faultless control. In addition, a little fluid usually escapes from the tip of the penis before ejaculation, and this sometimes contains sperm.

While not considered a particularly reliable method of contraception (see p.34), withdrawal certainly decreases the risk of pregnancy when compared with using no contraception at all.

Barrier methods

These methods prevent sperm from entering the cervix.

Condoms

One of these thin, disposable, rubber latex sheaths is placed over the man's erect penis before it enters the woman's vagina. They protect against pregnancy, and also give good (but not perfect) protection against a wide variety of sexually transmitted infections, including the HIV-AIDS virus.

Condoms do occasionally burst or tear or come off. They may also perish if kept in a hot place, or if used with any oil-based lubricant such as Vaseline.

Condoms come in a variety of brands and styles, and can be bought at chemists, supermarkets and vending machines. They are also available on prescription. Female condoms, designed to be worn in the vagina, are available overseas but are not readily available in New Zealand.

Diaphragms

A diaphragm is a reusable circular device with a firm edge, which is placed in the woman's vagina to cover the cervix before intercourse takes place. It must be used with a spermicidal cream, and left in place for at least six to eight hours after intercourse. It can remain in place for up to 24 hours, although fresh spermicide needs to be used if intercourse takes place more than two hours after insertion.

Diaphragms come in different sizes, and need to be fitted by a doctor or nurse skilled in their use. It is also really important to learn the correct insertion technique to ensure that the diaphragm covers the cervix.

Diaphragms provide some protection against infection, but they do not protect against HIV-AIDS. (See also p.395.)

Cervical caps and vault caps

These are small rubber caps that can be placed over the cervix and left for a day or so. Again, they need to be fitted carefully, and patience is required when learning the insertion technique. They should be used with spermicidal cream. The cap is held on by suction, and some women find that their cervix is not a 'good shape' for wearing one. For these reasons, caps are used less often than diaphragms.

Spermicides

Spermicides come in different forms: cream, foam, jelly and pessaries. They most commonly contain a chemical called nonoxynol-9, which kills sperm immediately on contact.

Spermicides are not recommended for use on their own. However, when combined with a diaphragm or cap, they greatly improve reliability. Rarely, people may be allergic to one or other of the preparations, in which case they should not be used.

A vaginal sponge containing spermicide is also available, but it is less reliable than the other barrier methods.

Intra-uterine contraceptive devices (IUCDs or IUDs)

These are small plastic devices, usually coated with a little spiral of copper wire, and attached to a monofilament nylon thread. Some types, such as the Mirena, have a small amount of hormone incorporated in the stem, which is slowly released over the five-year lifetime of the device. IUCDs need to be inserted into the uterus by a trained doctor (or occasionally a nurse), using sterile technique.

Multiload IUCD

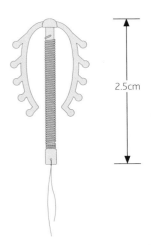

2.5cm

Once inserted, the IUCD prevents pregnancy by impairing fertilisation and implantation. The devices are very reliable and can remain in place for up to five years, depending on the type, after which they need to be changed. IUCDs tend to make periods heavier, although the type containing the hormone progestagen (synthetic progesterone) is designed to make periods lighter, and some women will get no periods at all. With this type, most of the hormone is released in the uterus, but a few women may get other troublesome hormone effects such as acne or vaginal dryness.

When IUCDs are used, there is an increased risk of pelvic inflammatory disease (PID) if an STI is present. This may lead to the fallopian tubes becoming blocked and result in infertility. IUCDs are therefore not recommended for women who have, or have had, a pelvic infection, or are likely to come into contact with a partner or partners who may have one. IUCDs are most suitable for women in a mutually faithful relationship with one partner, who have had at least one pregnancy. They may also be suitable for women who have not yet had children, but the potential risk to future fertility should be carefully thought through. Other methods of contraception should be considered first.

IUCDs are a reliable method of contraception (see p.34), but if pregnancy does occur, there is a greater risk of miscarriage, ectopic pregnancy and infection. This risk can be reduced if the IUCD is removed as early as possible in the pregnancy. If you are contemplating having an IUCD, it would be advisable to discuss your particular situation carefully with a health professional first.

Sometimes IUCDs can be used as a 'morning after' method of contraception. If inserted within five days of unprotected intercourse, an IUCD will effectively prevent pregnancy. However, the above warnings about the risk of pelvic infection still apply.

Hormonal contraceptives

The standard (combined or ordinary) pill

In New Zealand, this is by far the most commonly used reversible (as opposed to permanent) method of contraception. It is called the 'combined' pill because it combines a dose of two hormones – oestrogen and progestagen (synthetic progesterone) – in each pill. It is taken every day for three weeks, followed by a week off. In some packs, inactive pills are provided; these are taken in the week off. The pill must be taken every day at about the same time, and it's best to start at the beginning of a period, although there are exceptions.

The pill prevents pregnancy by stopping the release of eggs from the ovaries. In addition, it alters the lining of the uterus and the mucous at the cervix, which also helps prevent pregnancy. It is a very reliable method of contraception when taken correctly, and also makes periods regular, lighter, shorter and less painful. Precautions need to be taken if a woman misses a pill, uses antibiotics, or has an episode of severe diarrhoea where the pills might not be absorbed.

There is a wide variety of pills on the market, and not all types suit all women. The choice of pill is a complex decision, best made in consultation with a doctor or nurse skilled in their use.

The combined pill is generally not suitable for women who smoke (especially if over the age of 35) or are very overweight, those with a history of blood clots, those with liver disease, or those with high blood pressure or other illnesses associated with the heart or the circulation. Women who get migraine-type headaches may not be able to take the combined pill. A personal or family history of blood-clotting disorders can sometimes be a problem. If you are on regular medication (for example, for diabetes or epilepsy), you need to check whether you can take the combined pill safely and effectively.

The combined pill affects your whole body, not just the genital tract, so you may experience some side effects. If you are concerned about any symptoms that occur when you are on the pill, seek advice from your doctor, practice nurse or family planning clinic. In many instances, a change of pill may solve the problem.

All women taking the combined pill should have their blood pressure and weight measured at least once a year, as well as having a regular cervical smear (see p.28).

The combined pill has been found to protect against cancer of the ovary and cancer of the main part of the uterus. Its relationship to breast cancer is not yet certain, but most of the evidence so far suggests that it does not increase the risk. The combined pill also reduces the risk of iron depletion and anaemia due to menstruation, the most common reason for iron deficiency in women.

Some problems that may be helped by changing pills

- 'break-through bleeding' (menstrual bleeding at the wrong time of the month)

- slight nausea, especially on the first one or two packs

- weight gain (this is much less of a problem with modern pills)

- 'thrush' infection (see p.87)

- headaches (sometimes these make it necessary to stop taking the pill altogether)

- vaginal dryness, decreased interest in sex

- depression or negative mood changes

- acne

The mini-pill or progestagen-only pill (POP)

This type of pill contains only one of the hormones in the combined pill, progestagen, and in a much smaller dose. It prevents pregnancy by altering the cervical mucous, although it also has some effect on the uterus, and stops ovulation in some 40 per cent of women.

The mini-pill is slightly less reliable than the combined pill, so it must be taken very carefully, within a three-hour time span every day. There are no pill-free days. Because of its low-dose, one-hormone action, it is generally suitable for older women, women who are breastfeeding, and women who cannot take the combined pill for various reasons.

The most common problem encountered with the mini-pill is irregular menstrual bleeding, although this does tend to settle with time.

Depo-Provera ('contraceptive injection')

This progestagen-only contraceptive is given once every 12 weeks by injection. The progestagen is slowly released from the injection site to give very reliable contraception by preventing the release of eggs from the ovaries.

Over 50 per cent of women don't have any periods at all while on Depo-Provera: the lining of the uterus doesn't thicken up each month, so there is no blood to lose. A small number of women, however, get irregular bleeding while on the injection, particularly in the first three to six months. This often settles with time, although occasionally it requires the use of other medication. Some women gain weight while on the injection, but others are unaffected.

Because it can take several months for periods to resume once the injections are stopped, Depo-Provera may not be a good choice if you are planning to get pregnant within the next 6–12 months. Normal fertility will return after stopping the injections, but this can take time in some women.

Occasionally, Depo-Provera will cause vaginal dryness, decreased interest in sex or depression. In any of these instances, another form of contraception should be considered.

There is also some concern that women who have no periods while using the injection may be at risk of premature osteoporosis (permanent thinning of the bones). More research needs to be done to determine what this risk might be, but continuous use for two years or less does not seem to be a problem.[19]

Emergency contraception ('morning-after pill')

If unprotected intercourse occurs unexpectedly, emergency contraception can be used within three days (72 hours). At present, the most common method consists of two pills containing progestagen. One is taken as soon as possible after intercourse, followed by the other 12 hours later. An alternative regime is now being recommended, where both pills are taken together.[20] Either regime is effective if taken within 72 hours of unprotected intercourse, although within 48 hours is even better. The method is not perfect, but will prevent pregnancy in 97–98 per cent of cases.

Emergency contraception can be used after a condom has burst or come off, after the regular contraceptive pill has been forgotten (although the need for this will vary depending on the time in the pill cycle), after sexual abuse, or at any other time when completely unprotected intercourse has occurred

– especially around the middle of the woman's menstrual cycle. It is, however, only an emergency method and is not recommended for repeated use. A pregnancy test should be done three weeks after using emergency contraception, just in case it has failed. IUCDs can also be used sometimes as a 'morning-after' method of contraception (see p.38).

Permanent contraception (sterilisation)

This is the most commonly used form of contraception (male and female) in New Zealand, if all methods and all people who are fertile are taken into account.[21]

Tubal ligation (female sterilisation)

This involves putting a band or clip across each fallopian tube so that eggs cannot pass down into the uterus and sperm cannot make their way to the egg. Alternatively, a piece of each tube can be cut out. Tubal ligation is very reliable – failures can happen, but they are rare.

Because the fallopian tubes are within the abdomen, an operation under general anaesthetic is necessary. This means you will usually have to stay several hours in hospital, or occasionally overnight.

Small cuts are made in the abdomen, usually just below the tummy button and above the pubic hair line. The tubes are banded, clipped or cut. Only a small piece of tube is involved, and no other organs are affected. This means that the ovaries and the uterus continue to function normally after the operation, and menstrual periods occur just as before.

Although, in special circumstances, the tubes can be rejoined surgically, this method of contraception has to be regarded as permanent. So you must be very sure that you don't want any more children. Reconstructive tubal surgery is complicated, expensive and successful only some of the time.

Vasectomy (male sterilisation)

The vas deferens is the tube that normally carries sperm from the testes to the urethra in the penis. In a vasectomy, the vas deferens tube is cut (and sometimes a small piece removed) on each side, and the ends are tied. This means that sperm can no longer pass into the penis, although the rest of the seminal fluid is produced quite normally. A vasectomy does not affect sexual function in any way.

Because the vas deferens passes quite close to the surface in the scrotum, the operation can be done under local anaesthetic. Vasectomies are done by some GPs, at some family planning clinics, and by surgeons at public hospitals or in their private rooms. The operation takes about 20 minutes, and involves making one or two small cuts on either side of the scrotum.

Most men find that they can resume normal activities within a day or so. It does take time for the vas deferens to clear completely of sperm after a vasectomy, so at least two semen specimens need to be clear of sperm to make sure there is no chance of pregnancy. This can take several weeks, so other contraceptive methods need to be used in the meantime.

Again, vasectomy has to be regarded as a permanent form of contraception. It can, in some instances, be reversed by surgery, but there is no guarantee of success.

Tubal ligation

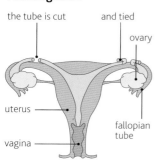

the tube is cut   and tied

ovary

uterus

fallopian tube

vagina

3. Deciding whether to have a child

With the advent of reliable contraception, most women can choose whether and when to get pregnant. While contraception and its use are by no means perfect, and unplanned pregnancies do occur, the majority of women now expect to control their own fertility. At the same time, changing social attitudes, greater financial autonomy, and the possibility of artificial insemination by a donor have given women greater freedom to conceive and raise children independently of marriage or even of heterosexual activity.

Do I want a child?

The answer to this question will depend on many factors, including how old you are, what sort of relationship you're in, what sort of work you do and what kind of life you lead. For the future of the population, it is obviously necessary for people in general to have children. But on an individual basis, there is great variation. Some people want to have children very much, some are easy one way or the other, and others are quite definite that they don't want children.

Traditionally, it was expected that everyone who married would have children if they could, as population expansion was considered critical to any society's progress. But this is clearly no longer the case, and most people now support the need to control global population growth. A wide variety of family types and living situations means that child-bearing and child-rearing are occurring in different contexts and communities; nuclear families, blended families, single-parent families, extended families, communal families, adopted families and same-sex parent families are all part of the mix.

An increasing number of people in New Zealand also actively choose to remain child-free. For a wide variety of reasons, they do not want children and may well contribute to the community in other, equally valuable ways.

If you think you might prefer to be child-free all your life, consider this carefully and make an active, informed decision. Women have fewer reproductive years than men, and it is better to make an active decision about whether to have children before those years are suddenly over. That way, you are more likely to reach the end of your reproductive years feeling happy and fulfilled as a child-free woman.

When is the best time?

On balance, the safest and easiest time to have children is somewhere between 20 and 35 years of age. Before 20, the bones and ligaments of the pelvis may not be fully ready for pregnancy, and there tend to be more complications with premature labour and babies that are smaller than usual. Nor are the nutritional needs of growing teenagers ideal for pregnancy. If you are a teenager, you may still be coming to terms with your own identity and independence; you are likely to be at school, polytechnic or university, or working towards a place in the workforce. Teenage relationships are often not stable, and pregnancy may ask a commitment that neither you nor your partner are ready for.

After the age of 35, the problems are different. It may be more difficult to become pregnant, as fertility in women tends to drop off slowly after the age of

'Although our baby was unplanned, she is a very welcome addition to our rather small extended family. The nicest thing about having her here now is that she can spend time with her great-grandmother – my maternal nana, who is 91. It is so incredibly special for them both. Nana was certain that this baby was a girl and although we had no preference and kept her gender a surprise, it is really neat to have four generations in the maternal line together. I try to get Isabel and her great-grandmother together at least once a week because they both really enjoy their cuddles. I am so glad that Nana is still here and that our "waiting for a couple of years, when we'll be in a better position" came to an end before we missed out on this.'

'I think a three-year gap works well. By three they're out of nappies, can eat and sleep independently, and will listen to stories while you feed the baby.'

30, especially among those who have not been pregnant before. Male fertility also declines with age, although at a very much slower rate. (On an individual basis, however, this pattern certainly cannot be relied on for contraception.) Miscarriage, premature labour and heavy bleeding after delivery are also more common beyond the age of 35.

The chance of having a baby with abnormal chromosomes increases as a woman gets older. The most common of these abnormalities causes Down syndrome (previously known as Down's syndrome), a condition resulting in characteristic facial features, varying degrees of intellectual disability, and sometimes heart and hearing difficulties. If the woman is aged 25–29, her risk of having an affected baby is about 1 in 1350; if she is aged 35–39, the risk increases to about 1 in 260; if she is over 45, her chances of having a Down syndrome child are approximately 1 in 50.[22] Tests are now available to detect such chromosomal abnormalities during pregnancy (see p.105).

It is important to remember that all these statistics do not necessarily apply to any one woman, but serve only as a guide to what is more likely to happen in each age group. If you have any choice in the matter, it does make sense to plan your pregnancies to occur somewhere between the ages of 20 and 35; if you want several children, then having your first child before the age of 30 is biologically sound.

The median age of first births for women has risen significantly in the last 40 years: in 1968, the median age was 25 years; in 2008, it was 30 years, with many more first-time mothers aged over 35 years.[23]

As many New Zealand women delay their child-bearing, more are having trouble getting pregnant when they do want to have children. This trend has seen a rise in the number of people attending fertility clinics. That said, there are many women who have borne children successfully at 18 or at 40. If your circumstances are such that you want to get pregnant earlier or later than the norm, be aware of the risks – and the benefits. Then make your decision.

'Emma and John are 15 months apart. Hard work for the first year and a half … but since then it's been easier I think. Now we think we might be ready for a third – six years later.'

Spacing between pregnancies

This really depends a lot on the support and help you have at home, and on how easy you find looking after one child. Many New Zealand families space their children about two years apart, with the idea that the children will 'play with each other', and that the child-bearing years 'won't last for ever'.

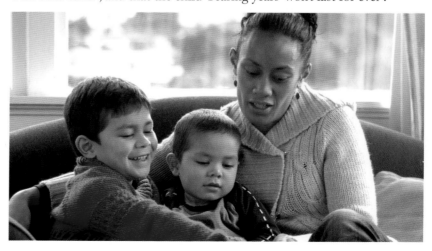

Pre-conception health check

If you are in good health, eat a well-balanced diet and do some regular exercise, planning for pregnancy should present few problems from a physical and medical point of view. There are, however, a few things that are worth checking before you begin.

Folic acid

Generous amounts of folic acid are necessary in early pregnancy to complete the proper development of the baby's brain and spinal cord. There is good evidence that the incidence of severe brain malformation and spina bifida (also known as neural tube defects, or NTDs; see p.151) can be reduced if pregnant women take extra folic acid prior to conception and in early pregnancy.[24] A lot of this crucial development takes place before most women realise they're pregnant, so it's best to take a daily supplement all the time you're trying to conceive, even if you have a diet rich in folic acid. In some countries, such as the United States, flour is fortified with folic acid to reduce the incidence of NTDs; as this is not the case in New Zealand, it's especially important to start taking folic acid before you become pregnant (see below).[25]

If you are not already doing so, start taking folic acid supplements – in the form of folic acid tablets, not multivitamins or other supplements that contain only traces of folic acid – well before you become pregnant. Folic acid tablets are recommended for all women from four weeks prior to conception. Folic acid is naturally present in lots of fresh leafy vegetables, but even eating generous amounts may not provide enough dietary folic acid to meet the needs of a developing baby in the early weeks.

Folic acid supplements – current recommendations[26]

Start taking folic acid tablets (0.8mg) at least four weeks before conception (in effect, this means taking the supplements all the time you are planning a pregnancy) until the end of the 12th week of pregnancy. Supplements can be started any time during the first 12 weeks of pregnancy, but the earlier the better. After that time, extra folic acid will not be effective in reducing the risk of a neural tube defect (NTD). Continue taking a tablet every day until the end of the 12th week.

If you are at higher risk than usual because you have previously had a baby with an NTD, including spina bifida, have a family history of NTD, or are taking medications that affect folate metabolism (such as insulin, some anti-epileptic drugs, clomiphene or isotretinoin), you should take a higher dose of folic acid (5mg) from four weeks before conception until the end of the 12th week of pregnancy. The tablets are safe in pregnancy, with no significant side effects.

Rubella[27]

Have you had the rubella vaccination, and/or a blood test to show that you are already immune, prior to pregnancy? Although rubella is usually a mild illness for the mother, it can severely affect a developing baby, causing mental retardation, blindness or deafness. If you are already immune, then your baby will be protected from this risk.

Most New Zealand girls, and boys, will have had the rubella vaccination as a child, either at age 11, or more recently at 15 months and four years as part of the normal vaccination schedule (see p.396), but if you are planning a pregnancy you do need to be sure that you have been vaccinated. It's worth having a blood test to check that you have maintained your immunity after vaccination, and/or early exposure to the disease. If you do need to have the vaccination as an adult, make sure you are not pregnant prior to vaccination, then use reliable contraception so you don't fall pregnant for the next 28 days. Even though vaccination during pregnancy is not recommended, when accidental vaccination has occurred, there is no evidence to date that it has in fact been harmful. Since vaccination has become routine, rubella-affected babies have become rare, but if general vaccination levels drop, the risk is likely to rise again, so checking your own immunity will ensure your baby is protected (see also p.81).

Weight

Are you significantly overweight or underweight for your height? A common measure of ideal weight is the body mass index (BMI). BMI is calculated by measuring weight (in kilos) and height (in metres), and then using this formula: weight divided by height squared. For European and Māori, normal BMI is considered to be 20–25. The range is slightly higher for Pacific Islands people, and slightly lower for those of Asian origin. Although the BMI is only an approximate measure and does have some limitations (for instance, it cannot distinguish between fat and muscle mass), it is a good initial guide (see chart).

Height–weight chart

You can use this chart to find out if you are a healthy weight. First measure your height and measure your weight. Mark the point on the graph where your height and weight measurements meet, and then check your weight against the broad categories listed on the right.

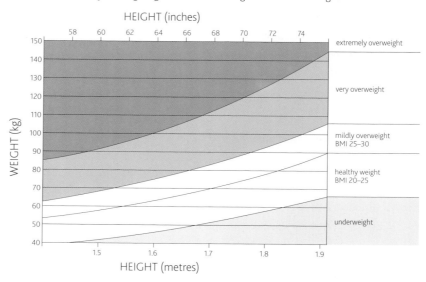

If you are overweight or underweight, falling pregnant and pregnancy itself will generally be much easier if you can lose or gain weight appropriately beforehand. Stringent weight-reducing diets are definitely not a good idea during pregnancy – it's better to see what you can do ahead of time.

Drugs and medicines

Any drugs or medicines, including alcohol, may affect pregnancy; likewise, pregnancy may affect the medication. As a general rule, it's best to avoid taking any drugs during pregnancy, especially in the first three months (including the time before you know that you're pregnant). This includes alcohol as well as medicines you can buy from the chemist such as cough mixtures and antihistamines for travel sickness or allergies.

However, there are some situations where drug-taking in pregnancy is unavoidable. For some women, underlying medical conditions mean that drugs must be taken throughout their pregnancy. Especially important are drugs for asthma, diabetes, epilepsy, schizophrenia and depression. Often these cannot simply be stopped, but need to be changed or the doses altered if you are pregnant. If you are on regular medication, discuss your plans for pregnancy with your regular doctor or health provider and/or the doctor who is prescribing your medication before you become pregnant. Before you take any drug, check that it is considered safe in pregnancy, and remind any doctor you see that you are, or may be, pregnant.

Addiction to alcohol, or to narcotics such as heroin, presents special problems to the baby as well as the mother. Babies born to addicted mothers suffer acute withdrawal after birth and need expert management if they are to survive.

Common drugs and substances to be especially wary of in pregnancy*

- ACE inhibitors (e.g. Quinapril)
- alcohol, tobacco, cigarettes, marijuana, 'P'(methamphetamine), Ecstasy and party pills
- anti-cancer drugs
- carbimazole (Neo-mercazole)
- chloroquin (Nivaquin) and other drugs used to prevent malaria
- lithium (Lithicarb, Priadel)
- metformin (Glucophage, Metomin), glibenclamide (Daonil) and other tablets for diabetes
- paroxetine (Aropax)
- phenytoin (Dilantin) and other drugs for epilepsy
- podophyllin
- radiation from X-rays
- roaccutane
- rubella, measles and yellow fever vaccines
- tetracyclines (Vibramycin, Minomycin and others)
- thyroxine (Eltroxin)
- warfarin (Marevan, Coumadin) and other anti-coagulants

Note: This list is not exhaustive.

Smoking

Smoking harms pregnant women and unborn babies in many ways (see p.23). While it is certainly best to give up smoking before getting pregnant if you possibly can, it's never too late to stop, and even cutting down a lot will help. Most midwives and doctors now offer special programmes for pregnant women who want to stop smoking, so ask about these if they haven't been mentioned yet.

Programmes for stopping smoking in pregnancy (or in preparation for pregnancy) are very similar to those used for non-pregnant people. Nicotine replacement therapy (NRT) can be used during pregnancy, and has been shown to be effective and safe; the risks to the baby from any NRT products are much less than those from smoking.[28] (See p.24.)

Illness and/or disability

There are not many illnesses or disabilities that absolutely preclude pregnancy. (Active cancer, with or without radiotherapy or chemotherapy, is one situation where pregnancy presents a grave risk to both mother and baby.) But ongoing illness often makes planning for pregnancy more important than usual; because of this, it may be best to delay conceiving until your particular condition improves or stabilises.

Sometimes it is not just a particular illness that has to be taken into account, but also the drugs or medicines used to treat that condition, which may need to be stopped or altered. If you have an ongoing illness or disease, it is worth discussing future pregnancy with your doctor well before making a firm decision to go ahead. It might be appropriate to talk about this when asking about contraception. And if you are, or intend to be, sexually active, it is even more important than usual to avoid unplanned pregnancy; you need to use the most reliable contraceptive method you possibly can.

Inherited conditions

Some conditions are carried in the chromosomes and can be passed from one generation to another via one or both parents. Some of these inherited conditions are well known, and it will often be obvious to those families who carry them which of their members are affected. An example is haemophilia, a disease where one of the factors responsible for the clotting of blood is absent or diminished. Most haemophiliacs are male, as the gene responsible is carried on their single X chromosome. (The other male sex chromosome is Y; see p.60.) Women with one affected X chromosome are said to 'carry' the gene; their other, unaffected X chromosome protects them from actually having the disease. Women have haemophilia only if they inherit two affected X chromosomes – one from each parent.

With other inherited disorders, people may not know that they carry the genes responsible until they have an affected child. In some cases, the disorder is not apparent at birth and may take months or years to manifest itself. If an abnormal baby has previously been born into your or your partner's extended family, it is worth finding out about the nature of the abnormality – it may be the first sign of an inherited condition that could affect some, but not all, family members.

Conditions where pregnancy will need special consideration

- cancers
- cerebral palsy
- diabetes
- drug addiction (including alcohol addiction)
- epilepsy
- genital herpes (only if active)
- heart disease (especially with valve replacement)
- high blood pressure
- HIV-AIDS
- kidney disease
- paraplegia
- syphilis
- tuberculosis

In any situation where an inherited disorder is known or suspected, it's wise to seek genetic advice. Sometimes this will be possible before a first pregnancy, but in other cases it may be suggested after a problem has occurred with a previous child.

Health professionals trained in the study of chromosomes (cytogeneticists and genetics counsellors) can advise you about the likelihood of having a baby affected by an inherited disorder. You can be referred through your doctor, either to one of the main genetics centres in Auckland or Wellington, to one of their regular clinics in other centres, or via email or post from rural areas. The consultation may involve chromosome studies being done on several members of your family.

Previous pregnancy complications

Again, there are not many complications that absolutely preclude another pregnancy, but previous complications may mean that particularly careful planning is required. A discussion with a health professional, with a review of your previous pregnancies, is well worthwhile. You will then be in a better position to decide whether to get pregnant again, and whether you can cope with the stress of another, possibly risky, pregnancy. You may even find that things are easier than you imagined.

Stopping contraception

Fertility returns quickly after you stop using most methods of contraception. If you are sexually active, pregnancy is perfectly possible during the very next menstrual cycle. This is especially true of all the barrier methods and natural family planning, and after the removal of an IUCD.

When you stop taking the pill, whether it's at the end of a packet or not, you will usually get a period. For most women, ovulation resumes rapidly and fertility returns promptly. There is some evidence now that, on average, women who come off the pill in order to conceive become pregnant even more quickly than those whose partners stop using condoms.[29] However, for some women, their first ovulation after stopping the pill takes a week or two longer than usual and the next period may be delayed. If conception intervenes, the expected date of delivery may be difficult to calculate accurately (see p.66). To avoid this problem, some women prefer to use a barrier method just for the first month or so after coming off the pill, although an early ultrasound scan can help confirm dates if there is any confusion.

A very few women find it takes several months for their periods to return after stopping the pill. In nearly all cases, periods do start again quite normally, given time. If you are particularly worried, or haven't had a period for over six months and you're not already pregnant, drugs can be used to 'restart' the menstrual cycle.

Depo-Provera is the only method of contraception where the return of periods is usually delayed. It can take up to a year for the menstrual cycle to resume, so it's not a good method of contraception to use if you then want to get pregnant quickly.

Previous complications to consider before you become pregnant again

- repeated miscarriage in first three months
- miscarriage/premature birth in second three months
- premature birth in the last three months (before 37 weeks)
- severe vomiting in early pregnancy
- intra-uterine death/ stillbirth
- abnormal baby
- more than two Caesarean sections
- severe bleeding, at any stage
- more than six previous pregnancies
- Rhesus disease
- post-natal depression

4. Trouble getting pregnant?

Not all women get pregnant as soon as they become sexually active or stop using contraception. On average, it takes several menstrual cycles to 'fall pregnant', even if both partners are normally fertile and they have regular sexual intercourse. So pregnancy may well occur in the very first month, but equally well it may not – a whole series of 'chances' are involved in any conception.

There is the chance that the woman produces an egg from her ovary and that it moves down her fallopian tube. There is the chance that the man produces sperm from his testes and that the sperm moves into the vas deferens (see p.40). There is the chance that the couple will have intercourse during the woman's fertile time and that the man's semen will arrive at the woman's cervix. There is the chance that the sperm will meet the egg and fertilise it. There is yet another chance that the fertilised egg will 'stick' (implant) in the wall of the uterus.

With so much left to chance, it's no wonder that pregnancy doesn't occur each cycle! Only about 65 per cent of couples become pregnant within three menstrual cycles, but approximately 83 per cent of couples become pregnant within a year.[30] This suggests that there is a range of fertility within our population, with some couples being more fertile than others.

If you want to fall pregnant sooner rather than later, there are several things you can do to maximise your chances.

Body weight

Being significantly overweight or underweight affects monthly ovulation in many women, so that some months an egg will not be produced and that menstrual cycle will not be a fertile one. If you are overweight, with a BMI (see p.44) of 27 or more, losing just a modest amount of weight will greatly increase your chances of ovulating every month. If you are underweight (BMI of 17 or less), gaining even a little weight will also help restore regular ovulation and increase fertility.[31]

Fertility awareness (natural family planning)

Each month, a woman can become pregnant at or around the time of ovulation. There are several fertile days and pregnancy is most likely to occur if intercourse takes place then. On the other hand, if intercourse is avoided on those days, pregnancy is unlikely to occur.

These fundamentals form the basis of the 'fertility awareness' approach to conception and contraception (also known as natural family planning). Successful use of this approach, either to achieve or to avoid pregnancy, relies on being able to detect ovulation as accurately as possible, and then having (or abstaining from) unprotected intercourse on the fertile days. The most reliable signs of ovulation are:

- the body temperature rises slightly after ovulation
- a positive result shows on an ovulation test kit

- the mucous released from the cervix becomes clear, thin and 'stretchy' during the fertile time
- the cervix becomes softer and slightly more open during the fertile time.

Following is a selection of methods that can be used to detect ovulation, with varying degrees of accuracy. The fertility awareness approach is most effective if several methods are combined. Used correctly, these methods can be reliable. However, it takes time, patience and motivation to learn how to use them accurately. It is best to learn from someone experienced, especially if you want to avoid pregnancy. Natural Fertility NZ Inc has trained teachers who can help. (See Appendix: Fertility awareness.)

Using fertility awareness

Basal body temperature

This used to be the only method of detecting ovulation, but it has largely been superseded by the use of ovulation detection kits (see below). The kits are not only more accurate but also much easier to use.

However, if you want to try the basal body temperature method, you need to take your temperature every morning as soon as you wake up, before you get up or have anything to eat or drink. It's best if you can use the same thermometer, take your temperature in the mouth or vagina (always use the same place), and record the temperature straight away on a specially made chart that you keep by your bed.

At the time of ovulation, your temperature may drop, and then rise by 0.2–0.5°C. It stays at this level until the next menstrual period. Once you have recorded five consecutive temperatures at this higher level, all of them above the previous six, the fertile time is *finished*. Intercourse after this point in the cycle will not result in pregnancy. While this method works well for some people, for many the temperature changes are just too subtle to record accurately, and mistakes can easily occur.

Ovulation detection kits

Special kits now available for use at home can chemically detect a rise in luteinising hormone (LH) in a urine sample. The level of LH rises dramatically just before ovulation. If you buy one of these kits, you need to use it for several days at what you think is your fertile time. They are fairly expensive, but are a reasonably accurate indicator that ovulation is indeed taking place.

Cervical mucous

You can learn to recognise changes in your own cervical mucous by observing the vaginal secretion. You can check the stretchiness with your fingers or with toilet tissue, and observe the mucous on underclothing. Record your observations each evening on a chart. (If you have recently had intercourse, this can confuse the picture.)

During the menstrual period there is usually no mucous, followed by a few 'dry' days when there is very little. Then the mucous returns and is often sticky, tacky and opaque. This mucous indicates that you are slightly fertile. If you want to avoid pregnancy, don't have intercourse on these days. The mucous then becomes thin, copious and clear, and stretches easily between the fingers.

This is the 'fertile' mucous, and it lasts for several days. The last day of fertile mucous is known as the 'peak day' (PD). The egg is usually released about 24 hours after the PD. Opaque mucous then replaces the clear mucous, although the fertile period lasts another three to four days.

If you want to get pregnant, having intercourse on alternate days during the fertile time immediately before the PD is most likely to result in pregnancy. If you want to avoid pregnancy, do not have intercourse until four days after the PD.

Cervical mucous at different stages of the menstrual cycle

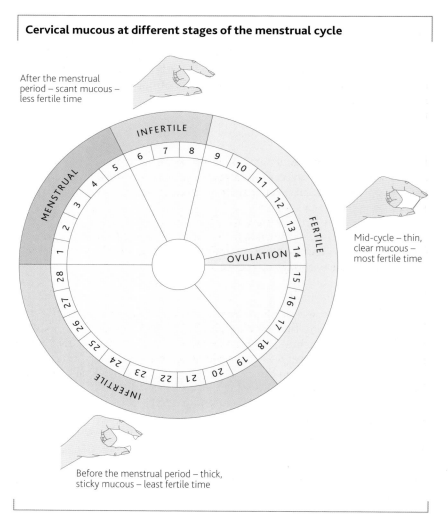

After the menstrual period – scant mucous – less fertile time

Mid-cycle – thin, clear mucous – most fertile time

Before the menstrual period – thick, sticky mucous – least fertile time

Cervical palpation

Many women can feel their cervix at the top of their vagina simply by inserting a finger as far as they can into the vagina. During the fertile phase of the cycle, the cervix can feel higher in position, softer and more 'open'. This too can be recorded on a chart each day, so that the changes become obvious.

Calendar method

This involves recording the start of every menstrual period on a calendar for at least six months. You can then calculate your average time of ovulation, using the 12–16-day premenstrual phase as a guide (see chart opposite). This method is not recommended for use on its own.

Intercourse

Frequency

Male fertility is dependent on the number of sperm in each millilitre of semen. The higher the count, the more likely it is that an egg could be fertilised if intercourse takes place. The count decreases with repeated ejaculation over a short time, and rises again within a couple of days. Having intercourse every alternate day during the fertile phase is recommended if you want to achieve a pregnancy.

Positions

There has been much speculation about whether different positions improve fertility. Some people feel that pregnancy is more likely if the man is on top and the woman underneath, but there is little evidence to suggest that this is really so.

A retroverted uterus (see p.349) was once considered to be a factor in infertility, in which case the woman on top would be a favourable position for intercourse. As knowledge about infertility has increased, the 'retroverted uterus' theory is now thought to be irrelevant.

Timing – a girl or a boy?

Obviously, it is necessary to have intercourse during a woman's fertile time for her to fall pregnant. But some couples believe that they are more likely to conceive a boy if intercourse takes place right on the day of ovulation, and a girl if intercourse takes place at either end of the fertile period. There has been considerable speculation on this theory over the years; at one time the theory favoured was the exact opposite of that described here.

If the baby is a boy, his sex chromosomes will have an XY pattern. A girl will have XX (see p.60). One of the sex chromosomes comes from the mother and is carried by the egg: it will always be X. The other sex chromosome comes from the father and is carried by the sperm: it may be either X or Y.

So while in one sense the father determines the sex of the baby, in another sense the mother determines the sex by perhaps favouring one or other type of sperm, depending on where she is in her cycle.

No one really knows whether the sex of a baby is purely a 50:50 chance, or whether those chances can be influenced significantly by the precise timing of intercourse. There are many other methods promoted for achieving a preferred-sex baby, but there are no foolproof recipes. Suffice it to say that most couples simply want to maximise their chances of a live, healthy baby – girl or boy.

And if I'm *still* not pregnant?

'We tried to get pregnant for a year, from the time I was 30, before we decided to go to a specialist. He did an internal scan and, bingo, he found polycystic ovaries. I was ovulating but the eggs were just turning into cysts on the ovaries – they weren't being released to get fertilised. I'd always had the condition and never knew; all those years I'd been trying to not get pregnant and really I needn't have bothered!

So many people have unexplained problems that mean they don't get pregnant. I was actually really happy to find that there was something wrong and that it could be dealt with.'

If you have not fallen pregnant within a year, despite having intercourse around the time of ovulation and using no method of contraception, then your chances of falling pregnant within the next year are small – not zero, but small. If you want to investigate why you're not getting pregnant, there is little point in waiting any longer than a year. Many couples want to find out earlier than this, and it's worth seeking advice any time after six months of trying to get pregnant, especially if you are over 35, or if it's beginning to worry you.

Your regular doctor or primary care provider is usually the first person to consult. Family planning clinics will also see you if you are having trouble getting pregnant after several months of trying to conceive. Either way, the doctor concerned will ask you about your past history and organise some basic tests and investigations. You may then be referred to a specialist, either a gynaecologist, a urologist and/or a fertility clinic, depending on what the issue might be. Most doctors – GPs, family planning doctors and specialists – will prefer to see you 'as a couple', except perhaps the first time. There are two reasons for seeing you together. First, the ability to get pregnant is dependent on two people, and even if only one appears to have a problem, both partners need to be checked out. Second, both of you can ask questions and listen to the answers.

Pregnancy for women not currently in a heterosexual relationship

It is increasingly common for some lesbians, and heterosexual women without partners, to seek assistance with donor insemination (DI) when they want to become pregnant. They may choose to approach a donor they know, or use the DI procedure described below. Of the various assisted reproduction techniques available, DI is technically one of the easiest and fertility clinics undertake it reasonably often. As with all decisions about having children, pregnancy in these situations deserves careful reflection about the implications of the particular technique being considered, as well as the implications of having a child.

Investigating infertility

A wide variety of investigations is possible, and just what is suggested will depend on your particular circumstances. Initially your doctor, whether a GP or a specialist, will probably want to do the following:

- Ask about your and your partner's medical histories (and your menstrual and contraceptive history), whether you are taking any medication, and whether you think you have any sexual problems.

- Ask about any previous relationships, sexually transmitted infections (STIs) and pregnancies. (This can be kept confidential, even between you and your partner if you wish, but you may need to arrange a separate consultation.)

- Examine both of you. For you, this will include weight measurement, a general and a vaginal examination, and an STI check (see p.31). You will be asked to have some blood tests to measure particular hormone levels, which must usually be done on a particular day in your cycle. Sometimes, an ultrasound scan will also be done to check the ovaries and uterus. For your partner, there will be weight measurement and examination of the abdomen, scrotum and testes. He will also be asked to collect two to three separate semen specimens (see box, right) and take them to a laboratory for analysis.

Your doctor will also probably want to talk with you about how you want to proceed with further investigations. The nature of some infertility problems will become obvious early on: sometimes treatment can be instituted relatively easily and successfully, but this is not always so.

In addition to the relatively simple tests already mentioned, one or some of the more complex and wide-ranging infertility investigations developed over the past 15 years may be suggested. Not all areas of New Zealand have access to the different types of specialist treatment, and travelling may have to become part of your commitment to treatment.

To collect semen specimens

- Abstain from intercourse for three days.

- Use a small sterile jar (usually supplied) with a wide mouth. The jar can be glass or plastic, but must have a non-metallic lid.

- Collect a specimen of semen, either by masturbation, or by intercourse using withdrawal (see p.36). Do not use a condom or any spermicidal product.

- Keep the specimen at room temperature. Do not warm it or carry it in the hand, but keep it in a bag and get it to the laboratory within two hours – the sooner the better.

- Put your name on the jar, and take it in with the form you have been given.

Infertility treatments available in New Zealand

- *Fertility clinic assessment*. There are both public and private fertility clinics in New Zealand, but only in the main centres. These clinics bring together multi-disciplinary teams of health professionals who can deal with the range of medical, social, emotional and psychological issues faced by people considering investigation and possible treatment of infertility.

- *Drugs, e.g. clomiphene, metformin*. These can help stimulate ovulation in women and sperm production in men.

- *Surgery*. In some women, micro-surgery can successfully restore function to the fallopian tubes. Very occasionally, surgery can help infertility in men.

- *IVF (in-vitro fertilisation)*. This method is suitable for women who have blocked fallopian tubes. Eggs from a woman's ovaries are removed from the body and fertilised by a man's sperm; the fertilised eggs become embryos. One or two embryos are placed within the woman's uterus at a precise time in her cycle. While two or three embryos give a greater chance of pregnancy, there is also a higher rate of multiple pregnancy (twins or triplets). As this creates greater risks for both babies and mother, single embryo transfer is increasingly preferred. Drugs and hormones are given to help stimulate egg production, and also to help the fertilised egg 'stick' within the walls of the uterus. Success rates (measured in terms of live births) of around 35–50 per cent are now being achieved at infertility clinics. However, success depends on a great many factors. Some women and/or couples face more barriers than others.

- *GIFT (gamete intra-fallopian tube transfer)*. This treatment is related to IVF. Here, the egg is removed from the ovary and can be placed into the fallopian tube, along with sperm from the man. Fertilisation takes place naturally within the tube. This method is used in some cases of male infertility or unexplained infertility.

- *ICSI (intracytoplasmic sperm injection)*. Again, the egg is removed from the ovary, but then a single sperm is injected directly into the egg cell, which is then placed in the fallopian tube. This is another useful method of dealing with some types of male infertility.

Continued on p.54

- *DI (donor insemination).* This treatment can be used when a man has a low or zero sperm count, or when sexual intercourse is not possible or acceptable. Here, semen from a donor is placed via a tiny tube into the woman's cervix during her fertile time. Donors are most often men under 45 years who have volunteered to donate to DI programmes to help infertile couples. Sometimes they will be personal donors (known to the woman or couple). All are screened as carefully as possible for disease, including hepatitis B and HIV-AIDS. They can donate only a few times. Donor programmes used to be deliberately anonymous, but since 2005, men who donate sperm (and women who are egg donors) are required to be identifiable to their offspring. The name of the donor is then recorded by the Registry of Births, Deaths and Marriages at the time of the birth.[32]
- *Surrogacy.* Occasionally, a woman may be able to have a baby on behalf of an infertile couple. IVF can be used to place an embryo into the surrogate woman's fallopian tube.

There are an increasing number of birth technologies, sometimes referred to collectively as assisted reproduction technologies (ARTs), available to help people achieve pregnancy. There are many differing opinions about their suitability, and the many ethical issues they raise present considerable challenges. The Human Assisted Reproduction Technologies (HART) Act, passed in 2004, provides a legislative and consultative framework within which such techniques can be considered, developed and delivered.[33] (See also Appendix: Infertility.)

'I went on a low dose of clompihene, which encourages the eggs to come out properly. This means the possibility of multiple births was quite high – the worst-case scenario was six babies!

I was on clompihene for a year before I got pregnant. Each month, I'd wait for my blood tests to come back and my hormone levels weren't going up very fast. I told myself that it was going to take time and I just carried on with my life really. I didn't let it take over: I always knew that what would be would be and it would work itself out. And it did – we had twins.'

Before embarking on intensive treatments for infertility, it is important to consider your own situation carefully. The complex process of investigation and treatment is not for everyone. At best, it is stressful, time-consuming and may be successful. At worst, it may be emotionally devastating, expensive, cause job losses and marital breakdown – and be unsuccessful.

Infertility affects 5–10 per cent of couples wishing to become pregnant, and this figure rises with increasing age.[34] (For women, fertility drops off steadily from 30 onwards; for men, fertility declines slowly but more variably after 50.) In some cases infertility is absolute – meaning that there is some clearly defined anatomical reason why pregnancy cannot occur (for example, congenital lack of a uterus).

But for most couples, this is not so; many simply have a much reduced chance of pregnancy. This means that they may, in fact, become pregnant without any active treatment, and may simply take much longer than usual to fall pregnant.

This uncertainty, together with the great uncertainty of treatment, is one of the things that infertile couples find hardest to cope with. The grief of infertility has been called the 'hidden grief'; society seldom recognises that infertile people have a right to grieve for the child, or children, they haven't been able to have. The New Zealand Infertility Society, also known as Fertility New Zealand, can provide information, support and advice. (See Appendix: Infertility.)

Adoption (see also p.71)

Some couples who cannot have children of their own feel that they would like to adopt. However, adoption cannot be regarded as 'just the same' as having one's own children, because the needs of the adoptive parent(s) have to be considered alongside the needs and rights of the child to be adopted. Birth parents also have needs and rights that need to be considered.

The number of children available for adoption in New Zealand is now very small, so it is not possible for everyone who wants to adopt to do so. Many adoptions in New Zealand today are private adoptions – that is, they take place within extended families or between people who know each other. Adoptions from other countries are also increasing, although these can be difficult to arrange, both emotionally and financially. They usually require the adoptive parent, or parents, to travel to the child's country, sometimes several times, with no guarantee of success. Increasingly, the extraordinary cultural challenges that inter-country adoption poses are being recognised; both host and recipient countries are also grappling with complex legislative issues.

If you are considering adoption, Child, Youth and Family (CYF, a service of the Ministry of Social Development) has information available about various types of adoption. (See Appendix: Child, Youth and Family.) If you wish to be placed on the service's list of prospective parents, you will need to supply quite a lot of information and compile a portfolio of photos and other details about yourself. The birth parent (or parents) makes the final decision about who will adopt the child.

Adoption can be a very positive and rewarding experience, but it is also a process fraught with potential difficulties and disappointments. CYF can provide more details, including information about overseas adoptions.

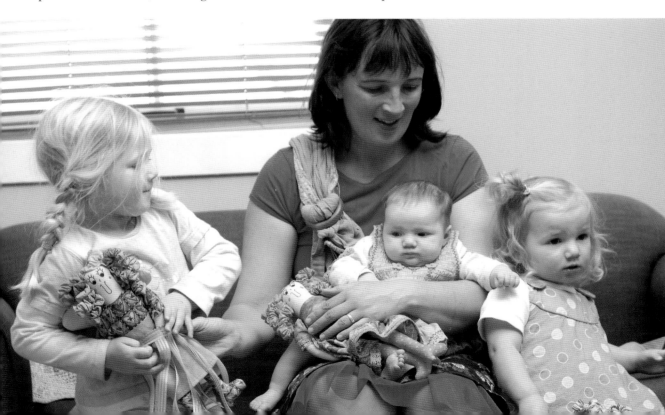

A Māori health professional's perspective

Dr Janice Wenn (Ngāti Kahungungu ki Wairarapa) is a Māori health specialist who has spent much of the past five decades working with women and families. She has been a 'bush nurse' in southern Tasmania, a public health nurse in the Wairarapa and Northland, chief nursing officer for the Taranaki Hospital Board, principal nurse for the Wairarapa Health Board, a member of the Wairarapa District Health Board, and founder of the Wairarapa-based community health service, Whaiora Whānui. In 2007, aged 74, Janice gained a PhD with a thesis exploring Māori concepts of kaupapa hauora (optimal health and well-being). She is currently a researcher at Massey University.

In many ways, I think the pregnancy and birth experiences of Māori women now are returning to the way things used to be. For example, there's now more recognition of the supportive role of whānau during the antenatal, birth and post-natal stages. That disappeared for a while. But the support of whānau is a really important component of care for Māori women, and needs to complement the care provided by their lead maternity carer. This means the LMC (lead maternity carer) needs to see a woman in her own environment, rather than expecting her to come to a clinic; that way, she can get to know the whānau and their way of doing things.

If you have been brought up as Māori, there's no question about many of the choices you will make about having a baby – where you give birth, who you want to be with you, how you want to handle labour. You know deep down that there are things that you must do, and you draw on your cultural values, your family history and the stories your nannies told you about pregnancy and childbirth.

For many women, mirimiri (massage) is important. Many new babies are massaged after birth by their nannies. Why? Because they were massaged by their nannies, and so on back in time. There are many other processes and rituals that have been handed down through the generations – saying karakia (prayers) over the whenua (placenta), the use of traditional pain relief in labour, various rituals and chants. Some of the early chants tell stories of what to do in specific situations. One I know describes how in prolonged labour, hot stones, steam and herbs can relax the woman's muscles and progress labour. Not all Māori will know these traditional rituals, but there are some Māori midwives who use them.

I've noticed a growing trend among many young urban Māori to take their baby's placenta back to their family land, as is customary. Some Māori midwives have developed the art of making beautiful containers for mothers to bury the placenta in, or they'll plant them in a big pot with a native tree over it. One young man I knew phoned his father to say he and his partner wanted to bring their baby's whenua out to the farm. Dad was delighted, but asked where the whenua was now. 'Oh,' said the young guy, 'it's in the deep freeze.' The father was a very spiritual person and was really quite shocked – but it shows that young Māori are modernising and adapting traditions to their own circumstances.

Other Māori don't believe in those sorts of practices, or don't care about them, and they seem to me like lost people really. They don't know what to do or who to relate to, and they can be very lonely.

But many young Māori women want to reconnect with their traditions when they're pregnant. They especially want to reconnect with their mothers and grandmothers, and for them to be part of the whole birth process. One very young girl I knew of was having a baby, and her grandmother and lots of other whānau were able to be present at the birth. In fact, the father of the baby ended up feeling rather excluded. The whānau was very focused on the girl, and protected her to the point where he was a bit left out – but that changed after the birth. The delivery of the placenta was a very special moment, which I felt privileged to witness. The kuia (women elders) examined it much more intricately than any midwife would have done, and said karakia over it. Then they took it and buried it on their family land.

The health services now are more responsive to these kinds of practices, and not just Māori health providers. There are no Māori midwives in this area, but I've noticed that the midwives generally are much more culturally responsive than they used to be. The hospitals have opened up their doors to different cultural values too, so women feel quite comfortable doing whatever they feel is important around the birth – whether it takes place at home or at hospital. Most midwives and GPs seem to be happy to work alongside whānau or Māori healers.

Another big change I've seen is the growth of Māori health providers, including those providing services for pregnant women and their families. The care they offer is based on kaupapa Māori, on values that Māori believe are important and want integrated into any health organisation – whether it's providing infant welfare services or surgical services. My research has identified eight core values that are especially important to Māori – whakapapa (a person's genealogical roots, which give them a sense of where they belong and their place on the earth), wairua (their spirituality), whenua (the land they belong to), whānau (the extended family to which a person relates), tikanga (the correct protocols and processes for doing things), te reo Māori (the language), tinana (physical health) and hinengaro (emotional and mental health).

Over time, I've seen the importance of these values to people. As a Māori health worker helping Māori, you pick up the cues – maybe this is a person who's not living on their own land and therefore they may be feeling a bit lost. People will mention where their baby's whenua is buried, so you know that this is a person who's spiritual, that they relate to the whenua and that their whānau's important to them. Or they might tell you how they were taught to fish, and to return so much of their catch back to Tangaroa. And you know then that they've got a really deep feeling about the land and about things that are Māori.

The Māori organisations that provide services to families and babies are making a huge difference. They're stepping in to fill the gaps, and giving people choices again. Interestingly, the services they provide are basically very similar to the services that were provided back in the 1960s by public health nurses.

For example, in this area, a Māori organisation is contracted to deliver Family Start [an intensive, home-based support service for families with high needs, funded by the Ministries of Education and Social Development] and offering really good support – not only to the child and the mother, but to the whole whānau. I met a group of young solo mothers in the Family Start programme a while back. Of the six, four had really good whānau support throughout their pregnancy and afterwards. But two didn't, and were very much on their own. It was Family Start that gave them the ability to trust themselves, and take responsibility for their babies and give them positive experiences. It was really lovely to watch.

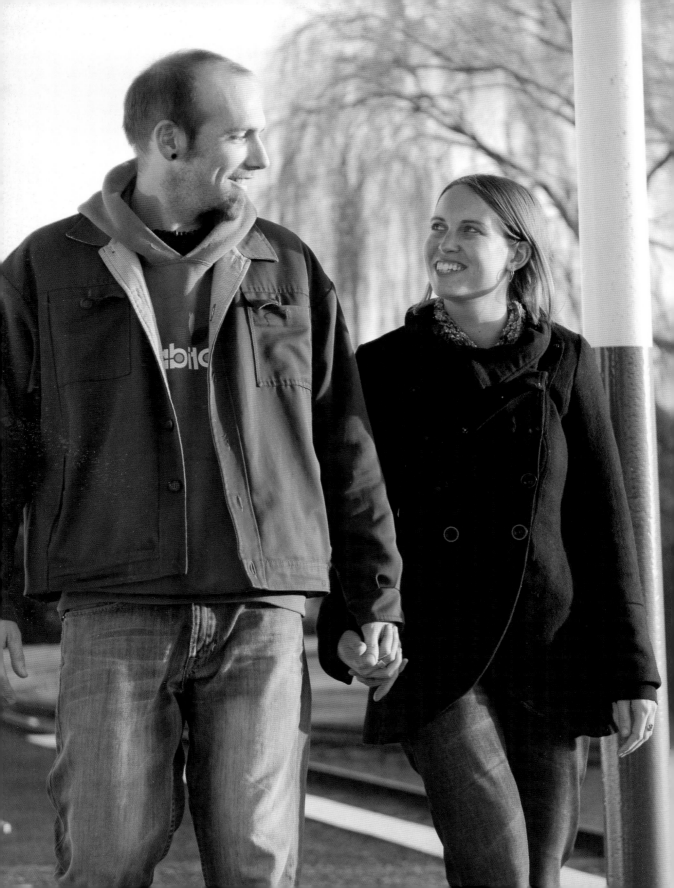

CHAPTER 2

Suspecting and confirming pregnancy

1. What's happening?

Fertilisation

After the egg is released from a woman's ovary at ovulation, it passes into the fallopian tube. A fluid-filled sac, known as the corpus luteum, is left behind in the ovary.

Once it has passed into the fallopian tube, the egg can be fertilised if it meets a healthy sperm from a man. The sperm penetrates the outer covering of the egg, and biochemical changes take place quickly so that no more sperm can penetrate.

Despite the fact that millions of sperm are deposited at the cervix during intercourse, only a few thousand manage to swim up into the uterus. Probably only a few hundred ever make it to the fallopian tube, and only one will actually fertilise the egg.

Fertilisation

egg

one sperm successfully penetrates the outer covering of egg

rapid biochemical change prevents other sperm entering egg

egg nucleus combines with sperm

The 23 chromosomes within the egg then fuse with the 23 chromosomes within the sperm to form the first cell of a new human being with 46 chromosomes. All the information necessary to determine every feature of this new person is contained in these 46 chromosomes. Every time a new cell is formed within the body, these 46 chromosomes are faithfully replicated.

Two of the 46 are known as sex chromosomes, and they determine whether the baby will be male or female. The sex chromosomes have a characteristic X or Y pattern. Eggs are always X, but sperm may be either X or Y. If the sex chromosomes of that first cell are in the XX configuration, the baby is female; if they are XY, it is male. The sperm thus carries the genetic code that determines the sex of the new human being.

Chromosome patterns

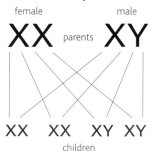

female   male

XX parents **XY**

XX   XX   XY   XY

children

Implantation

Once the egg has been fertilised, it moves down the fallopian tube towards the uterus, helped by tiny 'hair cells' on the lining of the tube. While this is happening, the single cell within the fertilised egg divides several times to form a blastocyst, which consists of two groups of cells and some fluid.

Now the blastocyst must stick to the inner lining of the uterus. This happens around 8–10 days after fertilisation, normally before a menstrual period is even missed. Some of the cells in one group then start to form placental tissue, and a link with the maternal blood supply is established. The other group of cells starts to form the embryo, or future baby. Pregnancy has begun.

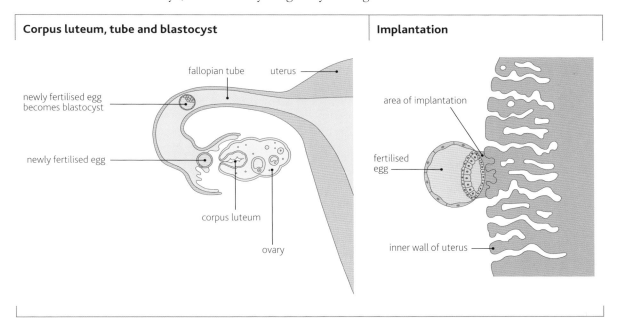

Corpus luteum, tube and blastocyst

fallopian tube   uterus

newly fertilised egg becomes blastocyst

newly fertilised egg

corpus luteum

ovary

Implantation

area of implantation

fertilised egg

inner wall of uterus

Hormonal changes

Once ovulation has occurred, the woman's body establishes the hormonal balance needed to maintain pregnancy should the egg become fertilised. This balance is maintained for about 14 days after ovulation, and then ceases abruptly. This change is marked by the onset of menstruation.

During the premenstrual phase, the corpus luteum produces the hormones progesterone and oestrogen. They maintain the lining of the uterus ready to receive a blastocyst.

When the blastocyst does implant in the inner wall of that lining, a new hormone, human chorionic gonadotrophin (HCG), is produced, at first in tiny amounts and then in greater quantities. HCG acts within the body to keep the corpus luteum intact for the first 8–9 weeks of pregnancy, producing a good supply of oestrogen and progesterone until the placenta takes over hormone production.

In a woman who is not pregnant, the corpus luteum normally collapses and ceases to function once the next menstrual period begins.

2. Finding out if you're pregnant

Earliest symptoms and signs

Missed menstrual period

A missed period is usually the first obvious sign that you may be pregnant – especially if your periods are usually regular and you are sexually active. If you are using contraception, then pregnancy is less likely, depending on what method you're using. But no method of contraception is absolutely perfect, so pregnancy is a possibility if you have missed a period for no other apparent reason.

In women who have irregular periods, a missed period is more difficult to interpret and may or may not mean pregnancy. (Periods can be delayed or missed for other reasons, such as stress, huge amounts of exercise, hormonal upsets, or some types of contraception, but pregnancy always needs to be considered.) Sometimes a very light period (compared to what is normal for you) can also indicate pregnancy. A very few women can continue to have menstrual periods when they are, in fact, pregnant. These periods are usually much lighter than normal, and it would be very rare to have two during a normal pregnancy. If you have ever had a period when you were pregnant, this is likely to happen again in future pregnancies.

If you have not been sexually active at all within the last ten months, then you cannot be pregnant, no matter how many periods you've missed. But remember that although pregnancy primarily occurs when the penis fully enters the vagina before ejaculation takes place, pregnancy can very occasionally result even if the penis does not fully enter the vagina; there are sometimes sperm in the small drop of fluid that gathers at the tip of the penis before ejaculation.

'My breasts were very sore and tight feeling; at first I thought it was just a premenstrual thing – but they got more and more uncomfortable ...'

Sore breasts

Many women notice breast changes in early pregnancy. The breasts may become very sensitive, particularly in the nipple area, even before a period has been missed.

Nausea

Not all women suffer from nausea in early pregnancy, and it is unusual for it to be the very first symptom of pregnancy. It is most common for nausea to become a problem around six weeks from the start of your last menstrual period (LMP).

Some women find that their sense of taste and smell alters dramatically within a few days of conception. With experience, these women can detect their own second and subsequent pregnancies very early.

'I get this taste in my mouth. It's a definite metallic taste; gets into everything. It tends to get better around four months, for me anyway.'

Tiredness

Excessive tiredness is often a feature of the early months of pregnancy – but again, it is most likely to be noticeable from six weeks onwards.

Other early symptoms

Different women experience other early signs of pregnancy in different ways. Some notice that they need to pass urine more often than usual; others describe changes in sexual desire or experience. Some women say that sex is better in pregnancy; others say exactly the opposite.

The nipple area may become darker very early in pregnancy, and women who have been pregnant before may notice a drop or two of milk appearing at the nipple.

Some women describe a bloated feeling in the abdomen early on in pregnancy. This is caused by hormonal changes. The uterus containing the growing baby is not normally big enough to be felt until you are about three months pregnant.

Pregnancy tests

Tests that measure hormones in the urine are often used to detect early pregnancy. Those most commonly used can detect pregnancy accurately 14 days after conception. The test is not reliable if done before this time, although a positive test is more likely to be correct than a negative one.

Pregnancy tests measure levels of the hormone HCG (see p.61), which is not normally produced by non-pregnant women. The hormone is produced once a fertilised egg implants in the wall of the uterus. Around 14 days after conception, enough is being produced to be reliably detected by a urine test.[1]

GPs, practice nurses, midwives and family planning clinics keep pregnancy test kits on hand, and can do a test and have the result ready for you within a few minutes. They can also offer appropriate advice at the time, which can be helpful if the results are unclear or unexpected. Some laboratories also offer pregnancy tests, but any advice will need to be sought elsewhere. Blood tests are available as well, but are no more reliable than modern urine tests (except in some unusual circumstances, such as after treatment for infertility).

Home tests

If you buy a do-it-yourself pregnancy test kit from a pharmacy, you need to follow the instructions exactly if you want an accurate result. Some home tests are not reliable until six weeks after your LMP, although most are now just as accurate as those used by health professionals. Whatever the result, you should have pregnancy confirmed by a doctor, nurse or midwife, either by examination and/or another pregnancy test, as soon as you reasonably can.

Ultrasound scans (see pp.107, 114 and 150)

Early pregnancy can also be detected with high-quality ultrasound scanning. This is sometimes done if very early detection is important – for example, after some infertility treatments. Otherwise, scanning is not generally used to detect pregnancy, but rather to confirm an unexpected pregnancy test result, or in other unusual circumstances. Scanning is very helpful in determining how far advanced a pregnancy is, especially if this is uncertain. In cases of suspected miscarriage or ectopic pregnancy, ultrasound scans can be invaluable. Transvaginal scans, where a small, smooth probe is placed in the vagina,

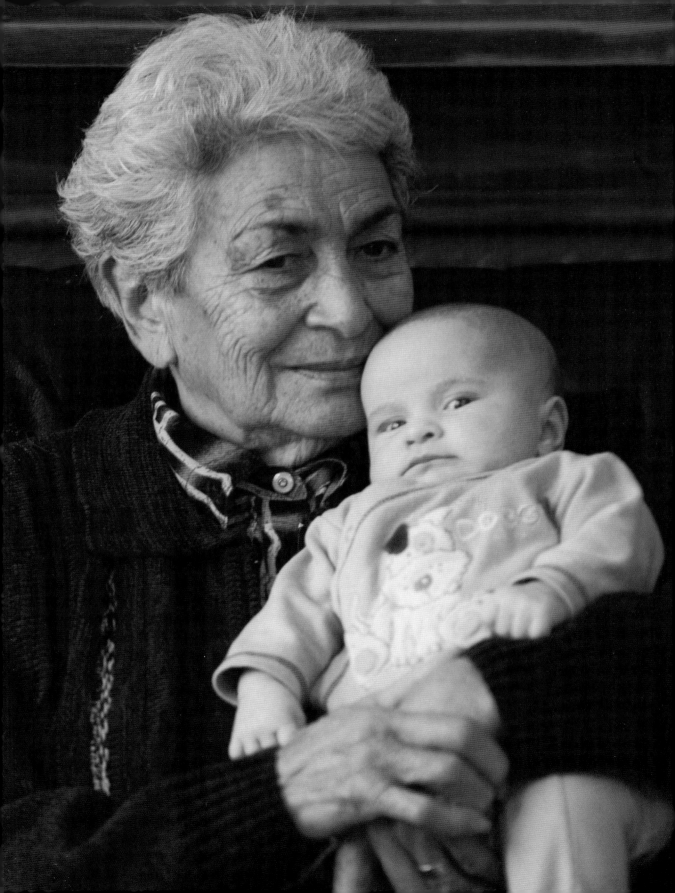

can be more accurate in these situations, and will sometimes be suggested by the ultrasonographer at the time.

First visit to a primary care service, doctor or midwife

If you suspect that you may be pregnant, a practice nurse, GP or midwife can confirm this with a pregnancy test. If the result is positive, you should see a GP or midwife within a week or two, or earlier if you have any special concerns. If the result is negative, but you still think you might be pregnant, a visit to a health professional may help sort this out for you. A false negative result can occur if the pregnancy test is done too early, if the urine specimen is not collected properly, or with a threatened miscarriage or an ectopic pregnancy.

Before your visit, work out as accurately as you can when you think you might have become pregnant. Think back to your last period, and see if you can remember which day it started. Even if you can't recall the exact date, get as close as you can (for example, 'the first week in October'). If you know the date on which you might have conceived, take this information along too. It will give an even more accurate guide to how pregnant you are, and whether the pregnancy test will be reliable. If you are likely to go ahead with your pregnancy, and are not already taking folic acid tablets, you should start these as soon as you suspect you are pregnant – the earlier the better (see p.43).

At this very first visit, your GP or midwife may do a full first antenatal check (see p.100). However, it is more likely that they will simply confirm that you are indeed pregnant, by doing a pregnancy test (if you have not already had one) and/or a vaginal examination to check that the size of your uterus fits with your calculations. If you have had any pain or bleeding, an examination may be necessary to check for a possible miscarriage or ectopic pregnancy. The doctor or midwife may then discuss with you how you feel about being pregnant, and ask you to come back for a more detailed visit. Once your pregnancy has been confirmed, all subsequent visits to do with the pregnancy are free unless you choose to go to a private specialist (see p.97).

If for some reason you do not want to go to your usual GP or primary care service about a suspected pregnancy, you can go to any other GP, an independent midwife or a family planning clinic. But don't just 'not go' – *especially* if you are unsure about what you want to do if you are pregnant.

3. Normal pregnancy

How long does pregnancy really last?

Strictly speaking, a woman is pregnant from the time a fertilised egg is implanted in the wall of her uterus until the moment the baby is born. But because it is difficult to know exactly when conception and implantation take place, pregnancy is usually regarded as starting on the first day of the last menstrual period (LMP) and finishing, ideally, 40 weeks later. The estimated date of delivery (EDD) – sometimes referred to as the estimated date of birth (EDB) – is calculated on this basis.

However, if a woman normally has a long menstrual cycle (for example, 35 days), ovulation is likely to have taken place later in the cycle than in the more usual 28-day cycle. Therefore the EDD is probably up to a week later than the standard 40 weeks.

If the date of the LMP is uncertain or unknown, the EDD is also likely to be uncertain. This may happen if the pregnancy is unplanned, or if conception occurs immediately after stopping the contraceptive pill or injection. An uncertain EDD can usually be sorted out by physical examination of the uterus and/or an ultrasound scan.

Pregnancy is often talked about in weeks rather than months, allowing your progress during pregnancy to be more precisely assessed. 'How many weeks are you?' becomes a common question for pregnant women. If a health professional writes '12/40', it means you are 12 weeks pregnant out of an expected 40 weeks of pregnancy.

Traditionally, however, pregnancy has been regarded as nine months in duration, and many women find it easier to think in months rather than weeks. This historical perspective has given us the concept of three phases of pregnancy, each lasting three months and known as a 'trimester'. This concept is also useful, because it recognises the three major milestones for the developing baby:

- being fully formed
- being able and likely to survive outside the uterus (womb)
- being born.

Just as importantly, talking about trimesters recognises that there are three maternal phases to pregnancy:

- 'non-visible' pregnancy – a time of mixed emotions, tiredness and, sometimes, sickness
- 'more visible' pregnancy – a time of adjustment and acceptance
- 'very visible' pregnancy – a time of waiting and slowing down.

The following three chapters are about each of the trimesters in turn. But of course there is considerable overlap, and some topics covered in one chapter will also apply to other phases of the pregnancy.

All these different ways of talking about pregnancy – whether in weeks, months or trimesters – are convenient labels to help describe particular stages. Remember, though, that pregnancy is a continuous process of growth and development, which doesn't stop or start in neat weekly or monthly blocks.

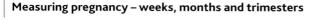

Measuring pregnancy – weeks, months and trimesters

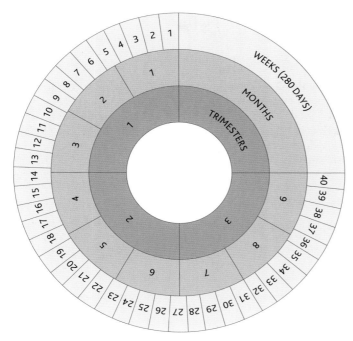

What is antenatal care?

Antenatal (or prenatal) simply means 'before birth'. Antenatal care (routine pregnancy care health checks by a midwife and/or doctor) is available to all pregnant women in New Zealand. Nearly all pregnant women in this country take advantage of these services, and this tradition is well established. For some women, having regular ongoing health checks may be a new experience, and most women find that it is easier if they see a health professional they know each time.

Nevertheless, even though you need to choose one nominated person who will coordinate your care (your lead maternity carer, or LMC), pregnancy care often requires a team approach. This allows you to get the benefit of the different skills each health professional, and each health service, can provide. An LMC is most commonly a midwife who is registered to provide full pregnancy care (see p.95). Everyone looking after you should work together to make sure you are treated with care and appropriate skill.

For most pregnancies, antenatal care is routine and does not interfere with the pregnancy; it simply provides the opportunity for health professionals to observe what is already happening and to detect any potential problems early. Often, but not always, complications can be averted or at least minimised by appropriate action. More detail on potential problems is provided in the chapters that follow, and information about choosing antenatal care is included in Chapter 3.

The Code of Health and Disability Services Consumers' Rights[2]

As a health consumer you have important rights, which are detailed in the Code of Health and Disability Services Consumers' Rights. The Code, and an easy-to-follow summary, can be found on the Health and Disability Commissioner's website (see Appendix). A useful pamphlet about the Code of Rights is also available from the website, the Health and Disability Commissioner's office, and health providers.

The Health and Disability Commissioner is charged with upholding the Code and improving the quality of health and disability services. The Commissioner's office can help to resolve any problems between consumers and health and disability services.

If you have any concerns about the care you are receiving, or if you think that any of your rights have not been respected, in the first place it is best to try and raise it directly with the person or organisation providing the service (such as a midwife, doctor or hospital). Often they will welcome your complaint as it will help them to improve their service or to uncover a problem.

You can take a relative or friend for support if you need to meet any of the above groups. You can also have the support of an independent health and disability advocate who is trained to help people in your situation. The service is free of charge.

Contact phone numbers:

- National Advocacy Service 0800 555 050

- The Health and Disability Commissioner 0800 11 22 33.

'My husband and I didn't do any of the conventional things like going to antenatal classes. Our midwife took us through a lot of the things we needed to know. I have a huge family and lots of nieces and nephews, so I guess I was a bit arrogant and thought, "Oh, it will be sweet, I already know how things go." And in the end it was fine, though there were things like tired signs and breastfeeding techniques I wished I'd learnt earlier.'

Education for pregnancy and parenting (antenatal education)

Many kinds of parenting education are available to pregnant women in New Zealand. In recent years, partners, friends and relatives have been able to attend classes too.

Antenatal education is, in fact, anything that enables you to learn about pregnancy, childbirth and caring for a baby. It can include advice from health professionals, books, pamphlets and chats with friends, but it commonly involves going to a series of classes where trained childbirth educators teach many of the things you might want to know.

Nowadays, both health professionals and women themselves recognise the importance of women knowing as much as they can about pregnancy and childbirth. Individually and collectively, women have demanded more information about the whole process of reproduction, so they are better able to make safe decisions about the care they receive. Choices about antenatal education are fully discussed in Chapters 4 and 5.

4. Unplanned pregnancy – your options

Despite the widespread use of contraception, unplanned pregnancy is still quite common. It can happen to any fertile woman who is sexually active with a man, at any stage – from the time of her first period to the time of her last.

Since most women are fertile and most are sexually active, it is not surprising that unplanned pregnancies continue to occur, despite the availability of better and more reliable contraceptive methods than ever before. Contraception is not absolutely foolproof and, for a variety of reasons, is not always used when needed (see diagram, p.34). The number of unintended pregnancies can certainly be greatly reduced by using good contraception, but will never be entirely eliminated.

Today, New Zealand women who find themselves accidentally pregnant have three main options: going ahead with the unplanned pregnancy, terminating the pregnancy, and/or adoption. Each of these options is discussed briefly below. However, if you are considering termination or adoption, you will need more detailed information than is provided here. A number of support services are available, although they vary from region to region. (See Appendix: Unplanned pregnancy.) Seek help as early as you can.

Going ahead with an unplanned pregnancy

Some women, finding themselves unexpectedly pregnant, continue with the pregnancy and accommodate the many changes that this entails. For some, this is not too difficult a choice at that particular stage of their lives. Their contraceptive use may have been rather haphazard, with the almost subconscious knowledge that an unplanned pregnancy was a possibility.

But for other women, dealing with an unplanned pregnancy is not so easy. Women who have had children recognise only too well the responsibilities another pregnancy and another child will bring.

Some women take a while to realise they are pregnant. If you're not planning to get pregnant and you're using some form of contraception, you may attribute the usual signs and symptoms to other causes – or the usual signs and symptoms may not be there.

Termination of pregnancy (abortion)

For some women, an unwanted pregnancy presents a potentially disastrous life situation. The current law in New Zealand (the Contraception, Sterilisation and Abortion Act 1977, and the Crimes Act 1961, Amendments 1977, 1978) makes provision for pregnancy to be terminated if a woman's physical or mental health is at risk because of the pregnancy.

If you are considering a termination, you need to confirm that you are indeed pregnant and to request a termination as soon as possible. To do this, you need to visit a doctor – either your own regular GP, another GP, or a

'My pregnancy was unplanned and was quite a shock. We had been married for just over five years and had talked about starting a family but had decided to wait a couple of years so that we could do a bit more travel and be in a better financial position. This was the one time in my life that I had unprotected sex and I just didn't think that it would result in a pregnancy. I guess we just got careless and assumed that we were safe – I really didn't give it another thought until a few days before my period was due and I didn't feel as I usually did at that time.'

'Once the pregnancy was confirmed, I knew that I had to go through with it and have the baby. Even so, we had a lot of worries about whether we were ready or would even make good parents. It really helped us both to talk to people together and separately. Having a trouble-free pregnancy probably helped a lot, especially as I felt absolutely wonderful once the morning sickness passed.'

doctor at a family planning or sexual health clinic. Check with them what abortion services are available in your area. (See Appendix: Termination of pregnancy.)

All doctors are legally required to refer you for further consideration of your request if this is what you definitely wish to do. If a doctor has a moral objection to arranging a referral for termination, they must provide you with accurate and timely information as to where you can consult a doctor promptly who will refer you for consideration of termination. If you have trouble getting referred for a termination, you can phone the nearest family planning or sexual health clinic for advice.

Two doctors, one of whom is a specialist obstetrician and gynaecologist, must agree that you have sufficient legal grounds for an abortion before you can have the procedure or operation. In the larger cities, there are dedicated clinics where you can talk to a counsellor, see the two doctors, and have the procedure all at the same place. In other areas there are different arrangements, and you may have to travel between appointments. Some clinics are private and a charge will be made. At the time of writing, the services provided by the public health system are free for New Zealand citizens. If you are an international visitor, temporary worker or here on an international student visa, you will have to pay the full cost of the termination procedure, even in a public hospital.

Up until the late 1970s, women seeking a termination of pregnancy in New Zealand had to go overseas, or seek help from illegal and often unscrupulous operators, where conditions and techniques were often dirty and dangerous. A significant number of women died from infections and haemorrhage after these procedures. Today, legal terminations are available in safe conditions.

There are now two methods available for carrying out terminations in the first trimester (the first 12 weeks of pregnancy): the medication method, where a combination of specific drugs are taken to induce abortion, and the surgical method.[3]

Although the *medication method* is more commonly used for abortions carried out after 12 weeks, it may also be suitable for women who are ready for a termination before the end of the eighth week of pregnancy, providing there are no other complications (not all clinics offer this option). Some medication is taken to soften the cervix, followed by a second medication that acts to empty the uterus. These special medications are available only through a certified clinic, and the usual requirements for legal abortion must still be met.

Termination by this method can take a day or two, so although one or two clinic visits are required, most women complete the process at home. Good follow-up from the clinic is important; for some women, the process may be incomplete and a surgical procedure may also be required.

Surgical abortion can be most safely performed within the first 12 weeks of pregnancy. During this time, the pregnancy sac and other material in the uterus can be sucked out through a tiny tube inserted into the cervix. The procedure takes about 20 minutes. Good technique under sterile conditions must be maintained throughout, so terminations are carried out only by doctors and nurses properly trained in the procedure. A surgical termination can be done under local or general anaesthetic, and an overnight stay is not usually necessary.

'There was no way of going ahead with pregnancy for me. I had just started a new job after months on the benefit, and was living at home with my dad ... and he's got problems ... I couldn't have coped, and nor could Dad ... I know I will live with that decision for the rest of my life ... and I have no regrets.'

'It has been very difficult for me since the abortion. I think about it a lot. Was I really too old (43)? Was my partner really that adamant?'

Once you are more than 12 weeks pregnant, this procedure is no longer suitable. Termination after 12 weeks requires admission to hospital, or to a clinic fully equipped to deal with this procedure. The process takes much longer and may involve having medication, vaginal pessaries, an injection into the uterus or a drip (see p.275) – all of which artificially trigger a mini-labour. This type of termination is to be avoided if possible, as it is an unpleasant experience and the risks of bleeding, infection and other complications increase as pregnancy progresses.

So if you do find yourself accidentally pregnant and want to request a termination, you need to act promptly – as soon as you suspect that you might be pregnant. You may have to wait two or three weeks to be seen at an abortion clinic or by a specialist, and may be refused a termination if you arrive more than 12 weeks pregnant. You can change your mind at any stage, right up until the time you have the operation or take the first tablets. But if you are unsure about a termination, it pays to leave all your options open.

Deciding to have a termination is never easy. It helps if you can talk it through with a trusted partner, friend or relative. You may feel that you should make this decision on your own, but most women faced with the possibility of a termination say they find some support from a good friend or family member very helpful. Whatever the situation, professional counselling is recommended, and is available from social workers, family planning clinics and at termination clinics, as well as from other agencies. Get as much information as you can about termination, and on what the options could be for going ahead with pregnancy, before you make your final decision. (See Appendix: Unplanned pregnancy.)

You will also need to review your current contraceptive method. A change may be necessary to avoid another unwanted pregnancy.

Adoption (see also p.55)

Some women wanting to go ahead with an unexpected pregnancy, but unable to provide the care they want for their baby, find that the best course is to give their baby up for adoption. If you are considering adoption, you may find it helpful to talk to a social worker from Child, Youth and Family (CYF) who is experienced in adoption procedures (see Appendix: Adoption). Do so early in the pregnancy, before you make any final decisions.

You may wish to have your baby adopted within your family, or by someone you know. CYF does not have to be involved at all in a private adoption, although in practice its social workers may sometimes take on an advisory role. But for a private adoption to be legal and binding, it must go through the court via a lawyer.

In adoptions arranged through CYF, as a birth parent you can choose what sort of people you would like as adoptive parents for your child. Factors such as ethnicity, family background, physical characteristics, occupation, religion and location can all be taken into account, and you will often get the opportunity to see some photos of prospective parents before making your decision.

It is important to remember that adoption means ultimately giving up your rights and responsibilities as a parent. In general, CYF encourages 'open' adoption (where some contact is maintained between the birth parent(s) and the child), but this is not compulsory.

'I gave up my baby for adoption when she was four months old. It tore me apart at the time … it was a terrible time … but I knew I couldn't look after her, either. It was the right decision. I feel happy for her now – and I never did when she was with me.'

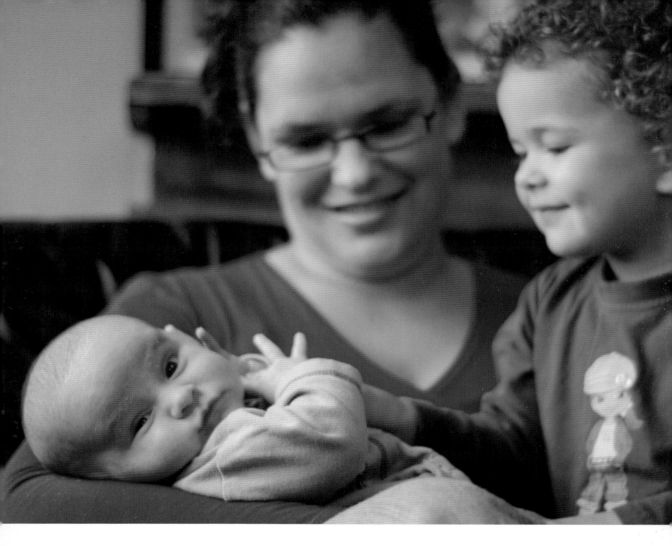

The decision to give up a baby for adoption is complicated. It is also permanent. Nevertheless, it is an option chosen by a small number of women who are unable to bring up a child at this time in their lives. By doing so, these women give a precious opportunity to other women and men to become loving parents, as well as considering it the best possible option for their baby.

Whāngai

Whāngai is a unique Māori child-placement practice that is likened to adoption although it is not the same. 'Adoption or foster care tends to be mainly focused on the interests of the child. The institution of whāngai, while being cognisant of the interests of the child, is weighted more towards establishing, nurturing and cementing relationships between individuals, families and wider relational networks.'[4]

If you are considering whāngai as an option, it is important to talk to your whānau, so they can give you the support you need, and help you make considered decisions.

Hope Tupara

A Pacific health professional's perspective

Violani 'Ilolahia (Lani) Wills was a midwife in Tonga and New Zealand before becoming charge nurse of the neonatal unit at Wellington Hospital, a role she held for 26 years. She was a founding member of the New Zealand Council of Tongan Women, and the national president (now patron) of the Tongan Nurses' Association. In 1999, she was awarded the MNZM, for services to nursing and the Pacific Islands community. She is now a community nurse for Pacific Health Services Wellington.

Suitable midwives

For Pacific women, finding a midwife they can communicate and feel comfortable with is one of the biggest challenges. I know of only three midwives in the Wellington area who work primarily with Pacific women. In the past, I have seen Pacific women arrive at hospital in labour, without a midwife. Today, there is government funding to ensure an adequate supply of hospital midwives is always available for these cases.

Any pregnant woman has to be completely comfortable with her midwife; she wants to feel that the midwife sees her as a person, and is prepared to 'work outside the box'. Not everyone will fit the same box! Not only is each individual different; there are also important differences between the various Pacific ethnic groups and how they think about pregnancy and childbirth. Among Tongans, for example – which is the community I know best – women do not usually go back to work until the baby is at least six months old. The babies are to stay home and not to venture out until baptism around three months. Tongans will never take their baby to a crèche or childcare centre: the baby will always be looked after by a grandmother or another female relative.

Barriers to care

Language barriers affect Pacific women's relationships with their midwives, and may be the source of misunderstandings that create unhappiness and tension. In turn, this tension may prevent the woman from sharing her concerns with her midwife, or asking questions about matters she is unsure of. Cultural awareness is essential in midwives working with Pacific women; its absence is the reason that many Pacific women appear not to communicate or show their real feelings and moods. Many Pacific people are very good at hiding what they really feel. To avoid sounding critical, a Pacific woman may simply say what she thinks the midwife wants to hear. The midwife needs to be aware of that, to be alert to possible misunderstandings, to look around and to ask the right questions.

Safe choices

There are other issues affecting Pacific women in pregnancy. Some migrants do not know how the maternal healthcare system works and what sort of care is available to them. Many midwives now require patients to visit them at their clinics, rather than seeing them in their own homes. But this does not suit most Pacific women, especially if they are reliant on public transport, do not know their way around, or have small children to care for as well. These are all reasons why not so many Pacific babies are seen by Plunket nurses, too. Financial costs and timing as well as difficulties in navigating the Pākehā system are real additional issues for Pacific people.

Hospital or home?

As in the wider community, there are many different views among Pacific women about whether to give birth at home or in hospital. Unfortunately, when they are considering where to have their babies, the issue of safety is not always adequately discussed. Because of language difficulties, some midwives find it hard to hold meaningful conversations with Pacific women about the options and the safety implications of each. For the same reason, women may find it hard to ask questions that elicit the information they need to make their choice. Similarly the issue of informed consent is questionable under this circumstance of variable comprehensions.

Some Pacific women find home birth convenient, because there is no need to travel across town or make arrangements for older children to be looked after. But some women may feel that their home is not good enough; perhaps the facilities are not suitable, or the house is overcrowded and there is no privacy. Others choose to give birth in hospital because they think it is better to have all the medical back-up if they need it. Considerably more Pacific women living in New Zealand give birth in hospital than at home. Either way a comprehensive dialogue in an appropriate language needs to take place before reaching a satisfactory decision.

It is not uncommon for many people to be present at the birth itself. Usually the husband or partner attends, and perhaps the grandmother or another female relative to help the midwife. The health professionals need to be aware of any language barriers, and recognise that the woman may be reluctant to ask for pain relief or other intervention; they should be prepared to take the initiative if they think intervention is the right thing to do. Pacific women are sometimes seen as 'bad' patients. We may be seen as too obliging, or else not obliging enough!

Placenta/fonua

After the baby is born, different families will have different wishes about what to do with the placenta. Even though burying the placenta and umbilical cord is part of traditional Pacific cultures, Pacific people living here in New Zealand will not necessarily want to. If they do not own their house, they would not want to bury it and then leave it behind, unattended, when they move. That would never happen in the Islands.

Postnatal and maternal care

Traditionally, a woman who has just given birth will be nurtured both by her family and by her community – they will bring her food, and look after her in many ways. That nurturing attitude continues among Pacific communities in New Zealand, but there are important differences. New mothers may miss out on the support and shared knowledge that other women can offer, especially if the local Pacific Islands community is small. For these isolated mothers, there is only the midwife to fulfil that role; therefore, it is even more critical that they have a good relationship based on mutual understanding. The level of Pacific community support available to new mothers is also different in New Zealand because older relatives are usually still in the workforce, meaning they are unable to help out as much as they might like.

Breastfeeding

The rate of breastfeeding in the first six months is reasonably low among Pacific women. There are many reasons. When the mother has to go back to work soon after her baby is born (which happens in most cases), it is simply not possible. Alternatively, she may not have the support and resources she needs to breastfeed, especially if she has older children. Again, these point to the need for good communication in the appropriate language with the midwife, so they really understand what is going on in the home and can make suggestions. As long as the mother and the midwife have tried as best they can, a mother who cannot breastfeed should never feel like a failure.

Bed-sharing

It is still very common among Pacific families for babies to share a bed with their parents. In traditional village life, in a warm climate, the whole family often sleeps in the same area on mats and without heavy bedding, so there is no risk of suffocation or smothering. Mothers often find breastfeeding is much easier to manage. But the situation here, where mattresses and blankets and cots are used, is very different. It is sometimes necessary to make people aware that there are real risks associated with bed-sharing in these conditions, especially for smoking and alcohol-imbibing parents or caregivers.

A settled baby, a happy family

Another issue that midwives need to appreciate is that Pacific mothers do not like to hear their baby cry. In the first few days, before her milk comes in, a mother may prefer to give her baby a complementary bottle-feed rather than having him cry from hunger. But she will still want to breastfeed once her milk supply is well established. I feel that this Pacific cultural attitude to breastfeeding does not always meet the expectations of western midwives. In our culture, when the baby is happy and settled, the whole family is at peace.

Summary

I have highlighted the key factors in midwifery best practice that contribute to a healthy pregnancy and the best possible outcomes for both mother and baby.

The maternity services need to be delivered as an ethnic-specific service and drive away from the economy-of-scale model. New Zealand needs to recognise its multiculturalism and train ethnic-specific midwives with strong cultural competency and high social literacy to maximise pregnancy outcomes for all New Zealanders.

Growing up in Tonga, I was privileged to be a recipient of, Kaliloa and eyewitness to, the best maternal care and baby healthcare delivery. As a nurse and midwife, I was mentored by my own mother and by a generation of wise Tongan midwives from a previous era. Their wisdom about how to nurture and deliver the best maternal and child care is their legacy. We left the Islands to come to New Zealand with the expectation of better healthcare for everyone. The dream remains – the best health outcomes for the Pacific mother and child in Aotearoa and Oceania.

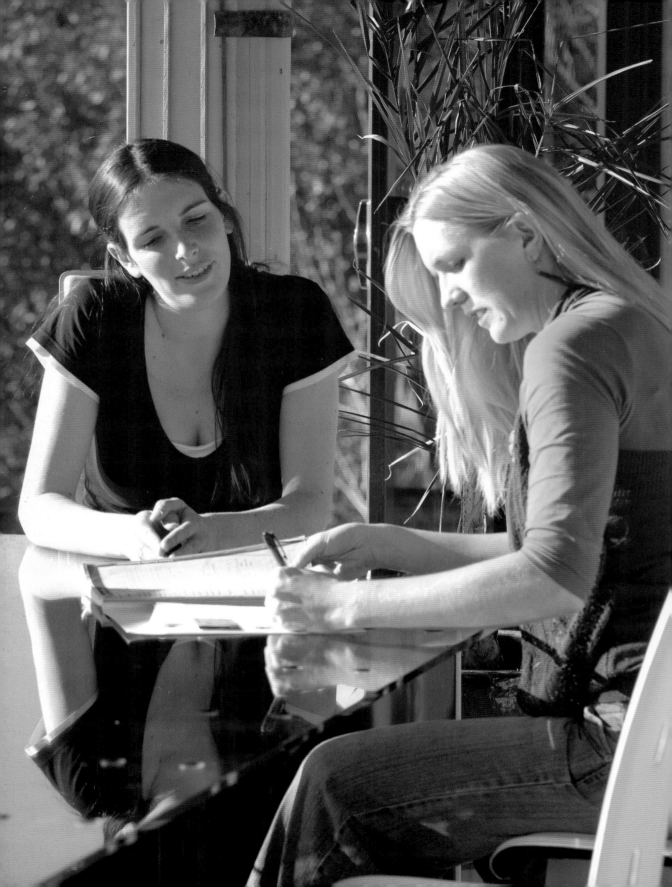

CHAPTER 3

The first
three months

(Weeks 1–13)

1. What's happening?

Foetal development in the first three months of pregnancy

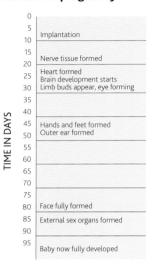

In this first trimester, a process of dramatic growth and change takes place as the fertilised egg develops into a fully formed embryo with its own support system within the womb.

Once the blastocyst (see p.61) has firmly attached itself to the wall of the uterus, it continues to grow rapidly. It is made up of two main groups of cells. At first, the group destined to become the placenta grows more quickly and starts to produce the special pregnancy hormone, human chorionic gonadotrophin (HCG). The other group of cells develops into the embryo, your future baby.

Hormones in pregnancy

- HCG (human chorionic gonadotrophin) is produced within two days of implantation and is important in early pregnancy (see also p.61).

- Oestrogen is produced in the ovary during a normal menstrual cycle (see p.26) and in much greater quantities from the placenta throughout pregnancy. It helps the breasts to grow and develop, and enables progesterone to do its work – protecting the pregnancy and kick-starting the maturation of the foetus.[1]

- Progesterone is produced in the ovary and later by the placenta (see p.61). It helps maintain early pregnancy and keeps the uterus relaxed, while also being responsible for other effects later in pregnancy (such as constipation).

In the next weeks, the embryo develops a heartbeat and circulation, and the brain and spinal cord complete their development (see also p.151). Limb buds form and grow. By the end of the eighth week, all the main organs are complete and the embryo becomes known as a foetus. By 12 weeks, the foetus is perfectly formed and is attached by a distinct cord to the placenta, which has developed next to the wall of the uterus.

Twins occur quite commonly in New Zealand (about one in every 80 pregnancies), but triplets or more are rare.[2] Twins or triplets are more common when in-vitro fertilisation (IVF) and some other assisted reproductive technologies (ARTs) are used to achieve pregnancy, but steadily improving techniques are helping to reduce the incidence of these multiple births (see pp.52–54). Although multiple pregnancies are usual for many animals, they are not the norm for humans.

With very few exceptions, twins are either fraternal (where two separate eggs are fertilised simultaneously), or identical (where one egg is fertilised but then divides into two embryos). The potential for conjoined or Siamese twins exists, but is exceedingly rare.

Fraternal twins have separate placentas and separate sacs, and may be of different genders; identical twins share a common placenta, although they may have separate sacs, and they are always the same gender. Only fraternal twins run in families (see p.203).

What controls your baby's amazing development in these first few weeks? As far as we know, there are two main factors. The first is the mother, and this chapter describes how her health and well-being can affect her developing baby. But the second factor is the foetus itself, which from the moment of

Pregnancy at 4 weeks

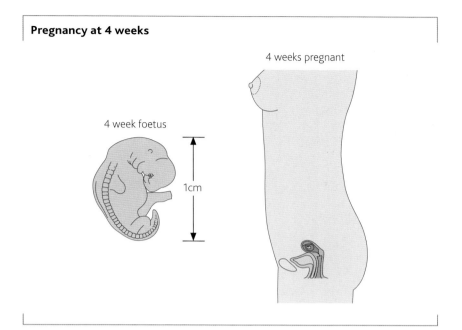

4 weeks pregnant

4 week foetus

1cm

conception has its own unique set of chromosomes that is reproduced without change every time cell division occurs. By 12 weeks, every cell in the foetal body carries the same chromosomal messages. Each message is known as a gene.

Somewhere in the myriad of messages carried by these unique chromosomes is the 'master plan' for this particular person. The master plan has lots of messages that are the same for everyone (meaning we all generally have four limbs, ten fingers, etc.) and other messages that are different (so that we may have black hair or blonde, a pointed nose or a flat one, and countless other unique characteristics).

Problems with development

Every once in a while, the chromosome master plan can be imperfect, and problems arise when this is translated into the different tissues that make up the foetus. When the early code for development is misread in this way, it cannot continue. This often results in spontaneous abortion, or miscarriage, and is quite common in early pregnancy.

The second major factor controlling foetal development is the mother's body. The fertilised egg must stick firmly to the wall of the uterus to enable it to establish a good blood supply and room to grow. Miscarriage may result if that position is not suitable in some way.

Sometimes the mother may pick up an infection that causes foetal abnormality. A small number of drugs are known to cause abnormalities in the foetus, and more are suspected of doing so. In addition, several drugs and viruses are known to affect the uterus in ways that cause early miscarriage.

But considering the number of pregnancies that occur every year, those with significant problems are remarkably few. Most pregnancies, and most babies, are destined to be absolutely normal. It's just that the 'odds' are not necessarily evenly distributed.

Pregnancy at 8 weeks

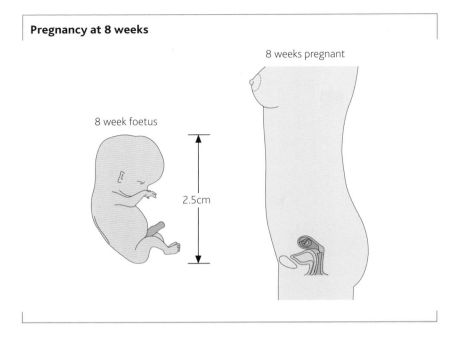

8 weeks pregnant

8 week foetus

2.5cm

Causes of problems in early pregnancy

- *Infections known sometimes to cause early miscarriage and/or foetal abnormality:* toxoplasmosis, rubella (German measles), cytomegalovirus (CMV), herpes, listeriosis, campylobacter, salmonella, bacterial vaginosis and occasionally some other viral infections (see opposite page).

- *Drugs known to cause foetal abnormality:* phenytoin (Dilantin), lithium (Priadel, Lithicarb), carbimazole (Neo-mercazole), isotretinoin (Isotane), alcohol (see p.45).

- *Drugs known to cause early miscarriage:* Ergometrine, oxytocin (Syntocinon), prostaglandin F2 (Dinoprost), prostin E2 (Dinoprostone), mifepristone (Mifegyne).

Precautions that can reduce the risk of infections[3]

While infections are responsible for only a very small number of abnormalities or miscarriages, it makes sense to avoid them if you can. Sometimes, exposure is unavoidable, but there are some precautions you can take to reduce the risk:

- Wash and dry your hands well after handling all pets and farm animals (all animals can carry campylobacter and salmonella).

- Avoiding handling cat litter or cleaning out litter boxes (toxoplasmosis).

- When gardening, wear gloves and avoid touching your face, mouth and eyes. Wash your hands well afterwards (toxoplasmosis).

Pregnancy at 12 weeks

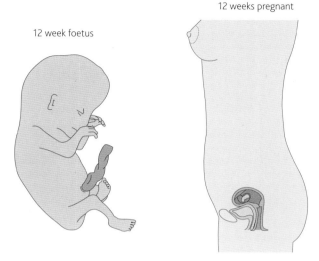

12 week foetus

12 weeks pregnant

- On farms, avoid handling silage and stillborn animals, and buy pasteurised milk to drink (listeriosis, toxoplasmosis).
- Check that you are immune to rubella before you get pregnant. If you're not immune, get vaccinated at least 28 days before falling pregnant or, if you are already pregnant, immediately after your baby is born (see also pp.43 and 44).
- Avoid eating any shellfish (cooked or raw); pâté; soft cheeses such as Brie, Camembert, ricotta, feta and processed cheeses; ready-made salads and coleslaws from salad bars; aioli or mayonnaise, especially if they have been pre-prepared and kept chilled (listeria, unlike many other harmful bacteria, will live at fridge temperatures and may cause listeriosis).
- If you are not in a stable, mutually faithful relationship, avoid unsafe sex by using condoms every time to avoid sexually transmitted infections such as chlamydia and gonorrhoea (see pp.31–32).

If you're already pregnant and not immune to rubella

- Stay away from children as much as possible, as they are most likely to have the illness.
- Find out if any child you may be going to see has a rash, a mild cough or a cold; stay away if that's the case.
- Tell your LMC or GP immediately if contact with rubella does occur, so that they can discuss your options with you.
- As soon as your baby is delivered, arrange to be vaccinated.

2. Feelings and changes

So, you're pregnant. Do you feel happy? Sad? Upset? Sick? Tired? Sexy? Lonely? Over the moon? Or all of these things – some of the time? Women experience every possible emotion in early pregnancy, and these mixed feelings are normal. So are the rapid changes from one mood to the next!

Nausea and vomiting ('morning sickness')

At least 50 per cent of women experience sickness during early pregnancy. Usually, the worst stage is at 6–12 weeks, but nausea doesn't necessarily occur in the morning. Many women experience a metallic taste in their mouth, and are less tolerant of the smell and taste of certain foods and beverages, especially coffee. But there is wide variation. Some women merely feel a little queasy for a week or two, while others vomit many times a day for several months.

Hyperemesis gravidarum

This is an unusual condition where severe vomiting in the first weeks of pregnancy causes dehydration and upsets the body's metabolism. Any woman who is unable to keep food or water down during pregnancy should be checked for dehydration. One way of checking is to measure products in the urine called 'ketones'. This is done by dipping a special test strip into a specimen of urine.

Giving intravenous (IV) fluids through a line (drip) – usually in hospital, and only very occasionally at home – will help restore the body's balance. Sometimes drugs such as metoclopromide (Maxolon, Metamide) or prochlorperazine (Antinaus, Buccastem, Stemetil) can be used in conjunction with other health professional advice.

Hyperemesis gravidarum seems to occur in women who are very sensitive to the hormonal changes in pregnancy. It may be worse if a woman is under physical or psychological stress, particularly if she feels unsafe in some way.[4] (See also pp.85–86.)

The growth of the uterus and common problems

The growth of the uterus. The uterus grows gradually but fairly constantly as the pregnancy sac containing the embryo gets bigger. At first this is hardly noticeable, but between 6 and 12 weeks the uterus more than doubles its non-pregnant size. It presses on the bowel and the bladder, often causing a desire to pass urine more frequently. Sometimes the urethra (the tube from the bladder to outside) changes shape, which makes urinary infection more likely.

Tiredness. After nausea and vomiting, the most common complaint is tiredness. Some women say that they feel more tired at the beginning of pregnancy than at any other time. They are often frustrated because there's no obvious reason, and find that no matter how much they rest, they're still tired.

Other problems. Sore and swollen breasts mean that sleeping can be uncomfortable. Women may also find they have to get up in the night more often to pass urine. Increased vaginal discharge is common, and some women have more trouble with urinary and vaginal infections, especially 'thrush' (see p.87).

Hormonal changes

Nearly all these symptoms – so dramatic in some women and hardly noticeable in others – are due at least in part to the remarkable hormonal changes that occur in early pregnancy.

The hormones produced from the ovaries, as well as the hormone of pregnancy (HCG), are largely responsible. Rising oestrogen levels tend to cause nausea and vomiting, swollen breasts, increased vaginal discharge, the tendency to get thrush, and increased sexual interest.

For most pregnancies, sex during the first three months of pregnancy is very unlikely to cause any problems, but see p.138 for more advice. However, if any bleeding or other signs of a miscarriage occur, or you have had recurrent miscarriages, it's wise to avoid sex until this settles, although intercourse is not usually the cause.

High progesterone levels in the first eight weeks or so can, on the other hand, contribute to a decrease in sexual interest and to constipation.

Hormonal changes are also thought to be responsible for the skin irritation, dryness and itchiness that some women experience during pregnancy.

Remember, though, that not every woman experiences all these symptoms. Women are all individuals, and vary tremendously in their sensitivity to the different hormones. For oestrogen to act in the body, it has to be attached to special 'oestrogen receptors' that occur in varying numbers in different parts of the body. It seems likely that different women have differing numbers of these receptors, and that this explains – at least in part – why some women feel so sick, and some so well, in early pregnancy. Although there is widespread agreement that the nausea of early pregnancy is hormonally related, exactly which hormones (and in what combination) are responsible is still under debate.[5]

'Even though this pregnancy wasn't entirely unplanned, I felt shattered by the news. How could I accommodate a child? My life was too busy as it was – and then, I hadn't expected to feel sick – I had thought that "sort of thing" only happened to the faint-hearted!!'

Places in the body where oestrogen receptors are concentrated

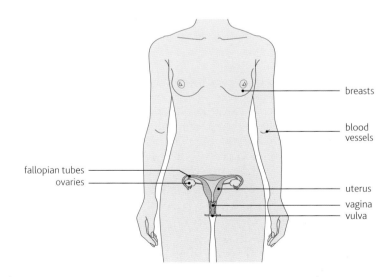

fallopian tubes
ovaries

breasts

blood vessels

uterus

vagina
vulva

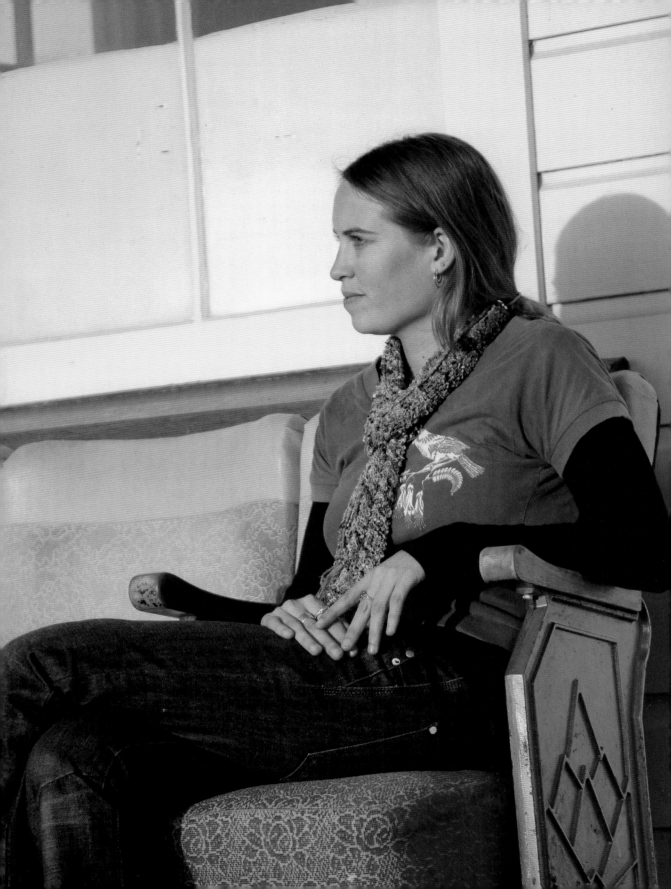

3. Helping yourself

Tiredness

It seems obvious – but first and foremost, give in and have more rest. Try to have a rest lying down every day. If you're at work, see if you can arrange to lie down for half an hour at lunch-time. If you're at home with children, rest when they do, or at least lie down on the floor with a pillow and a blanket while they play around you. It *does* make a difference, even if you don't actually sleep.

Go to bed earlier in the evening. If necessary, set the alarm for 9 p.m. and, when it rings, immediately stop whatever you're doing and *go to bed*. Get up later in the morning, if your lifestyle allows you this luxury – make the most of it while you can.

'There's nothing on earth like that tiredness of early pregnancy – I just want to sleep by ten o'clock in the morning.'

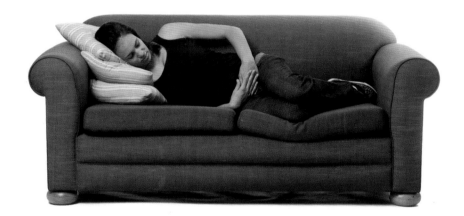

Nausea and vomiting

The following suggestions may help. However, if you are unable to keep anything down at all, even warm water, for 48 hours, contact your GP, or your lead maternity carer (LMC) (see p.94) if you already have one.

- *Have more rest.* The nausea and vomiting seem to be worse when you're tired. While a positive attitude will help to some extent, there will probably be good days and not-so-good days. Try to focus on getting through one day at a time.

- *Avoid alcohol in any form.* Even one or two drinks can precipitate severe vomiting if you have a tendency this way, and alcohol is not good for the developing baby (see p.24). Instead, try to drink some dilute fruit juice if you can; it contains potassium, which you often lose if you are vomiting.

- *Eat very small amounts quite often* – every two to three hours. Going for long periods without food often makes the nausea worse.

Food suggestions for early pregnancy

- *Items women commonly can't tolerate:* coffee, other caffeinated drinks, eggs, meat, beans and lentils, fried foods, take-aways, milk and cream, ice-cream, acid fruit (e.g. tomatoes, plums).

- *Items commonly found useful:* sweet fresh fruit (e.g. peaches), toast, cracker biscuits, plain sweet biscuits, warm water, stewed apple, potatoes, flat lemonade (all in small amounts).

- *Try eating a range of foods.* Women vary in what they can and can't tolerate, and only trial and error will sort this out for you personally. Leave out things you are not normally keen on – pregnancy is unlikely to whet your appetite for them.

- *Acupuncture and acupressure.* Some women find acupuncture very effective in easing nausea and vomiting, especially using the P6 acupressure point.[6] You need to find a person who is skilled in applying acupuncture, and you may have to wear a very small needle (or needles) for some time. Anti-seasickness wrist-bands purchased at a chemist can also be used to put pressure on the P6 point at the wrist, and some women find this helps their nausea.

- *Ginger and pyridoxine* (vitamin B6). Ginger has been known for centuries as a digestive aid, and many women also find it helpful for nausea in pregnancy. Pyridoxine and ginger have been well investigated and are considered effective and safe, but only in modest amounts. Pyridoxine can be obtained cheaply on prescription, but total intake should not exceed 40mg per day.[7]

- *Prescription drugs.* Obviously, drugs are best avoided entirely (see p.45), but in severe cases of nausea and vomiting there are some that may be used with caution. Metoclopromide (Maxolon) and prochlorperizine (Stemetil) are available on prescription, but should be used in conjunction with health professional advice. There is no evidence to date that these drugs cause harm to the developing baby. They are available as a tablet that goes under the tongue or is swallowed, a syrup, or a suppository (capsule inserted into the rectum or back passage). Some women find one form of the drug better than another, so it's worth experimenting.

- *Homeopathic remedies.* Some women get relief from taking remedies such as sepia, nux vomica, pulsatilla, colchicum and phosphorus.[8] You must be guided by someone trained in the use of homeopathic remedies so that correct doses are not exceeded. (See Appendix: Homeopathy.) It is important to remember that any substance that has a direct effect on the body is a drug, whether derived from plants or made synthetically in a laboratory. Homeopathic remedies are no exception, and should be used with as much caution as any other drug. There is no evidence to date that the remedies mentioned above cause harm to the unborn baby.

- *Feeling safe.* If you are feeling emotionally or physically threatened, this can make nausea and vomiting in early pregnancy much worse. If this is the case, try to think carefully about your situation. Pregnancy is a vulnerable time, and you need to feel as safe as possible; otherwise, not only your health but also the health of your unborn baby will suffer. No pregnant woman deserves emotional or physical abuse; if this is happening to you, or you are worried it could happen, then you may need help to get out of your current situation. No matter how hard it might be, try to talk to your midwife or doctor about what is happening. If you feel unable to do this, a list of other possible safe contacts appears in the Appendix (see Women's Refuge).

Breast tenderness

Wear a firm bra, even if you don't normally wear one. It may also help to wear it at night for a week or two. Tenderness usually subsides quite quickly, even though your breasts will remain enlarged throughout pregnancy.

Skin itchiness and dryness

Water-based skin washes and moisturising creams may be of some help. However, simple warm water – with nothing added at all – is often best for cleansing. If your skin remains irritated, it's worth considering whether your usual soap and/or washing powder may be responsible.

Vaginal thrush and bacterial vaginosis

Vaginal infections are common in pregnancy because of hormonal changes or if certain antibiotics are taken. The following precautions may help you avoid such infections:

- Wash the vaginal area gently with warm water two to three times a day. Soak in a bath if possible. It's best to avoid soap completely – even the mildest can be irritating. Sometimes a bath oil can be useful, but beware of the slippery bath. Douches (vaginal washes) are unnecessary, as they upset the natural balance of normal bacteria in the vagina. They can be quite irritating to the delicate vaginal walls.

- Wear light cotton underwear, or none at all, and avoid tight jeans, panty-hose and wet swimming gear.

- If you are prescribed antibiotics, check if they are likely to cause thrush. This may be the case with 'broad spectrum' antibiotics (those that cover a wide range of possible organisms), but to some extent you can minimise the risk of thrush occurring by maintaining the 'good bacteria' in your gut with a healthy diet (see p.18). Products are also available from pharmacies to boost gut health.[9]

Breast changes in early pregnancy

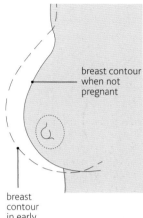

breast contour when not pregnant

breast contour in early pregnancy

Treatment

If you do get a very itchy, thick white vaginal discharge, despite taking all the precautions suggested above, this is likely to be a 'thrush' infection. Seek professional advice, as it is important to be sure that this is thrush, and not some other infection.

Your GP, or LMC if you have one, will probably do a gentle vaginal examination and take some swabs (see p.30). Treatment for thrush usually consists of a vaginal cream and/or pessaries, both of which can safely be used throughout pregnancy.

The lactobacillus present in natural unsweetened yogurt is an 'anti-thrush' agent. Eating yogurt may help to keep the bowel free of thrush, and for some women this also helps keep vaginal thrush at bay. Some women get relief from the itchiness by applying natural yogurt directly to the vulval area – messy, but perhaps worth a try. However, if you find the application of food such as yogurt unacceptable, make this clear to anyone who might suggest it, so they can respect your preference.

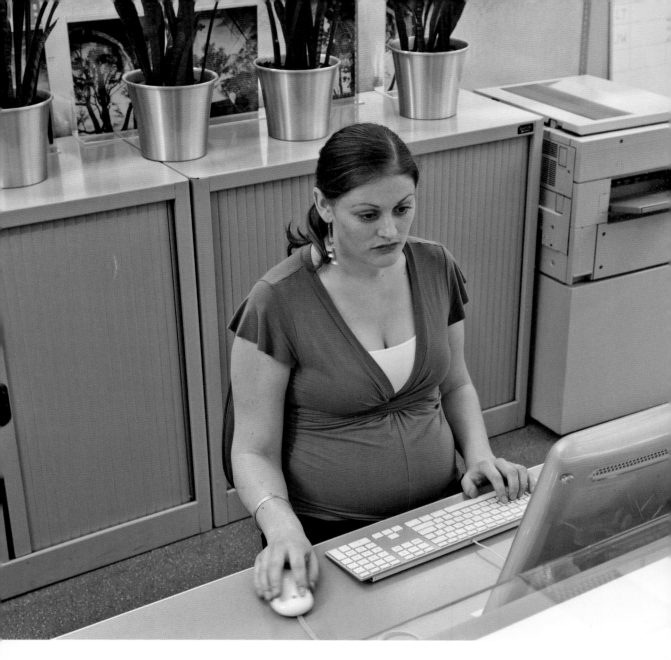

Similar symptoms may occur with another infection known as bacterial vaginosis. This is thought to be caused by bowel organisms getting into the vagina and upsetting the normal vaginal bacteria. It is not necessarily sexually transmitted (that is, passed from one sexual partner to the other), but it may be; treatment is sometimes recommended for both partners. Bacterial vaginosis can also be present without any symptoms, and may be picked up at a routine visit when a swab is taken.

It is important that this infection is detected, as it can sometimes bring on miscarriage or premature labour if left untreated. For this reason, it is usually checked for at the first antenatal visit (see p.103). Bacterial vaginosis can be treated effectively with antibiotics, either in pessary or tablet form.

Urinary frequency and infection

There is little you can do about the frequency, which will improve after about 12 weeks. But it may be necessary to plan regular toilet stops and carry a spare pair of pants when you're at work or out and about. Go when you feel the urge, or even before. 'Holding on' may well result in an accident. If the worst happens, try not to feel too bad; pregnancy can take the blame. Pelvic floor exercises may help (see p.126).

Urinary infections become more likely in pregnancy because of pressure on the bladder and urethra, and the relaxing effect of some pregnancy hormones on the tubes taking urine from the kidneys to the bladder (the ureters). If you suspect you might have an infection, take a urine specimen (see p.104) to your primary care provider, GP or LMC for testing. Urinary infections need to be treated, first to relieve the symptoms, but also because they sometimes spread to the kidneys and cause an infection known as pyelonephritis (see p.117). This is more likely in pregnancy, because the ureters are softer and more dilated than usual. Urinary infections are also associated with premature labour, so it is important to detect and treat them as quickly as possible. Not all antibiotics may be safe in pregnancy, so it is essential that the person treating you knows that you are pregnant.

It also helps to drink plenty of fluid (2 litres a day, preferably water) to help flush the bacteria out of the bladder.

Signs of urinary tract infection (UTI)

If the infection is in the bladder, you may have:

- no symptoms at all
- a burning sensation when passing urine
- pain during or after passing urine, but be otherwise well.

If the infection has spread to the kidneys, you may have the following symptoms as well as, or instead of, those above – if so, get them checked promptly:

- fever (temperature usually over 38°C), shivering or sweating, feeling unwell
- loin pain, or low central abdominal pain.

Constipation

Again, it seems obvious, but the first thing to do is drink more fluid. Water is best, but weak fruit juice, tea or a little soft drink are fine. Drinking plenty of fluids helps to keep the bowel motion soft.

Eat prunes, raisins, fresh fruit, and cereals that contain bran (for example, muesli or All-Bran), or try sprinkling bran flakes on your usual cereal. Cut down on fatty foods, including cheese.

Don't worry if you don't move your bowels every day – if you're not eating much, you may not need to. Don't strain when on the toilet, as this will only make any tendency to piles worse (see p.195).

It's best not to use laxatives – the bowel very quickly becomes reliant on them. If you do feel really constipated and uncomfortable, discuss this with your midwife or doctor. They may be able to give you a tablet or granules containing fibre that are safe in pregnancy. Kiwifruit have also been found to be very helpful: eat them in the usual way or in the form of a fruit drink.[10]

4. Miscarriage

Miscarriage, or spontaneous abortion, means that a pregnancy is lost without any intervention. It occurs quite commonly in the first 13 weeks, and much more rarely after that.

It is estimated that as many as 30 per cent of pregnancies are lost within the first trimester (13 weeks), although many of these occur even before the woman is able to confirm pregnancy. About 20 per cent of all confirmed pregnancies are lost.[11] The reasons for these losses are varied (see box), and most cannot be prevented. If foetal abnormality is the cause, there is little that can be done to avert a miscarriage. However, maternal causes may be treatable so that even if that pregnancy cannot be saved, the next will not be at risk.

If the fertilised egg implants in the wrong position (for example, in the fallopian tube or very low down in the uterus), or if the uterus has an unusual internal shape, the foetus may not have room to grow properly and spontaneous abortion will occur. Accidents and/or shock are sometimes blamed for early miscarriage, but unless they are life-threatening, they don't usually cause miscarriage at this stage of the pregnancy. Only the direct introduction of an instrument into the uterus itself through the cervix is likely to do this.

Possible reasons for miscarriage

Foetal causes

- neural tube defects (impaired brain and spine development, see p.151)
- empty pregnancy sac
- multiple pregnancy (twins or more)
- chromosomal defect(s) and other abnormalities

Maternal causes

- drugs
- infection
- intra-uterine contraceptive device (IUCD) still in place
- past pelvic infection
- uterus an unusual internal shape
- cervical incompetence
- ectopic pregnancy
- severe accident

Unusual shape within the uterus

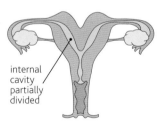

internal cavity partially divided

Suspecting miscarriage

The most common warning of miscarriage is vaginal bleeding. It may be only a few spots, or heavier than a normal period. It is often accompanied by painful cramps in the lower abdomen and/or lower back. If bleeding is heavy, faintness or nausea may occur.

What to do

Lie down; if possible, go to bed. If the bleeding and pain subside, your pregnancy may well continue normally. It is best to presume that this is so, but you need to report what happened to your GP, or your LMC if you have one. An ultrasound scan will often be arranged within the next few days to check that the foetus is alive and well, and in a satisfactory position in the uterus.

If things don't settle down within a few hours, or the bleeding and pain are getting worse, it's advisable to contact your LMC or GP promptly. If the bleeding is heavy, or the pain severe, contact them straight away. (If this is not possible, seek immediate help from an after-hours medical service or a local doctor. There will usually be no charge.)

An inspection of the cervix using a speculum will be needed to determine whether the cervix is open or closed. If the cervix is open, miscarriage is inevitable. If it is closed, there is a possibility the pregnancy will continue. Again, an ultrasound scan will often be arranged to give more accurate information.

If miscarriage is inevitable, then the more quickly the uterus empties its contents (known as 'products of conception'), the more quickly normal function can return. The cramping pains experienced by some women are an indication that the uterus is contracting to expel its contents. Before 7 weeks, and after 13 weeks, complete clearance often takes place naturally.

Signs of miscarriage

- vaginal bleeding
- abdominal cramps
- backache
- faintness

Inevitable miscarriage

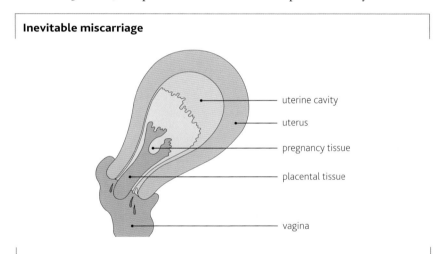

- uterine cavity
- uterus
- pregnancy tissue
- placental tissue
- vagina

However, between 7 and 13 weeks, or sometimes later, the uterus may empty only partially and continued heavy bleeding and/or infection may result. This can be avoided if the uterus is cleared in a sterile procedure known as a 'D & C' (dilatation and curettage). In a D & C, the cervix is opened sufficiently for a curette (a small, narrow, spoon-shaped instrument) or a small suction device to remove blood and tissue from the inside of the uterus. This is a skilled procedure that needs to be performed by a trained operator, usually a specialist obstetrician. Because it is an invasive procedure, and has the potential to damage the uterine lining occasionally, a D & C is to be avoided if possible, although the complication rate is low and the results good in skilled hands. It is always done under a general anaesthetic, as it would otherwise be quite painful, and generally takes only a few minutes.

After a miscarriage: feelings

Nearly all women feel some sense of loss after a miscarriage, even if the pregnancy was unplanned. In a wanted pregnancy, these feelings can be very intense and quite overwhelming for several weeks.

'I hadn't told very many people that I was pregnant – and when I lost it I felt like I had no one to turn to. In the end, my doctor was the most helpful. He took my feelings of despair seriously. That surprised me. Yes, it was good to talk about it in the end.'

Coming to terms with miscarriage

Miscarriage has been described as both the birth and the death of a baby,[12] and the feelings that surround it are similarly contradictory.

As with any death, reactions to miscarriage are very often a mix of numbness, grief, isolation, confusion and anger – intense emotions that may affect you simultaneously or in turn, and physically as well as mentally.

But miscarriage is an especially complicated kind of death to deal with. Despite it being so common, it is seldom talked about. Other people who have not experienced it themselves – perhaps even your partner or close family members – may find it hard to understand why you are so upset and unable to 'get over it' quickly. If your pregnancy was unexpected or unplanned, others may find your grief incomprehensible; even you may be shocked by the strength of your feelings. Depending on the stage at which you miscarried, few people may have known you were pregnant; even if they notice that something is wrong, you may not feel like explaining. Some women find it is simply easier to 'carry on', at least in public.

For all these reasons, miscarriage remains a hidden experience for many women. Miscarriage is also a hard death to deal with because, very often, there is no baby to bury. There is no funeral, no notice in the newspaper, no sympathy cards or flowers. There is only an absence.

There may also be shame and guilt after a miscarriage. Some women describe a sense of failure at being unable to carry a child to full term, especially when 'everyone else' seems to do it so easily. They may be jealous and resentful of pregnant women or those with new babies, and then feel guilty for having such thoughts.

The partners and family of women who have miscarried may also experience a blur of emotions. An expectant father or grandparent may grieve both for the baby they have lost, and for the woman they love. Older women who have themselves experienced miscarriage may find it an especially emotional time, particularly if they have never grieved properly for or talked about their own loss.

Coming to terms with miscarriage may take a long time. Many things can help – talking with other people, expressing yourself in writing or art, farewelling your baby with a special ceremony or ritual, or professional counselling. However, it is important to remember that the ways in which we grieve, and deal with our grief, are as individual as we are. (See Appendix: Miscarriage.)

'I miscarried for the first time at 12 weeks, the day after my mother's funeral. I never found out why it happened. I ended up in hospital, and needed a D & C. Afterwards, I just felt completely emptied. I lay in bed for a week and watched a cricket test on TV, day after day, every excruciating ball. I felt that if I stopped watching, I would be engulfed by something dreadful. I didn't want to talk about it either, certainly not with strangers. I just went back to work and eleven months later, my son was born. Somehow, I'd healed myself.'

Because a miscarriage in the first three months is a very private loss for the woman concerned, it can be hard for other people, even a loving partner, to understand the bereavement she is experiencing. But it does help to know that this is a normal reaction, and that the grief will ease with time. Sometimes talking with other women who have suffered a miscarriage can help.

Some women find it helps to acknowledge the loss of their baby in some visible way – naming them so they become part of the family, planting a tree in their memory, painting pictures or creating murals that refer to the baby they have lost. These are all ways that different women have found to deal with their grief.

If you continue to feel really bad after a miscarriage, consider asking your doctor, midwife or practice nurse for advice. Counsellors are available through abortion clinics, antenatal clinics and, in some areas, through infertility groups. (See Appendix: Infertility; Miscarriage.)

Pregnancy after miscarriage

Women have varied feelings about getting pregnant again after a miscarriage. Most will want to conceive again – some straight away, and others not for several months. Some women experience a delay in becoming pregnant, particularly if the miscarriage has been complicated by infection, heavy bleeding at the time, or continued bleeding afterwards. These problems are less likely to occur if the uterus empties quickly and completely.

The chances of getting and staying pregnant after one miscarriage are good. Studies suggest that there is no increased risk after one miscarriage, and a slightly increased risk after two consecutive miscarriages. However, once a woman has had three consecutive miscarriages (which occurs in about 1–2 per cent of fertile couples), her chances of miscarrying again are higher. There are some special investigations that can be done (usually by a specialist obstetrician or gynaecologist) to determine a recurring cause, but most of the time nothing specific can be identified. Sometimes treatment is available and warranted, but more often successful pregnancy can still occur with no intervention.[13]

Ectopic pregnancy

This type of pregnancy, which fortunately is rare, occurs when the fertilised egg gets stuck on its way down the fallopian tube. It tries to grow in the tube, instead of in the uterus. This pregnancy cannot continue, as sooner or later (usually six to eight weeks after the LMP) the tube and/or pregnancy sac will burst, causing sudden and severe bleeding and pain. The bleeding may be internal or vaginal, and the pain low down in the abdomen, usually on one side.

If you have severe abdominal pain, possibly worse on one side, after a missed period, you should immediately contact your LMC (if you have one by then) or seek medical advice (your GP, an after-hours centre or a hospital emergency department) and ask if it could be an ectopic pregnancy. If an ectopic pregnancy has occurred, an operation is necessary to remove the pregnancy sac and to repair or remove the affected tube before heavy internal bleeding puts the woman's life at risk. Occasionally a drug (methotrexate) can be used instead of surgery to stop the ectopic pregnancy growing.

The chances of getting pregnant again after an ectopic pregnancy are lower, but vary with each individual case. If you can, discuss this with the doctor who did your operation.

Conditions making an ectopic pregnancy more likely

- previous pelvic infection, especially more than one episode
- previous infertility
- becoming pregnant with an IUCD still in place
- becoming pregnant while on the mini-pill
- previous ectopic pregnancy
- previous tubal surgery

Ectopic pregnancy – most common sites

end of fallopian tube near ovary

middle of tube

end of tube near uterus

5. Choosing a system of antenatal care (see also p.156)

You should decide who will be your lead maternity carer (LMC) as early as is practicable within the first three to four months of your pregnancy. An LMC is most commonly a midwife who is registered to provide full pregnancy care. This includes care during labour and birth, and after the baby is born (for up to four to six weeks). Currently, about 80 per cent of lead maternity care is provided by midwives. A small number of GPs (known as GP obstetricians) and specialist obstetricians are also registered as LMCs; this means they are trained and registered to provide primary antenatal care, care during labour and birth, and post-natal care until four to six weeks after the birth.

However, before you choose and register with your LMC, you can get early antenatal care from your own GP, another GP, a registered midwife, a family planning doctor or a specialist obstetrician. This is known as 'non-LMC first trimester care'. As long as this care starts within the first 12 weeks, it can extend up to 14 weeks, or later under urgent circumstances. It is funded by the government to ensure all pregnant women have access to initial pregnancy care, free of charge and regardless of their circumstances.

You can register with your chosen LMC as soon as your pregnancy is confirmed. As soon as you are able to do so, you should transfer all your antenatal care to that person so that you have good continuity of care throughout your pregnancy, labour, birth and with your new baby. Once you have registered with your LMC, you should contact them first about any pregnancy-related concern, no matter what your stage of pregnancy. Your LMC should be the first person you contact in any urgent circumstances from then on. Even if you are away from home, make a phone call to her if at all possible.

There is a shortage of LMCs in some areas, so it is advisable to seek one early. If possible, interview a few people to ensure you find the LMC who best meets your needs.

Section 88

In New Zealand, all maternity care provided to women must meet requirements set by the Ministry of Health. These are contained in Section 88 of the Public Health and Disability Act 2000. (See Appendix: Section 88.) This section specifies what health professionals (midwives, GPs and obstetricians) must do as 'lead maternity carers' (LMCs) , as 'first trimester carers' and as other pregnancy carers. Maternity care providers must be authorised (or registered) and, as such, receive payment to enable women to access pregnancy care free of charge.

After your pregnancy has been confirmed, you should not be charged for your antenatal care (unless you see a specialist obstetrician for private, not primary, maternity care). The LMC you register with will be paid by the Ministry of Health for the care they provide. Your pregnancy care will continue to be fully funded by the government, even if you have to transfer later to a specialist because of some problem that needs further attention. If your care becomes unexpectedly complicated and needs to be managed by a specialist obstetrician in a fully equipped maternity hospital, the hospital team then becomes your LMC, at no charge to you.

While your LMC has overall responsibility for your care, they will work with other health professionals to provide all the services you need. For example, if your LMC is a GP or specialist obstetrician, they will always work with a midwife around the time of your labour and birth, and often during your pregnancy as well. If your LMC is an independent midwife, she may share your care with another midwife during your pregnancy, labour and birth. Other health professionals, such as anaesthetists, paediatricians and lactation consultants, can also be called in if necessary.

A midwife as your LMC

Midwives are fully educated and trained in all aspects of normal pregnancy care, labour, delivery and post-natal care. Many handle both home and hospital births. They are also educated to detect problems and complications, and to seek help when dealing with such cases. Some midwives work as hospital employees on a 'shift' basis, while others are employees who manage caseloads of women – they provide all their antenatal, labour, birth and post-natal care as part of a team of midwives. Other midwives choose to be self-employed and provide all maternity care to a caseload of women, working with other health professionals as required.

For specific pregnancy problems, your midwife will usually refer you directly to a specialist obstetrician, using the referral guidelines set out in Section 88 (see box opposite). In certain circumstances, especially in rural areas, she may work with a GP obstetrician. For other medical problems, particularly those unrelated to pregnancy (such as a chest infection), you will need to see a GP. But because apparently unrelated conditions may in fact affect pregnancy, and pregnancy may affect a medical condition you already have, you should seek your midwife's advice if you are in any doubt. For example, a woman with asthma would normally see her GP about the condition but, because pregnancy may make the asthma change, both her doctor and midwife need to know about any problems or changes in medication.

Qualifications required for midwives[14]

A midwife must either

- be an NZRN fully registered nurse (three- to four-year nursing degree) with a Bachelor of Midwifery degree (another two to three years) (total nursing/midwifery education at least five to six years);

- **or** have completed a Bachelor of Midwifery degree (three years of full-time study), and passed the National Midwifery Exam (total education at least three to four years).

The qualifications of midwives with overseas training may vary from the New Zealand regime, but all have to meet the training and experience requirements of the Midwifery Council of New Zealand. This will usually involve undertaking additional study, sitting additional exams and having supervised experience in New Zealand.

Further information about midwifery education and qualifications is available on the Council's website. (See Appendix: Midwives.) The site includes an online register listing all midwives registered to practise in New Zealand.

A GP obstetrician as your LMC

GP obstetricians are fully qualified general practitioners (GPs; see p.28) who have extra education and training in all aspects of obstetric care. They work with a midwife to provide care during pregnancy, labour and birth, and after the baby is born. Some may assist at home births. Although the number of GPs in New Zealand is stable (and many are able to provide early antenatal, or first trimester, care), the number of GPs who are also practising GP obstetricians has rapidly decreased in the last ten years.

GP obstetricians are trained to cope with most of the common situations that arise in pregnancy. But with more complicated problems, your GP obstetrician will arrange (with your consent) for you to be seen by a specialist. This specialist care is free of charge if arranged through the local hospital's obstetric service, but you may have to pay if it is arranged with a private obstetrician.

Qualifications required for doctors practising obstetrics[15]

- *MBChB*. Basic medical education. Fully qualified doctor but no advanced training (six years at medical school, plus two years as a junior hospital doctor). Total medical education at least eight to nine years.

- *RNZCGP*. Vocational training to be a fully qualified GP (minimum three years of training in addition to above to gain FRNZCGP; see p.28). Total medical education at least 11–12 years.

- *Diploma of Obstetrics*. Extra training and education in obstetrics. Minimum qualification for GP obstetricians (six months in addition to above). Total medical education at least eight to nine years.

- *RANZCOG (Royal Australian and New Zealand College of Obstetricians and Gynaecologists) Part 1*. Specialist in training (four years in addition to above). Total medical education at least 12 years.

- *RANZCOG Part 2*. Fully qualified specialist obstetrician (two to four years in addition to above). Total medical education at least 14 years, often longer.

The qualifications of doctors with overseas training may vary from the New Zealand regime, but all have to meet the training and experience requirements of the Medical Council of New Zealand. This may involve undertaking additional study, sitting extra exams and having supervised experience in New Zealand.

All doctors registered to practise in New Zealand are listed on the medical register, with details of their 'vocational scope' (the particular area of work in which they specialise). Fully qualified general practitioners are registered under the vocational scope 'General Practice', and specialist obstetricians are registered under the vocational scope 'Obstetrics and Gynaecology'. Doctors who do not have a vocational scope listed beside their name are usually still undergoing postgraduate training to become fully qualified in their field (such as general practice, obstetrics and gynaecology, or paediatrics). All these details can be viewed in the 'Find a registered doctor' section of the Medical Council of New Zealand's website. (See Appendix: Doctors.)

A specialist obstetrician as your LMC

Specialist obstetricians are fully qualified to deal with all complications arising in pregnancy and birth, including Caesarean sections (see p.282). They work in maternity hospitals and many also have private practices offering pregnancy care. They do not, except in very exceptional circumstances, assist at home births, since their expertise is in dealing with abnormal pregnancies and complicated deliveries that are best dealt with in hospital.

A specialist obstetrician acting as your LMC will work with a midwife or midwives to provide all your pregnancy care. The obstetrician will arrange for a colleague to look after you if they themselves are ill, or away. They will initially see you in their private rooms, or surgery. In most places, you can have your baby in the local hospital, with your specialist in charge of your care. In a few areas, private hospital care is an option.

Specialist obstetricians working in a private capacity are able to apply a part charge that you will need to pay. Charges vary widely, so check this out before deciding on this type of care.

How to decide?

First and foremost, it is important to find a midwife and/or doctor you get on well with, and can talk to openly and easily. So it pays to check out whether their philosophy on pregnancy and childbirth is compatible with yours.

> **Questions you could ask when choosing your LMC**
>
> Some, but not all, of these questions come from the list supplied in the Ministry of Health's booklet, *Your pregnancy: Tō hapūtanga.*[16]
>
> - What is your philosophy on pregnancy care, childbirth and post-natal care?
> - Will you provide all my care or will others be involved?
> - How can I contact you if I need help or advice?
> - Who will provide back-up care if you can't be there?
> - What birthing options do you offer?
> - Do you offer home birth and what happens if I need hospital care?
> - Where will my antenatal visits be? In my home? At a clinic?
> - How many antenatal visits can I expect to have?
> - What happens if I need specialist care during my pregnancy or labour?
> - Who would you consult first if any problems arose during pregnancy and/or birth?
> - Will you visit me in hospital? What will your role be?
> - Are you likely to be away when I'm due?
> - How many post-natal visits can I expect, both in hospital and at home?
> - How will you communicate with my primary care provider?

'I didn't even have a midwife until I was about four months pregnant, just because I was quite confident in the process and knew that it would happen how I wanted it to happen. Of course, I didn't understand then how in demand midwives are. I ended up having to ring quite a few and they were either full or didn't do home births. Finally, I found one through a work connection and she was perfect – an independent Māori midwife with years of experience in home birth delivery.'

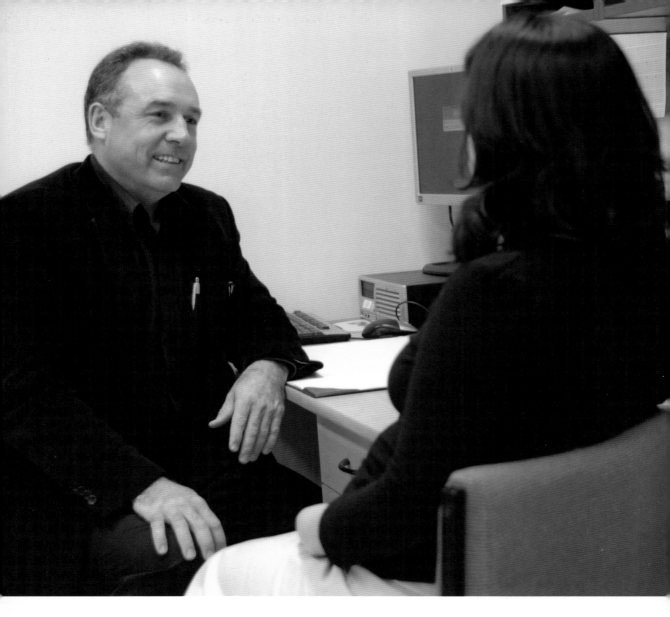

Your LMC should also be someone whose professional expertise you respect. That doesn't necessarily mean you will agree with everything they suggest, but there may be times during your pregnancy, labour or birth when you need to have faith in advice or recommendations from your LMC. Ultimately, the decisions made at such times need to be negotiated between you, your LMC and often those closest to you. Ask about your LMC's training and experience if you are not sure (see opposite).

If, like the majority of women, you anticipate a fairly normal pregnancy and delivery, the LMC midwife and/or GP obstetrician service works very well. However, if you run into complications, your LMC may have to work in consultation with an obstetrician, or hand your care over to a specialist at the hospital.

A small number of women feel happier seeing a specialist obstetrician privately for their pregnancy care. Whether or not problems are anticipated, you may feel you want to see the same highly qualified person throughout your pregnancy and delivery, without having to worry about being transferred to someone else's care if complications arise. Specialist obstetricians in private practice often work closely with two or three midwives, and you will have the opportunity to get to know them well over the course of your pregnancy. In some areas, this care will continue through labour, birth and afterwards; in other places, you may be cared for during labour by several midwives in the hospital, some of whom you may not have met before. However, all midwives, whether they know you well or not, will do their very best to give you the care and attention you need. Remember that using a specialist obstetrician may be a costly option, because this type of private care is only minimally subsidised by the government.

Questions you could ask an LMC about training and experience

Some, but not all, of these questions come from the list supplied in the Ministry of Health's booklet, *Your pregnancy: Tō hapūtanga*.[17]

- What sort of training have you had? What are your qualifications? What level of care are you able to provide? (Ask to see a certificate if you are not sure about their answers.)
- How long have you been caring for pregnant women, attending births, and looking after women after they have had their babies?
- About how many births a year do you attend?
- Have you had an annual standards review, or an audit? Is your recertification up to date?

Changing your LMC

Remember that you *can* change your LMC if your circumstances change or you're not happy with your existing arrangement. This might be because you move house, because you may want to switch to a different system of care, or because you simply don't 'get on' with your LMC. Before you do change, consider your reasons carefully. Remember that your new LMC will need time to get to know you, and vice versa.

Whatever you decide to do, make sure you're satisfied with the new arrangements before getting your records transferred. If possible, give your present LMC some advance warning, and tell them why you want to change. This can be useful feedback for your LMC, who may be oblivious to any problems you have with them. It is important to let your LMC know if you change to another LMC. Under Section 88 you are entitled to hold a copy of your own notes; this makes transferring to another LMC a bit easier, as you can show the new LMC your records to date. Notes held by women should replicate those held by their LMC, but because this is not always the case, records may need to be sent straight from one LMC to another.

Your present LMC may write a letter of introduction for you. Whatever the circumstances, continuity of care is your choice, but also your responsibility.

'My first midwife and I just didn't click. She was a lovely lady in her own way, but I knew right away that I wouldn't be comfortable with her. Also, I had to go to her clinic. With my second midwife, I liked the fact that she would come to my house. Especially towards the end, you feel so much more comfortable. I enjoyed having her here. She gave me this great confidence – I just really enjoyed working with her.'

6. The first antenatal visit with your LMC

Usually, you will already have seen your primary care provider (GP or practice nurse) to confirm that you are indeed pregnant, so that is not the purpose of this visit. Rather, it's your first formal antenatal appointment with the midwife or doctor you have chosen as your LMC. If this first meeting is occurring later in pregnancy, things may be done a little differently from an early pregnancy appointment. Sometimes, this thorough visit will be with your GP who is providing first trimester care only. But most often (and ideally) it will be with your LMC, so the term LMC has been used exclusively in this section for the sake of simplicity.

This is an important visit for both you and your LMC, and there are lots of questions and answers to get through on both sides. If you make your appointment through a receptionist, it's a good idea to let them know that this is your first antenatal visit, so that enough time can be allocated.

Because it's a longer visit, now is the time to ask any questions you may have about your pregnancy, to discuss where you want the birth to take place (see p.156), and to talk about your preferences and concerns. It often helps to write down all the things you want to ask about, and to take your list along to refer to. If you wish, take your partner or support person with you too – not only can they give you moral support and remember things you may forget to mention, but it also helps them to feel involved right from the start. It's also important at this visit to bring the results of any blood tests or swabs your GP may have requested when your pregnancy was confirmed. You should pass these on to your LMC as soon as you register with them, or at this first antenatal appointment.

This visit should give you both a good chance to get to know each other and find out whether you're going to get on together during the next nine to ten months. Some midwives may also want to meet you even before this first formal appointment to ensure that you both understand each other's require-ments and needs. This is very important: the best antenatal care – care that gives you and your baby the best possible chance of health and happiness – lies in the partnership between you and your midwife and/or doctor. And it is a partnership: you both have responsibilities (see box below).

Responsibilities during pregnancy and birth

Your responsibilities:

- to come to or be available for appointments as arranged (or to ring and change the time if it's unsuitable)
- to ask your questions clearly and openly – including questions about costs, and approaches to different options during pregnancy and birth (make a list so that you can remember to ask them at the time of the visit)

- to give honest answers to questions asked of you
- to express concerns as they arise, preferably at each visit (your LMC, or a practice nurse at your GP/primary health provider's clinic, is usually also available for advice over the phone)
- to report anything you've been asked to report on
- finally, to place some trust in your LMC/doctor and/or other midwife, so that they can make supportive decisions in your best interests, in consultation with you.

The responsibilities of your LMC (and other health professionals where applicable):

- to be appropriately qualified and competent in practising the art and craft of maternity care, soundly based on current best practice that is supported by the best scientific evidence available
- to explain the system of care they offer during pregnancy, labour and birth, and after the birth
- to see you at appointments as arranged, or to arrange for a responsible back-up LMC to see you in their absence (your LMC or back-up LMC is required to be available 24 hours a day, seven days a week, to provide phone advice and assessment for urgent problems)
- to inform you of your progress, including test results, honestly and with appropriate sensitivity
- to maintain confidentiality at all times (this may include not giving sensitive information to your partner)
- to discuss with you options for your care that are appropriate for you and your particular pregnancy
- to be available for your labour and birth, or to arrange for a back-up LMC you are happy with to attend
- to place trust in you, and respect your decisions.

Things your LMC will want to know

- Name(s) by which you wish to be known. Use the same name(s) from then on, so that your records can be found quickly.
- Partner's name(s), address and phone numbers (day and night), or, if that is not appropriate, those of a key support person (e.g. mother, sister, close friend).
- Next of kin's name, address and phone numbers, if different from above (in case of emergency).
- Age and date of birth – yours, and that of the baby's father. This is important information: the older the mother (and, to a lesser extent, the father), the greater the risk of problems. Teenage mothers are also at greater risk.
- Nationality and place of birth. All New Zealand citizens and residents are entitled to free maternity care (see p.94).

- Previous medical history. Details and dates of events are helpful, especially those involving heart conditions, high blood pressure, circulatory problems including thrombosis (clots) in the legs, abdominal operations, blood diseases, diabetes or epilepsy. Also, any history of smoking, alcohol and/or drug use (prescribed, non-prescribed or illegal).

- Family history – your own family. Any history of blood clots, heart problems, strokes or high blood pressure in parents, brothers or sisters may make these more likely in your pregnancy, depending on your age. Your mother's and/or sisters' obstetric history, any history of twins, and any history of significant conditions known to be passed on in families (e.g. haemophilia) are also relevant. Some conditions are also more common in particular racial groups, so you may be asked about your wider family and background.

- Family history – on the father's side. Inherited conditions can also be passed on through the paternal side of a family, so check if the father of your baby has any significant diseases and/or birth abnormalities among members of his family.

- Past pregnancies. Details of all your previous pregnancies, including terminations and miscarriages. Dates, duration of pregnancy, any complications, labours and birthweight of babies. (This information can make a difference to the management of this pregnancy.)

- Previous contraception, as this may affect the calculation of dates.

- Any regular medication, including tablets, medicines, patches, pessaries and inhalers. Any medication taken early in pregnancy. Some medication does have to be continued during pregnancy, despite the risks, but most does not.

- Your social/economic situation. Emotional and financial support is very necessary to new mothers. Some support is available through a variety of agencies for those who need it – for example, Working for Families and the Citizens Advice Bureau. (See Appendix: Financial support/advice for families.)

- Details of your menstrual cycle, especially the date of your LMP (first day of your last menstrual period). Try to be as accurate as you can. Mark on a calendar when you think it might have been – even being able to say 'the last two weeks of October' is better than 'I don't know'. Other important information includes whether your period was light, heavy or normal, and the length of your cycle (i.e. how many days between the start of one period and the next). This allows your LMC to calculate how many weeks pregnant you are, and the expected date of birth.

After going through these personal details, your LMC will need to do a physical examination. This will vary according to your particular history, but the checks may include those listed in the box opposite. Once the examination is completed, your LMC will be able to answer most of your questions, so take this opportunity to ask them if you haven't done so already.

There are also some tests to organise at this first visit – be sure you know where to go and what to do before you leave the appointment.

Your first antenatal physical examination – checks that may be included

- Blood pressure, heart, lungs and abdomen are checked, looking for signs of any pre-existing problems.

- A vaginal examination (VE) is carried out (see p.30). If your first visit is before about 12 weeks (which is the ideal), this may be done to estimate the size of the growing uterus, especially if you have no particular reason to have an early ultrasound examination. A vaginal examination gives a far more accurate assessment of how many weeks pregnant you are than looking at your tummy later on. It's also an opportunity to check that the other organs in the pelvis are normal, and to take swabs to check for infection. Chlamydia is a particularly important infection to check for, as it is common in New Zealand, may produce no symptoms, and if left untreated can seriously affect your newborn baby (see p.32).[18] Your LMC may discuss with you the possibility of having a sexual health check done with your primary health provider, or occasionally at a sexual health clinic. A cervical smear can also be done if you are due for this, but will otherwise be deferred until well after your baby is born.

- A breast check is carried out. This may not be done at this visit but later in the pregnancy. Lumps and scars are best detected before the breasts swell in preparation for breastfeeding. Nipples that are inverted may need extra preparation for successful breastfeeding.

- Other checks may be necessary, depending on any particular problems you may have. If you are not sure why something is being done, ask for an explanation so that you are quite clear what is being asked of you. You have the right to have full information before you consent or decline to have particular tests or examinations done. You also have the right to ask about tests that are not being offered when you think they should be.

Tests for checking on the mother's health

A number of fairly simple investigations can give a lot of information about a pregnant woman's health and well-being, particularly any conditions or problems that might cause concern during pregnancy, and that may directly or indirectly affect her baby. The following tests will be organised at your first antenatal visit (if they have not already been requested by your GP prior to your first antenatal visit to your chosen LMC).

Blood tests

Blood tests are done in pregnancy (with your consent) to check for several different things. It pays to check what you are being tested for, so that you are prepared for any unexpected results. This particularly applies to conditions such as HIV-AIDS, where a positive result would obviously have major consequences. Your LMC, doctor or midwife may actually do the blood test, or will give you a form to take to the nearest medical laboratory.

- A full blood count (FBC) checks for several things, including anaemia, infection and other rarer blood diseases.

- Blood group and maternal antibody tests determine whether you are Rhesus negative (see p.206), and potentially at risk of being 'blood sensitive' to your baby.
- The hepatitis B test indicates whether you are a carrier of the disease, which can be passed on to your baby and/or the staff who attend you, unless vaccination and other precautions are taken. (Vaccination of the baby is usually done in the first 24 hours after the birth.)
- The venereal disease research laboratory (VDRL) test (now called syphilis screen) checks for the sexually transmitted disease syphilis. A woman with syphilis may have few symptoms but can pass it on to her baby, who may be severely and permanently affected. Although syphilis is uncommon in New Zealand, its early detection and treatment is very effective, curing the disease in the woman and preventing it from passing to her baby.
- The rubella (German measles) test determines whether you are immune to this viral disease. A high proportion of the New Zealand population is immune because of the national vaccination programme that has been in place since 1970.[19] But even if you have been vaccinated, it is possible that your immunity is no longer sufficient to protect you from developing the disease again, because immunity declines naturally but variably over time. For this reason, testing is recommended with each pregnancy; even though you should not have the vaccination while you are pregnant, you can at least have the vaccine after the birth to protect the next pregnancy (see p.44).[20]
- An HIV test has recently been introduced, to be done along with the other initial antenatal blood tests.[21] While the disease is still uncommon in pregnant women in New Zealand, early detection can help the mother with treatment and, even more importantly, prevent her baby from getting HIV-AIDS (see p.32).
- First trimester serum screening tests (see opposite).

Urine test

A urine specimen is often checked at the laboratory when your blood tests are done. It is tested for infection and for protein and sugar levels (see p.139). Ideally, it should be mid-stream urine (MSU), which provides as clear a specimen as possible.

Collecting an MSU specimen
- Collect a sterile jar and container from laboratory staff. Wash your hands.
- Wipe the vaginal area gently but thoroughly with toilet paper.
- Start to pass urine into the toilet.
- Then pass a small amount into the clean container provided (10ml, or 2 teaspoons, is enough).
- Finish passing urine into the toilet.
- Pour the collected urine carefully into the jar, taking care not to touch the inside of the jar, and close the lid firmly. Wash your hands.
- Return the filled jar to the laboratory staff.

Tests for checking on the baby's development (prenatal diagnosis)

Over the last 25 years, more complex investigations have been introduced that provide information about the baby's growth and development during pregnancy. These prenatal screening and diagnostic tests can include special blood tests (serum testing) at different times in pregnancy (see below), three main types of ultrasound scans (see pp.107 and 150), chorionic villus sampling (see p.110) and amniocentesis (see p.147). In general, prenatal screening tests are relatively safe, simple tests that can give an indication of a possible problem, whereas prenatal diagnostic tests, although much more accurate, carry a small risk for both the woman and her baby.

Abnormalities can be chromosomal, where the replication of the chromosomes is faulty (for example, Down syndrome), and/or structural, where major organs fail to develop properly (for example, heart defects, or spina bifida and other neural tube defects; see p.151). Some types of chromosomal abnormality can cause structural abnormalities.

Different tests are used to detect different types of problem, but no test is perfect and some have significant associated risks. All the tests need careful consideration. They may put a normal pregnancy at risk, or detect problems for which there is no treatment; they may also raise the question of possible termination of pregnancy if a major abnormality is found. On the other hand, valuable information may be found that reduces the risk of miscarriage or a sick baby.

Screening for Down syndrome during pregnancy

As New Zealand women are now older on average when they become pregnant, they face a somewhat increased risk of having a baby with a chromosomal abnormality. While a low risk is present for all women, it is higher for older women (see p.42).

The most common type of chromosomal abnormality is Down syndrome (also known as trisomy 21, because the problem involves an extra copy of the 21st chromosome). A number of tests have been developed that can help to detect a Down syndrome baby in the first three to four months of pregnancy. While these initial tests can be very useful, it is important to realise that they are screening tests, and as such will only give an indication of your risk of having a Down syndrome baby. On their own, they will not tell you whether your baby actually has the condition or not.

Further, the risks they show relate only to Down syndrome, even though sometimes other abnormalities will also be picked up. On the other hand, other chromosomal abnormalities that are much less common than Down syndrome may remain undetected.

Overall, while the Down syndrome screening tests can be very helpful, they do have limitations and you may decide not to have any of them, or to have only some.

The three main types of prenatal screening tests are:

- Special blood tests done within the first ten weeks of pregnancy, known as first trimester serum screening tests. These detect and measure two to three hormones that are present at higher levels in the mother's blood if her baby is affected by chromosomal, and occasionally other, abnormalities.

These tests have been more recently developed, and are not yet (as at 2008) routinely available in New Zealand.

- Nuchal translucency ultrasound scanning (NTS), done at 11–13 weeks of pregnancy (see opposite). This screening test has been available in New Zealand on a limited basis since the late 1990s, but has been more widely available from fully certified ultrasonographers since about 2002.

- Special blood tests done at 14–16 weeks of pregnancy, known as maternal serum screening (or the triple or quadruple test). These detect and measure three or four main hormones (different hormones from those in the early serum blood test) that are present at higher levels in the mother's blood if her baby is affected. These tests have been available for a number of years, but have always had the disadvantage of not giving a result until 15–17 weeks of pregnancy – about the same time that an amniocentesis can give results. However, for women who first come for pregnancy care at, or later than, 14 weeks of pregnancy, this test can still be extremely useful. Until recently, there was a still a charge for this test, but it is now fully funded.

Although the NTS is the most commonly used screening test at present, there are problems associated with it. More accurate results can be obtained by combining the results of first trimester serum tests with the NTS, and this is likely to be offered in New Zealand within the next few years as a nationally coordinated screening programme is developed.[22]

Getting the results of the initial prenatal screening tests

The initial screening result is computer-calculated by taking account of your age, the number of weeks you are pregnant, and the test results. The result is expressed as a risk ratio (for example, 1:500) and explained as a low, intermediate or high risk compared to the whole population. A ratio of 1:500 suggests you have one chance in 500 of having a baby with Down syndrome. A ratio of 1:1000 suggests you have one chance in 1000 of having a baby with Down syndrome, so 1:1000 is a much lower risk than 1:500.

The subsequent diagnostic test that can give a really accurate result is amniocentesis (see p.147), but unfortunately it carries a small risk of miscarriage – about one in 200 – over and above the very small miscarriage risk every woman has. If you get a low-risk result with the screening tests, then the risk of having the more accurate test will probably outweigh the risk of having an affected baby. In other words, it will be safer for both you and your baby to avoid an amniocentesis. However, because Down syndrome does occur at any maternal age, it is inevitable that a very small number of women with a low-risk result will nonetheless have a baby with Down syndrome (see p.42 for risk at different ages).

If, on the other hand, the results from the screening tests show you are at increased risk of having a baby with Down syndrome, then it may well be worth taking the small risk involved in having an amniocentesis in order to get a much more certain result. Even for women with higher risk results, such as 1:300 or 1:200, the most likely outcome of the amniocentesis is that the baby will have a normal result, because a risk of 1:200 also means that 199 times out of 200, the baby will not have Down syndrome. You pregnancy will continue uneventfully, and this reassurance can be tremendously helpful.

However, you do not have to proceed with any further tests if you do not want to. It is not uncommon for women with a higher risk result simply to continue with their pregnancy without further tests, and to accept, along with their families, that they just may have a baby with Down syndrome.

Ultrasound examination

This test is a method of examining the foetus and the pregnancy sac, using sound waves. The waves are emitted from a special machine, and bounce back to the machine at different times and frequencies from the different structures within the body. The information is collated into a picture that is shown on a screen, and gives valuable information about a pregnancy (or anything else it is applied to).

It has become common practice for women to have at least one scan during pregnancy, to check the size and growth of the baby and to pick up any major abnormalities.

Scans have now been widely used in developed countries for over 20 years, and so far they appear to be a very safe method of examining unborn babies. However, no one can rule out the possibility of some as yet undetected problem being discovered in the future. For this reason, it is prudent to limit the number of scans undertaken in any pregnancy. If everything seems to be going well, and you are sure about the dates for your pregnancy, an anatomy scan at 18–20 weeks and, probably, a nuchal translucency scan at 11–13 weeks are likely to be sufficient (see below). For authorised LMCs, the Ministry of Health regulations specify a limited number of reasons for requesting scans during pregnancy to ensure that unnecessary scans are not performed.

Ultrasound scans for routine observation (offered to all pregnant women)

Routine scans, sometimes known as 'morphology' or anatomy scans, are often done at around 18–20 weeks, because at this time the foetal anatomy can be clearly seen and dates can be confirmed (see p.150).

Ultrasound scans to screen for Down syndrome (nuchal translucency scan, or NTS)

Ultrasound scans can also be used to detect Down syndrome babies during pregnancy. A nuchal translucency scan has to be taken accurately as close as possible to the 13th week of pregnancy by an ultrasonographer specially trained and certified in the procedure. The ultrasonographer will look at the baby and measure the width of a fluid-filled sac at the back of the neck (nuchal) area: if more than the usual amount of fluid is present, there may be an increased risk of a chromosomal abnormality. This measurement, along with the maternal age and gestation, is entered into an internationally accredited computer program to determine the risk ratio discussed in the previous section.[23]

Ultrasound scans to check for particular problems

Where there are problems or suspected problems, 'diagnostic' ultrasound scans can be tremendously helpful; in such cases, the very small potential risk of having a scan is far outweighed by the valuable information gained about a baby who is, or might be, in trouble for some reason. In some particularly complicated pregnancies, a whole series of diagnostic scans may be suggested. These should never be regarded as just 'photos' of the baby; they should only be done to ascertain particular relevant and important information. Always ask if you are unsure why a scan is being suggested, and what difference it might make to your pregnancy care.

Some reasons to have an ultrasound scan in the first trimester

- uncertain dates
- in association with chorionic villus biopsy (CVS; see p.110)
- threatened miscarriage
- suspected ectopic pregnancy
- pelvic mass in pregnancy
- severe vomiting
- uterus not equal to dates, when there is a discrepancy of more than four weeks (e.g. suspected twins)
- follow-up of early test for chromosomal abnormality
- pregnancy following in-vitro fertilisation (IVF) or gamete intra-fallopian tube transfer (GIFT; see p.53)

Even though the scan may be undertaken for various purposes, the procedure is essentially the same and involves the same machine and equipment. An ultrasound scan takes 5–20 minutes, and is painless. During pregnancy, the cost of ultrasound scans is generally part of your antenatal care, and in that case there is usually no charge to you. However, some radiology providers may require you to pay a surcharge; if so, they should inform you or your LMC midwife or doctor when a scan appointment is made.

When you go for a scan

You will usually be asked to drink a certain volume of fluid in advance so you have a full bladder for the examination. In the first three months of pregnancy, the uterus is still quite small and positioned in the pelvis. A full bladder will push it upwards, enabling a clear picture to be obtained. Occasionally, in very early pregnancy, a vaginal probe can be used for scanning, and in this case there is no need to have a full bladder.

You will be asked to lie down on a firm bed, on your back, and expose your tummy. Some clear jelly will be squirted onto your tummy from a tube. Then the ultrasonographer, midwife or doctor will place a small hand-held device on your tummy and move it around. The sound-wave messages are transferred via a flexible tube to a small screen.

Preparing for a scan in early pregnancy

- Empty your bladder about an hour before your scan appointment, and then drink about a litre of water.
- Don't drink so much that you can't 'hold on' long enough and have to empty your bladder just before the scan. Drink a moderate amount, and remember that the ultrasonographer or doctor doing the scan is more likely to be running late than early.
- Arrive with your scan request form about ten minutes before your appointment (if you do not bring the request form with you, the scan may not be undertaken at that time).

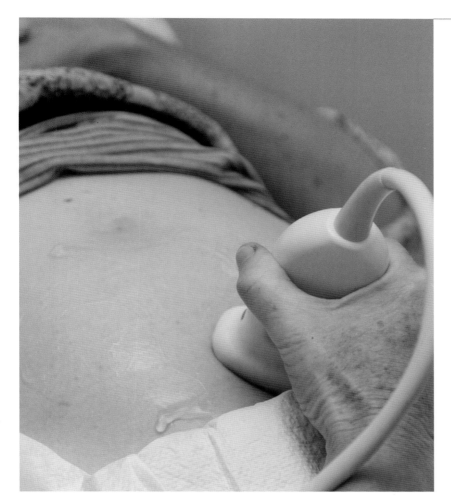

Just what can be seen, and what can be checked for, depends a lot on your stage of pregnancy. The pregnancy sac and baby (or, occasionally, babies) can be seen early on, and the heartbeat is often detected. But in the very early weeks, it is difficult to see other details of the baby's anatomy, which is why the routine (anatomy) scan needs to be done later (see p.150). In general, the earlier the scan is done, the more accurate the estimate of dates. This is because there is an ever-widening range of normal measurements as pregnancy progresses. The baby is measured from 'crown to rump' (head to bottom) up until about 11–13 weeks. If you have a nuchal translucency scan (11–13 weeks), the result will not be available at the time because of the complex calculations required.

X-rays in pregnancy

Since the advent of ultrasound scans, X-rays during pregnancy are rarely done. There is evidence to show that X-rays may affect the development of the baby, especially in the first three months of pregnancy. For this reason, always make sure that anyone organising an X-ray for some reason unrelated to pregnancy is aware that you are (or may be) pregnant, so that precautions can be taken to ensure your pregnancy is protected.

Chorionic villus biopsy (CVS)

This test can be done in early pregnancy to diagnose some chromosomal abnormalities, particularly those that may run in families. It may be recommended in specific circumstances, often after consultation with a genetics specialist. As with amniocentesis (see p.147), if you are thinking of having a CVS you need to weigh up the benefits and the risks carefully.

The procedure is similar to that used for amniocentesis, and is carried out at 10–12 weeks. But instead of taking a sample of amniotic fluid, CVS involves taking a minute piece of placental tissue, using a tiny instrument inserted through the cervix or abdominal wall under ultrasound guidance. The tissue is analysed for a variety of chromosome and other abnormalities. This procedure carries a higher risk of miscarriage (about one in 100) than the risk with an amniocentesis (about one in 200).[24]

The results can take up to two or three weeks, although urgent results for some tests may be provided within 24–48 hours. If a major abnormality is discovered, it is possible to consider terminating the pregnancy earlier than with an amniocentesis. If CVS is used, it is usually reserved for specific circumstances (mainly where an increased genetic risk to the foetus has been identified) and will, in those situations, be highly accurate. However, for general use, the results are not quite as reliable as those for amniocentesis. Moreover, because there is a higher miscarriage risk with CVS, amniocentesis is still preferred for most women if this type of accurate, but invasive, test is required.

Ongoing pregnancy care

If your first antenatal visit is with your LMC, this is the time to discuss and organise your ongoing pregnancy care. Your LMC will arrange to see you in about four weeks' time, unless you have any concerns before then.

But if this first comprehensive visit is with someone other than your eventual LMC, these arrangements will be deferred until you are actually enrolled with and under the care of your LMC. Instead, your GP or another midwife will talk with you about contacting an LMC, and will arrange to continue providing your pregnancy care until you have visited your LMC for the first time.

Lead maternity carers use a variety of maternity records. They may have developed their own records, or use those developed by a provider organisation such as the Midwifery and Maternity Provider Organisation (MMPO). Your LMC will start to fill in your pregnancy record during your first antenatal visit and use it throughout your pregnancy, labour, birth and post-natal period. Some types of pregnancy care records are designed to be held by the pregnant woman herself; these are particularly useful if care is complex and involves several health professionals.

Ting's story: Choosing a lead maternity carer

It was difficult for me to acclimatise to the totally different maternity care system in this country. In China where I came from, most people still use a medical, technical and mechanistic model of care. Women in labour are taken care of by whichever hospital doctors and nurses are on duty on that day. There are not many choices. However, things are simpler in some ways.

Here in New Zealand, the most important thing I needed to do was to choose an LMC as soon as I knew I was pregnant. At first, I thought of having a specialist obstetrician. That would have been my choice in China as a 36-year-old first-time pregnant woman. However, I soon found out that people in New Zealand are not too worried about the woman's age, as long as she does not have serious medical conditions. Not entirely comfortably, I decided to go with the more popular and economical option – to have a midwife as my LMC.

Finding my LMC was not a smooth process. At about eight weeks, I contacted the Ministry of Health who sent me a two-page list of all the midwives in my area. Every midwife warranted only one row in the list, with her name, contact information and what kind of delivery (normal birth, home birth, water birth, etc.) she provided. I would have expected to see at least a photo, a brief résumé, and a little self-introduction, as everyone agrees that having a midwife is such an important and personal choice!

I turned to the Internet to try to find more information about the midwives. Quickly, I realised that many other people were in the same situation and were anxiously seeking recommendations for 'good midwives'. I managed to find two names in my area that were recommended by somebody on an online forum. I rang one, and regrettably found out she was already booked up for the next year. I contacted the other one. She said she was going on holiday when my baby was due; she could hand me over to another midwife who was then on leave but would be back in two months' time. I was very hesitant about whether to go with her or not.

A nurse friend of my husband warned me that I needed to find someone soon in case I missed out on all the 'good' midwives! Finally she recommended someone who was the midwife of one of her friends. After talking to the midwife on the phone and then meeting her in person, I eventually decided that she would be my LMC. She was experienced, friendly and confident. Also, she visited me at home rather than getting me to visit her at a clinic. This made it so much easier for me as a non-driver.

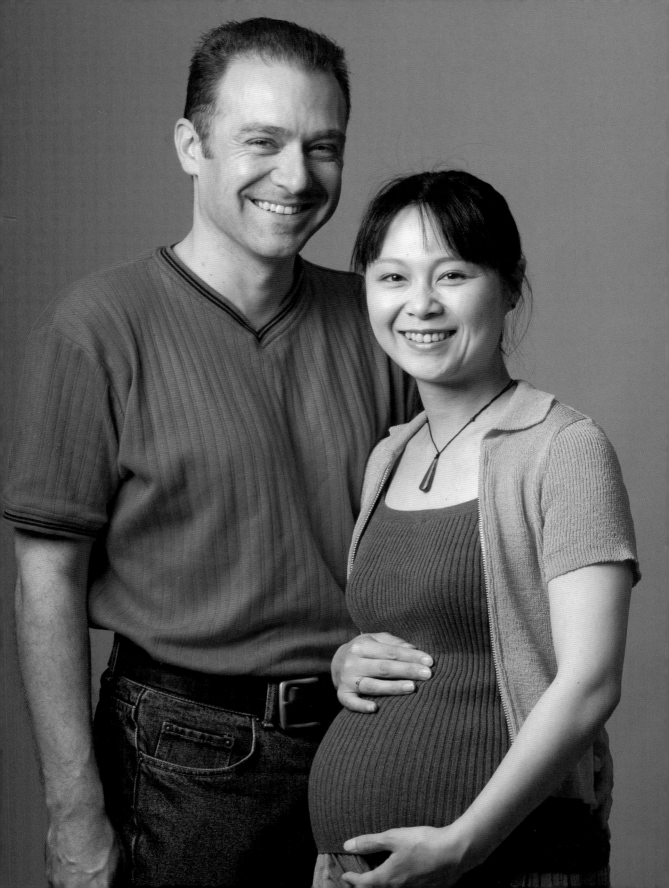

CHAPTER 4

The second three months

(Weeks 14–27)

1. What's happening?

The baby

By 14 weeks from your last menstrual period (LMP), the baby is virtually fully formed. He or she (and yes, 'it' is recognisably a 'he' or a 'she' by now) is still very small – about 12cm long, with an apparently huge head. The heart is beating strongly, and the legs and arms can move vigorously. The skin is transparent, and the blood vessels can be seen through the skin.

By 20 weeks, a fine downy hair has started to partially cover the skin. This is known as lanugo. The eyelids are still fused at this stage, although the eyebrows have started to form.

Ultrasound image

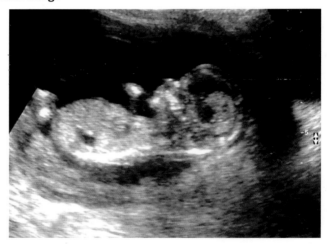

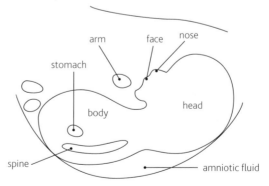

Foetus at 12 weeks and 6 days gestation.
At the beginning of the second trimester, the baby is fully formed.

Pregnancy at 16 weeks

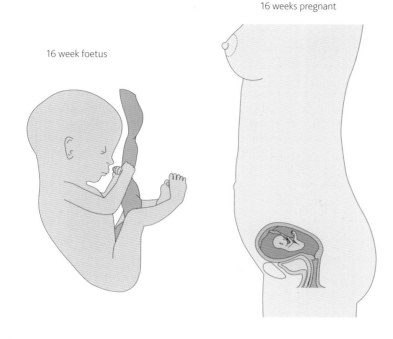

16 weeks pregnant

16 week foetus

At about 24 weeks, the skin has become thicker and less transparent, but is still wrinkled because there is no fat underneath it. The eyelids are now separated, and the baby is moving very strongly. There is still plenty of room for him to move, and he frequently changes position. He is also practising breathing and swallowing movements, even though his lungs are not yet functional.

By 28 weeks, the baby will be about 35cm long and weigh 1000–1200g. Never again in his whole life will this human being grow so fast!

The placenta

What makes this fantastic growth possible? It's easy to forget the importance of the placenta, or whenua, which started to form along with the baby a few days after implantation. By 14 weeks, it is a separate organ, connected to the baby via the umbilical cord and 'stuck' to the inner wall of the uterus.

The placenta is really a complex exchange system, organised so that the mother's blood system and the baby's blood system come into very close contact but never actually mix. The contact is so close (just a thin membrane separates the two systems) that oxygen and food can pass from the mother to the baby, and carbon dioxide and waste products can pass from the baby back to the mother.

Placental transfer

Things transferred from the mother to the baby via the placenta:

- heat
- oxygen
- food (as amino acids, simple sugars and fatty acids)
- some drugs and some viruses.

Things transferred from the baby to the mother via the placenta:

- heat
- carbon dioxide
- wastes (as urea)
- some blood antigens.

Placental circulation

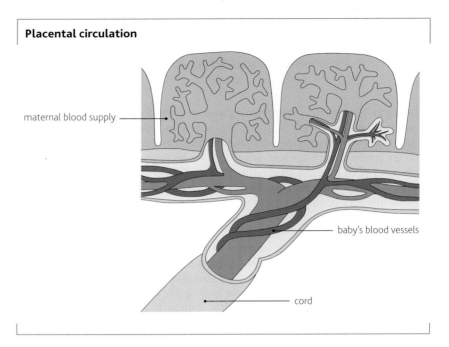

maternal blood supply

baby's blood vessels

cord

The baby's body heat is controlled entirely by the mother's circulation. Heat is exchanged, and cooling and heating allow the baby to remain at a very even temperature. The mother's average body temperature, however, will rise a degree or two by late pregnancy. That's why pregnant women 'feel the heat', and find it more difficult to cool down in hot weather.

This delicate temperature balance can become upset if the mother has a very high temperature due to a severe illness such as pyelonephritis (kidney infection; see opposite), septicaemia (infection of the blood) or peritonitis (infection around the bowel). If the baby's temperature is too disturbed by one of these infections, premature labour may occur. This can be prevented by good management in hospital and the appropriate use of antibiotics; together, they may save the life of the mother and/or her baby.

Maternal changes

So, the baby is growing, the placenta is growing, and the amount of amniotic fluid around the baby is increasing: how does the pregnant woman accommodate all this growth?

The hormones that prepare the pregnant woman's body for change are the same as those that control the menstrual cycle (see pp.26 and 61), allow fertilisation and implantation to occur, and maintain the pregnancy sac in the early weeks.

The uterus

The wall of the uterus softens and thins. As pregnancy progresses, it stretches and stretches – and stretches some more. The uterus also becomes heavier, but does not grow evenly all over. The lower part of the uterus stretches more than the upper parts, particularly later in pregnancy.

Pregnancy at 20 and 24 weeks

20 weeks pregnant

24 weeks pregnant

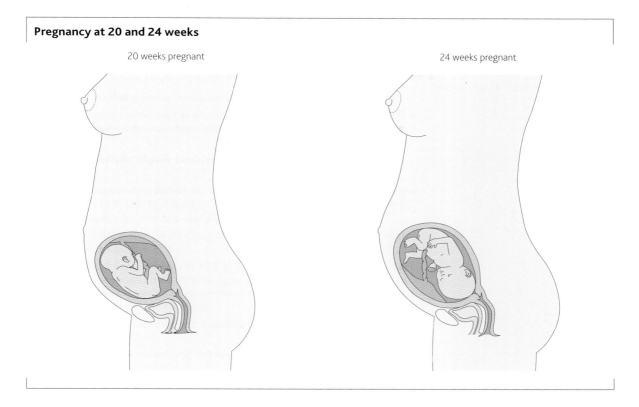

Ligaments in the pelvis

These also soften and stretch, so that the bones within the pelvic ring can make as large a cavity as possible. This softening and stretching can cause discomfort (see p.195).

Kidneys

Because of the increased amount of blood flowing to the kidneys, and the extra wastes from the baby, a pregnant woman produces a lot of urine. The ureters (tubes from the kidneys to the bladder) expand to cope with this increased flow, and so to a lesser extent do the bladder and urethra (tube from the bladder to the outside). This makes it easier for bacteria to get into the bladder and cause urinary tract infections. If an infection does occur, it usually affects the bladder only and can easily be treated, but occasionally the infection will spread up to the kidneys (pyelonephritis).

Pyelonephritis in pregnancy

When bacteria enter the bladder, usually from the skin around the opening of the urethra near the vagina, they can multiply very quickly and soon cause the typical symptoms of bladder infection (pain and stinging when passing urine). If left unchecked, sometimes these same bacteria will spread up the tubes (ureters) to the kidney on one or both sides and cause a much more serious infection. You may experience loin pain, fever, shivering and shaking, light-headedness and/or vomiting, and require prompt attention in hospital.

Bones and ligaments of the pelvis

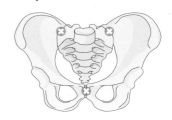

✪ ligaments

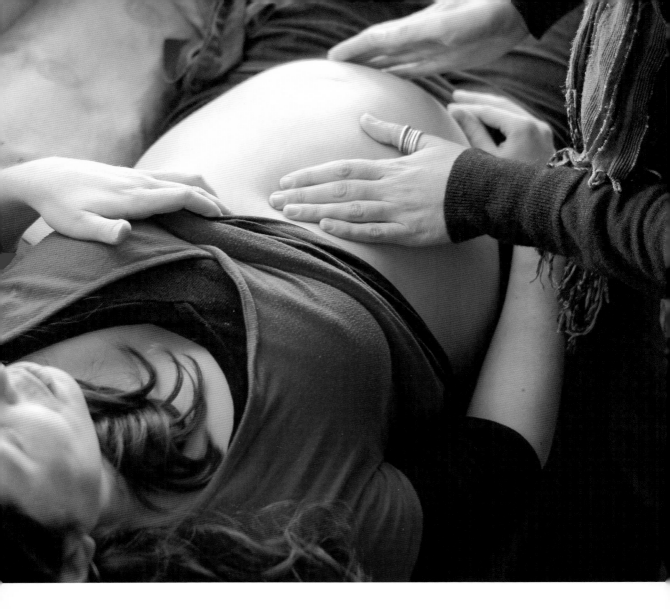

Fluids, painkillers and intravenous antibiotics will be used to treat the infection, relieve the pain, and avoid possible blood poisoning (septicaemia) and/or premature labour. To avoid this serious complication, have any symptoms of a possible bladder infection checked out and treated if they persist for more than 24 hours, or sooner if the pain is getting worse.

Renal colic in pregnancy

In about 5 per cent of the population, there is a tendency for small stones to form in the kidneys. These stones may lie undetected for years, but cause severe pain (colic) if they move into the ureters with the urine.

If you happen to have renal stones, they are more likely to move as pregnancy progresses, because there is more urine and the ureters are wider than normal. They can cause severe loin or abdominal pain, usually on one side. The stones will often pass with adequate pain relief and fluids; sometimes admission to hospital is necessary.

Weight gain (see also pp.134 and 402)

Weight gain is normal in pregnancy, although the amount varies. Most women in New Zealand gain at least 10–12kg over their non-pregnant weight, and much of this is accounted for by the growing breasts, the uterus, the placenta and of course the baby. In addition, fat does tend to get laid down in pregnancy in preparation for breastfeeding. Some women put on a lot of weight, while others gain only a relatively small amount. The biggest weight gain takes place between 20 and 36 weeks, so the increase is not spread evenly over your whole pregnancy.

While for most women it's sensible to try to keep the weight gain to around the 10–12kg mark, it's *not* sensible to starve yourself. Eating a balanced diet will help (see pp.18 and 134). But don't get too upset if you put on more weight than you'd like – moderate your food intake, and concentrate on losing weight after the baby is born.

Breasts

During pregnancy, hormonal changes prepare the breasts for producing milk once the baby is born. Two main hormones are responsible: human placental lactogen (HPL) from the placenta, and prolactin from the pituitary gland at the base of the brain.

Initially, the breasts may retain extra fluid, which makes them tender and larger than normal. During the second trimester this tenderness subsides, although the breasts will continue to be somewhat larger than usual. The milk ducts and collecting sacs within the breasts grow and develop, but after 20–24 weeks you will not notice much increase in breast size until the milk 'comes in' after the baby is born (see pp.305 and 327).

> **Sources of weight gain in pregnancy**
>
> - the baby
> - the placenta
> - the uterus
> - the amniotic fluid
> - increased blood volume
> - extra fluid in the tissues
> - breast development
> - extra fat deposited

Breast tissue development

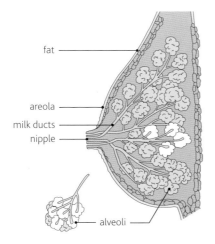
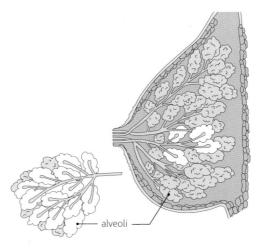

fat
areola
milk ducts
nipple
alveoli

alveoli

Non-pregnant breast   Pregnant breast

2. Feelings

'I found it hugely enjoyable. I loved the attention I got when I was pregnant – we'd be in a supermarket and I'd bend down to grab something off the shelf and someone would say, "Shouldn't your husband be doing that?" And I'd say, "Yeah, he should!" It was a wonderful, wonderful experience.'

Now you've been pregnant for three whole months. Does it seem that long? Are you still reeling from the realisation that you are actually pregnant? Or does the first trimester seem to have gone on for ever, and you're wondering if the nausea is ever going to stop? Some women find it does, quite dramatically, at around 12–14 weeks; for others, the nausea persists, gradually improving somewhere between 16 and 20 weeks. Most problems of early pregnancy settle down in the second trimester – if not completely, then at least to a more tolerable level.

Other problems that can emerge in these middle months, and sometimes continue, include constipation, heartburn, backache as the uterus and pregnancy sac grow larger, and aching legs (especially if you have a tendency to varicose veins).

Despite these, many women feel positive about their pregnancy during this time, even if it was unplanned or unexpected. The dramatic mood swings of the first three months tend to settle down. There are things to do and plan for. Many women have more energy; some have a lot more, and are full of projects and ideas – at work and at home. Try to take some 'time out' to do things you enjoy during these middle months, especially activities that will be more difficult with a small baby.

Expansion

'It seemed as if everyone in the world knew more about having a baby than I did – strangers in the supermarket even told me what I should be buying. I really resented it.'

How do you feel about that expanding tummy? Love it? Hate it? Proud of it? Resigned to it? Some women can't wait to look pregnant; others resent 'going public' and having people comment on what they feel is a very private matter. However you feel, you are likely to be sensitive about being pregnant – well-meaning remarks about your size often don't go down well, but do your best to simply ignore them.

Women vary remarkably in how they look during this time. Differences in body shape and weight mean that some women look quite pregnant by 16 weeks, while others start to look pregnant only at 24–28 weeks. If you really do think you are too big or too small for your dates, discuss this with your LMC at your next antenatal visit. They may want to examine your tummy, take measurements, and possibly do an ultrasound scan to check your pregnancy size against your dates.

Movements ('quickening')

Sooner or later, you'll feel the baby move. Some women don't really feel pregnant until this happens. Tell your partner or support person – they may be even more excited than you are. In first pregnancies, this quickening occurs somewhere between 18 and 22 weeks; with subsequent pregnancies it can be as early as 16 weeks. This is because the wall of the uterus is usually firmer in a first pregnancy, making early movements more difficult to feel.

You may not be sure about the movements at first, but they should become more frequent and obvious over the next couple of weeks. Keep a note of the date you think you first felt the baby move.

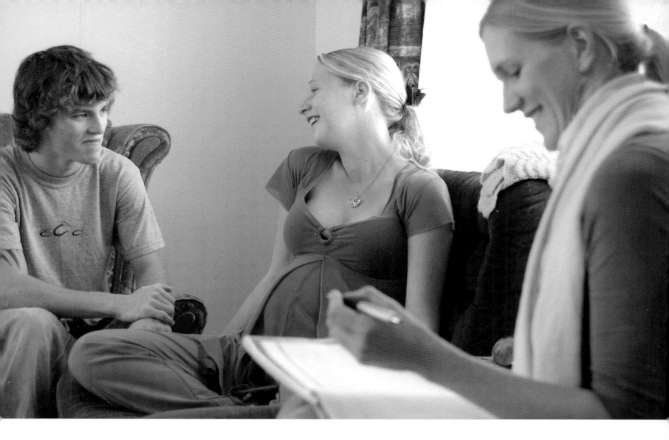

Travel during pregnancy

You might take the opportunity to enjoy some travel around this time – whether it be a weekend away with friends, a business conference, or some 'time out' from the children. Or you may find that you have to travel because of work or family circumstances.

When is the best time to travel when pregnant? During the first three months, the nausea of early pregnancy is likely to be aggravated by any sort of travel, especially by sea. (Even if you have never suffered from seasickness in your life, you may do so then. Anti-seasickness wrist-bands that put pressure on the P6 acupressure point have been found to be helpful for nausea and vomiting in pregnancy,[1] as well as for travel sickness whether you are pregnant or not.) Early pregnancy is also the time when miscarriage is more likely to occur, so if you are at a distance from health care services, this could mean significant delay in getting help if you need it.

The last three months of pregnancy, and especially the last six weeks, are not the best time for travelling either. Sitting in a cramped car or plane becomes more uncomfortable as each week of pregnancy passes, and further increases the risk of blood clots. Also, you may go into labour earlier than expected, and end up having to give birth in a strange hospital, possibly without the help of your partner or support person.

If you have any choice in the matter, the middle three to four months of pregnancy (between about 14 and 30 weeks) are the best time for any extended travel involving long journeys by plane, car or train. Discuss any international travel plans with your LMC, and if you have any particular problems with your pregnancy, discuss domestic travel as well.

'We walked the Routeburn when I was about 24 weeks. It was fine, but putting the pack on put me right off my balance! I got used to it, though.'

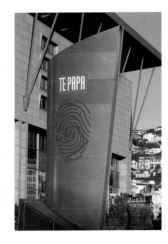

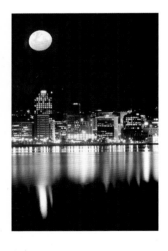

Travel tips[2]

Your trip can be enjoyable, safe and relaxing, as long as you bear a few points in mind:

- *Car travel*. Car accidents are a significant cause of injury during pregnancy, so wear a seat belt fastened firmly (but not tightly) either low in the pelvic area or across the shoulders. Unborn babies usually recover well from seat-belt pressure in mild or even moderate accidents. If you are involved in an accident, tell any emergency services that you are pregnant, and seek help and or advice from your LMC (or another appropriate doctor or midwife if you are away from home), regardless of how minor the accident may seem.

- *International travel*. Go with a companion, and make sure you have travel insurance that will cover you for pregnancy-related conditions and complications. Carry information with you about your expected delivery date (EDD), your blood group and contact details for your LMC. If your LMC routinely leaves your pregnancy notes with you, take those with you even if you are going away for just a short time. Travel medicine clinics are an excellent source of expert advice, especially if you are contemplating travel to a developing country.[3]

- *Travel sickness drugs*. It's best to avoid these altogether. Also avoid taking sleeping tablets.

- *Food- and water-borne illnesses*. Traveller's diarrhoea and/or vomiting may be difficult to treat when you're pregnant as dehydration is more difficult to correct and the range of safe, effective antibiotics is limited. Drink bottled water, and avoid putting ice in drinks.

- *Prolonged exercise at altitudes*. Undergoing prolonged exercise above about 3000m (12,000ft) is liable to cause intra-uterine growth restriction (IUGR; see p.142). However, there is little evidence that short-term exposure (with gradual acclimatisation over a few days to altitude) causes problems in healthy pregnant women who normally live close to sea-level.[4]

- *Vaccination*. This is best undertaken before pregnancy, so it makes sense for all women in their child-bearing years to keep up to date with routine vaccinations, and if travelling frequently, the more common traveller's vaccines (such as hepatitis A).

  During pregnancy, inactivated vaccines (e.g. hepatitis A, hepatitis B, inactivated influenza) are very unlikely to cause problems, and should be used unless the risk of exposure is very low or absent. However, pregnant women should avoid live vaccines (e.g. measles, mumps, rubella, yellow fever), although the risk of any adverse effects is still small.

- *Malaria prevention*. Malaria is a serious disease in pregnancy and carries risk for both mother and baby, so avoid travel to malaria-prone areas if at all possible. If this is unavoidable, extra care needs to be taken to avoid exposure to the mosquitoes that carry the disease. Some, but not all, anti-malarial tablets are dangerous for the baby.

- *Blood clots (deep vein thrombosis, or DVT)*. The hormonal changes in pregnancy make the blood clot more easily (see p.205). When you are inactive for a long time, your circulation is impaired and clots can develop in the veins of the legs or pelvic area. Guard against this by making more frequent stops on car journeys to get out and walk around. On planes or trains, stand up and move around for 15 minutes every hour. Special support stockings to aid circulation are also available. Drink even more fluids than you normally would, to reduce dehydration. Avoid alcohol completely; it is best avoided during pregnancy anyway (see p.24), and it will cause dehydration.

- *Airline restrictions*. Most airlines do not restrict pregnant women from flying until 36 weeks into a normal pregnancy, or four weeks before the EDD. Between 36 and 39 weeks, New Zealand airlines generally permit flights of less than five hours for normal pregnancies. But different airlines have different requirements, so if you are over 35 weeks pregnant, check with the airline when booking.

  A medical certificate from your LMC may be required if you take a flight of more than five hours in the four weeks before your EDD. Your LMC will be asked for information about the stability of your pregnancy. Decisions about flying are made on a case-by-case basis.

  International air travel is generally unrestricted for normal pregnancies up until four weeks prior to the EDD – but again, check with the airline. Beyond that time, a certificate is required from your LMC, and clearance on a case-by-case basis will need to be obtained from the airline. Most airlines will not allow you to fly within one week of your EDD.

  For multiple pregnancies, or those with other complications, earlier restrictions are likely to apply. If in any doubt, check with your LMC before confirming your booking.

- *Oxygen on aircraft*. Less oxygen is available in an aircraft when it is at cruising altitudes. However, breathlessness will not be a problem unless you exercise vigorously or are unwell in some way. The baby's oxygen supply is not affected at normal cabin pressures.

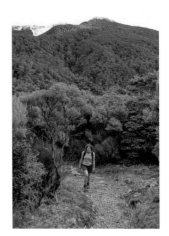

Problems that might preclude international travel

- multiple pregnancy
- placental problems
- incompetent cervix
- threatened miscarriage or vaginal bleeding
- high blood pressure, pre-eclampsia (toxaemia) or diabetes (in this or a previous pregnancy)
- miscarriage, premature labour or premature rupture of membranes (in this or a previous pregnancy)
- past or present blood clots (in legs and/or lungs)
- severe asthma or other lung disease
- heart disease
- kidney disease
- severe anaemia or other blood disorder

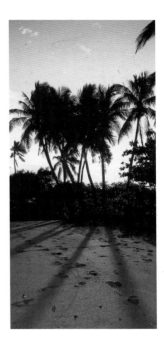

3. Helping yourself

Exercise during pregnancy

Regular exercise is part of a healthy lifestyle, including during pregnancy. Many women enter pregnancy with an aerobic and strength training programme already in place, and this is a great start. Other women use pregnancy as an opportunity to improve their health by developing good exercise habits. Whatever your situation, it's beneficial to do some regular exercise if you possibly can.[5]

Exercise will help prevent loss of fitness, too much weight gain and low back pain. It will probably also help prevent such things as pregnancy-induced high blood pressure, diabetes and varicose veins. It will make you feel better in yourself – exercise is proven to have a positive effect on people's moods.[6]

Mild or moderate exercise is best. Nearly all pregnant women (with the possible exception of those with very complex pregnancies or severe heart, lung or high blood pressure problems) can safely manage some exercise. If you have any particular problems, other conditions or concerns, discuss with your LMC how they might affect your ability to exercise.

Strenuous exercise is probably best avoided, as it will reduce the blood flow to the placenta. Whether or not this adversely affects the baby depends on a number of other factors related to the placenta. There may be exceptions to this general rule if you were very fit before becoming pregnant, so discuss this with your LMC or GP. You may also want to seek advice from a sports medicine expert if you are involved in top-level competitive sport.[7]

Precautions for exercise[8]

Because pregnancy causes changes to body mass and blood volume, there are some basic precautions to take when exercising:

- Drink more fluid than normal before and during exercise to prevent dehydration.
- Wear loose, comfortable clothing to avoid overheating, and don't exercise if you have a temperature. (There is some evidence to suggest that the baby's health is put at risk if the mother is overheated, either from vigorous exercise or from an illness that causes a fever.)
- Eat plenty of carbohydrates to replace your own energy levels quickly after exercise.
- Avoid exercising while lying flat on your back once you are more than 20 weeks pregnant.
- Avoid exercise where the oxygen supply can be severely compromised (e.g. scuba-diving, high-altitude climbing).
- Avoid exercise where you may get hit directly in the abdomen, especially later in pregnancy.
- Stop exercising if you get any vaginal bleeding, leakage of amniotic fluid or painful uterine contractions, or if you feel very faint, get chest pain or have excessive shortness of breath.

Recommended activities

Walking

This is a wonderful form of exercise. It is certainly the easiest and cheapest, and is available to everyone. Just 15 minutes of brisk walking, building up to 30 minutes three times a week, is helpful. Walking even a kilometre a day will ease aching legs and a sore back, and help maintain a degree of physical fitness. The 'talk test' is a good indication of whether your exercise intensity level is too high. If you can maintain a conversation while exercising, keep going; this is considered a comfortable intensity.[9] If you cannot do this, exercise less intensely. Take it slowly, have plenty of rests if you need them, but *walk*.

Jogging

This is less popular than walking, because it is a high-impact exercise, and as pregnancy progresses it puts extra strain on softened pelvic ligaments. If you want to run, take it more easily as your weight increases. Some women find it too uncomfortable as pregnancy progresses, and urinary incontinence may be a problem. But if you enjoy it, carry on gently as long as it's comfortable, and then do some other form of exercise such as walking instead.

Swimming

This is excellent for pregnant women and probably the perfect pregnancy exercise. It's relaxing – provided the water is neither too hot nor too cold – and the buoyancy of the water supports your increasing body weight. It's quite safe to swim during pregnancy, unless the amniotic sac around the baby has broken (see p.260), although this is very unusual until late in pregnancy. As your EDD approaches, swimming is also helpful to get your baby into a good position: the 'tummy down' position you use doing breaststroke or with a kickboard, for example, can help your baby's back to move forward rather than lying against your back. This posterior position often causes backache in pregnancy and labour, so anything you can do to relieve it is helpful (see box on p.225).

Aquarobics

Aquarobics classes are offered by many swimming pool complexes around the country, and involve a range of exercises done in the water.

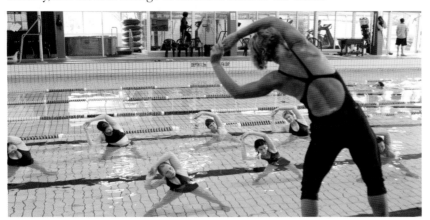

Many pregnant women find them relaxing and fun. Keeping fit in the water has a number of advantages during pregnancy:

- Every muscle in the body can be exercised in the water, either gently or more vigorously.
- The water takes some of the weight off your lower limbs, and is good for increasing the blood circulation in the legs, especially when standing and walking in the water.
- You can exercise quite actively in the water without overheating.
- Classes are a good way to meet other women who are pregnant, and those who already have children.

Exercise programmes

A variety of exercise programmes tailored specifically for pregnant women are available in some centres in New Zealand, and many commercial gyms now offer courses that take pregnancy requirements into account. Check out suitable classes offered in your area – yoga centres and physiotherapists are also worth trying, as some run excellent classes for pregnancy and in preparation for birth.

Essential pregnancy exercises (see also pp.323–326)

There are two muscle groups that need special attention during pregnancy and after birth: the pelvic floor muscles and the abdominal muscles. It helps to understand just what these remarkable structures do, so you can look after them well. Looking after these muscles will also help you look after your back, which has increasing strain placed on it as pregnancy progresses.

The pelvic floor muscles

The pelvic floor is a complex structure made up of layers of muscle and other tissue sitting in the base of the pelvis. If you cup your hands together, one on top of the other, this will give you some idea of its size. The pelvic floor passes from the pubic bone in front to the tail bone behind, and stretches side to side in the pelvis from one sit-upon pelvic bone (ischium) to the other.

Why is the pelvic floor so important? It provides support for the pelvic organs (the bowel, uterus, vagina and bladder), helping to hold them all in their correct place. As well, the pelvic floor is part of the closure mechanism for the bladder and bowel, so it plays an important part in keeping us continent, helping with both bladder and bowel control. The more superficial layer of the pelvic floor plays an important part in sexual function.

During pregnancy, the pelvic floor comes under increasing stress because of hormonal changes, weight gain, and increasing pressure from the growing uterus. The pelvic floor muscles need to be kept strong as pregnancy proceeds. But during labour, these same muscles must relax and stretch to allow the baby to pass through them and be born. That's why the pelvic floor needs care during pregnancy and after birth to restore good function.

Muscles of the pelvic floor

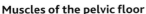

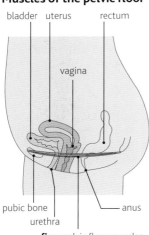

firm pelvic floor muscles

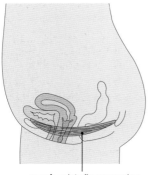

weak pelvic floor muscles

The pelvic floor muscles can be divided into three areas:

- Around the entrance to the anus or back passage. These are the muscles you tighten if you are stopping yourself from passing wind.
- Around the entrance to the vagina. To feel where these are, imagine you have a tampon in your vagina that is slipping out – tighten the muscles around the vagina as if to pull it up inside you.
- Around the urethra or bladder outlet. To feel these muscles, try stopping your urine flow mid-stream. Sit on the toilet with knees apart and a straight back. Start the flow of urine, and then try to stop it. (Do this as a test only, not as a repeated exercise.)

How to exercise the pelvic floor[10]

Getting started
- Try sitting with a rolled towel underneath your bottom and between your legs – the pressure on your perineum will make it easier to feel the muscles. It may not be very comfortable, but it will increase the sensory awareness of the muscles and give you something to lift off (see picture).
- Sit with a straight back. A rounded back will inhibit your pelvic floor function.
- You may notice that your tummy muscles pull in just a little above the pubic bone as you tighten the pelvic floor. This is good, as it shows this 'deep corset abdominal muscle' is working together with the pelvic floor muscles.

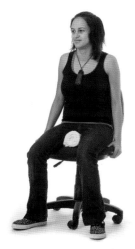

Sitting on a rolled towel

Putting it together[11]
- Tighten your muscles from the back forward, around the anus, vagina and urethra. As you tighten, feel that the pelvic floor is also lifting up inside you. Hold this position steady for two normal breaths. Concentrate on achieving a strong, steady, rock-like hold. If it wavers or fades, you need to practise so you are better able to hold it steady before increasing the number of times you repeat it.
- Totally let it go before repeating the exercise. This relaxation is as important as the tightening. As you relax your pelvic floor, think, 'This is what I need to do to give birth and allow my body to open up.'
- Pelvic floor exercises during pregnancy are best done regularly from 20 weeks onwards. Aim to get as close as possible to maximum contraction of the pelvic floor muscles, building up to 8–12 muscle contractions three times a day. It may help you to remember to do them regularly if you complete a set before leaving the table after every meal.
- If you have any problems with stress incontinence (a small leakage of urine with a cough or sneeze), train yourself to tighten your pelvic floor as automatically as you cover your mouth when you cough or sneeze. This is often referred to by physiotherapists as 'the knack'.

Pelvic floor exercises – points to remember

- Breathe normally, and avoid the natural tendency to hold your breath.
- Resist the temptation to bear down; instead, the pelvic floor must lift up.
- Don't tighten your seat muscles or pull your legs together; keep your seat muscles and inner thighs relaxed.

Deep abdominal muscles

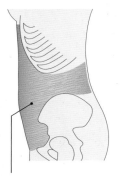

deep corset
abdominal muscle

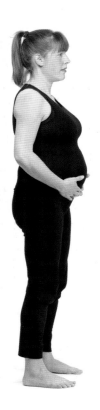

The abdominal muscles[12]

The abdominal muscles are like an elaborate corset. They support the abdominal organs, including the growing weight of the uterus and your baby. They also provide support for your back, and help you maintain good posture. The hormonal changes of pregnancy and the inevitable stretching of the abdominal muscles mean they need extra care.

You can protect your abdominal muscles if you:

- Avoid doing sit-ups in any shape or form.
- To get off a bed, roll like a log (see opposite). Use the bent knees and the upper arm pushing forward to create momentum.
- Do the 'tummy tuck' (below) often, and always when lifting.

Deep corset abdominal muscle

The 'deep corset' abdominal muscle is a big muscle that works in conjunction with your pelvic floor muscles. It's especially important to look after it, as it provides support for your expanding uterus. It can be exercised with the tummy tuck.

The tummy tuck

This exercise is also known as 'baby hugs', and works the deep corset abdominal muscle.

- Place your hands under your tummy as in the photo, or place your fingers gently on your lower tummy just above the pubic bone.
- Very gently pull your tummy in. The gentle movement inwards should be felt under your hands.
- Maintain normal breathing while you hold the tummy tuck.
- Take care that it is your abdominal muscles that are working, and that you are not just breathing in to get this movement.
- Contract your pelvic floor muscles and feel what happens to these lower abdominal muscles.
- Do a tummy tuck and see what happens to your pelvic floor.
- Remember when doing a pelvic floor exercise, it is a strong, steady lift of the pelvic floor that is needed, holding this for two normal breaths.
- When you do a tummy tuck, be very gentle – only about 10 per cent effort is required compared to the effort you use to do your pelvic floor exercise.
- Do this exercise gently but often. To remind yourself, try getting into the habit of doing a tummy tuck every time you walk down your hallway, up the stairs, down the street or from the car to the office.
- Whenever you lift, *always* use the tummy tuck exercise.

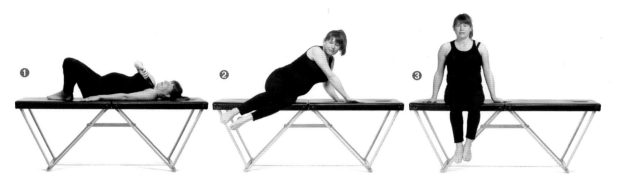

Separation (diastasis) of the long abdominal muscles

Sometimes, the long abdominal muscles, known as the rectus abdominis muscles (see diagram, below right), can separate in the midline. This is called diastasis, and happens to some extent to about 70 per cent of pregnant women.[13] When you sit up or slightly raise your head when lying down, you may notice that a bulge appears above your umbilicus (tummy button) in the midline of your abdomen. This is an indication that there is probably some separation. You can check by lying on your back with your knees bent up. Gently lift your head and shoulders off the pillow. Feel in the midline two or three finger-widths above and below the tummy button. If you can feel a gap in the upper and/or lower abdominal muscles, this is a fairly good indication that there is some separation.

Diastasis is not usually a problem unless it involves the whole muscle from top to bottom, if the separation is more than three finger-widths wide, or if you have significant low backache. If this is the case, speak to your LMC about getting an external support, or seek out a women's health physiotherapist for advice. (See Appendix: Physiotherapy.) Try to wear clothes that will give your tummy extra support. A physiotherapist may be able to provide a stretchy circular support made of soft but firm fabric to wear.

For most women, diastasis settles after pregnancy. But if the problem is significant, it can persist, be associated with pelvic floor dysfunction, and cause problems as women get older – so ask for help if you need it.

Roll like a log

❶ Start to roll, bringing upper arm over.
❷ Use upper arm to push forward, keeping knees bent.
❸ Ready to stand.

Long abdominal muscles

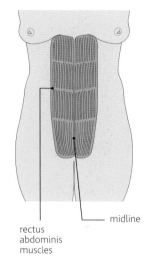

midline

rectus
abdominis
muscles

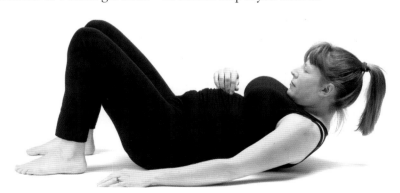

Checking for separation of the abdominal muscles

Looking after your back

As the ligaments of the lower back and pelvis soften and stretch to accommodate your growing baby, and to prepare the pelvis to open up to give birth, you may experience some aches and pains and feelings of pressure. Poor posture, stretched abdominal muscles, and lifting heavy loads (including children) can turn discomfort into quite severe pain in the lower back and even down the back of one or both legs.

The following measures can help:

- Don't overlook your daily rest.
- Take some regular exercise – swimming is especially good.
- Remember to do tummy tucks often. These help stop the tendency to increase the lumbar curve of the lower back, which in turn helps stabilise the pelvic joints and prevent low back pain.

Looking after your back

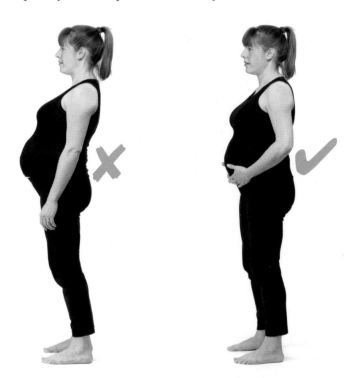

- Make sure your bed has a firm base. If it doesn't, you can either put the mattress on the floor, put boards under the mattress, or beg, borrow or buy a good-quality inner-sprung mattress with a firm base.
- Minimise lifting. At work, get others to lift heavy or awkward loads, or use mechanical help. At home, put commonly used items at bench height. If you do have to lift, always do the tummy tuck exercise shown on p.128, holding the muscle gently throughout. Bend your knees before you lift, then gradually straighten.

- Sit well at all times, maintaining your normal lumbar curve. Using a lumbar roll is helpful. Don't sit with a rounded back – it will give you backache. You may like to sit back to front on a chair so that the weight of your uterus is not resting on your back. Sitting on a Swiss ball helps to maintain a good posture and encourages the abdominal muscles to work well (see p.221).

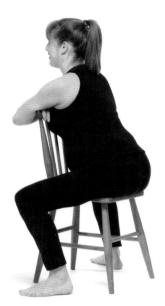

Sitting posture

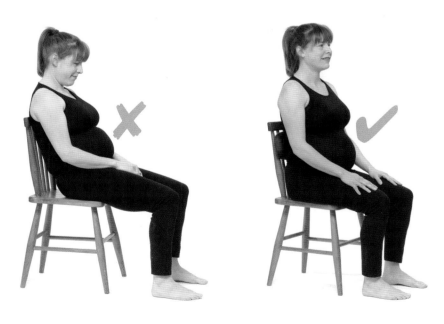

Looking after your legs

Your leg and bottom muscles also take extra strain as pregnancy progresses, as they bear much of the increasing weight. Their circulation can also be more sluggish as the growing uterus presses on the big veins in the pelvic area. Keeping these muscles exercised and supple not only keeps you more comfortable, but reduces the risk of clots in the leg veins. Get some daily exercise; walking and swimming are both excellent (see p.125). The stretching exercises shown below can also help if done regularly.

Calf stretch

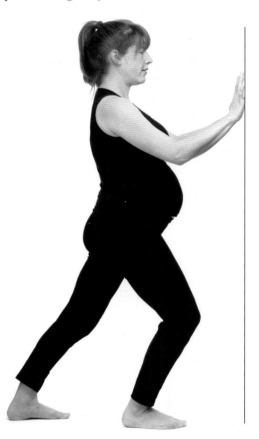

- Stand with one foot close to a wall, and the other a metre behind. Now, lean your forearms on the wall while bending the front knee. Keep both heels on the ground, and feel the calf muscles of the back leg being gently stretched. Hold this for about 20 seconds, then repeat with the other leg. If you are getting leg cramps, try doing this exercise morning and night.

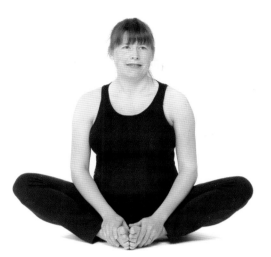

Butterfly

- Sit with your knees apart and the soles of your feet together. Pull your heels in towards your body and let your knees drop towards the floor. Keep your back straight.

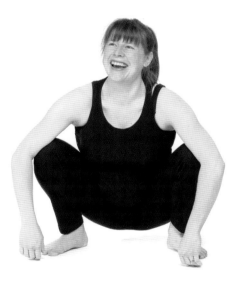

Squatting

- Try to incorporate some squatting into your day. It is especially helpful if you can do a full squat with your heels on the floor. (You should not do this if you have a cervical suture – see p.143 – or bad varicose veins.)

Nutrition[14]

Now that the first 12–14 weeks are over, and any nausea has at least begun to improve, it's a good time to think about the nutritional value of your diet. Many myths exist about what, and how much, pregnant women should eat. A lot of of them date from long ago when living and dietary standards were very different from what they are today. For the modern New Zealand woman, all the ingredients of an excellent diet are readily available.

Why is nutrition more important in pregnancy than at other times? Strictly speaking, it's not – ideally, we should all eat a balanced and nutritious diet throughout our lives (see Chapter 1).

However, during pregnancy, and breastfeeding, women have an increased need for:

- some extra calories as carbohydrates
- protein
- fluid
- iron
- folic acid
- vitamins B, C and D
- calcium, zinc and magnesium.

Most healthy pregnant women in New Zealand can meet nearly all these extra requirements simply by eating a varied, balanced diet; special supplements are not generally needed. Some exceptions are described below. All women should expect to gain weight during pregnancy, mainly in the second and third trimesters.

Some special situations

- Women who are underweight for their height at the start of pregnancy (anyone with a BMI of less than 18.5, irrespective of ethnicity) may need to increase the amount of high-energy foods and protein in their diet. Many thin women gain 12–18kg during pregnancy.
- Women who are significantly overweight for their height at the start of pregnancy (i.e. with a BMI of more than 30 for European women, more than 32 for Māori and Pacific Island women, or more than 27.5 for Asian women) will not need to increase their overall food intake very much, but will still need to pay attention to getting enough protein, vitamins and minerals in their diet. A balanced diet (see p.20) is important. This is not the time to go on stringent reducing diets, and a weight gain of 6–8kg during pregnancy is to be expected.
- Teenage women who are pregnant may well still be growing themselves, so will have higher energy requirements than older pregnant women. Teenagers of normal weight should aim to gain at least 10kg during their pregnancy, and preferably more.
- Women who have, or have had, trouble with an eating disorder can greatly benefit from a dietician's help.
- Women who are vegetarian may need to eat more iron-rich foods and/or take iron supplements.

- Women who are vegan (i.e. who eat no animal products at all) need to ensure that they eat a wide variety of foods containing protein, iron, calcium and vitamin B12. A diet that is rich in legumes, nuts, wholegrain breads and cereals contains many of these things, but supplements may still be needed.
- Women who eat a lot of processed or take-away foods need to increase their intake of foods rich in protein and folic acid.
- A multiple pregnancy (twins or more) does increase nutritional demand. It is much easier to become deficient in iron and folic acid than with a single pregnancy, and supplements are sometimes needed.

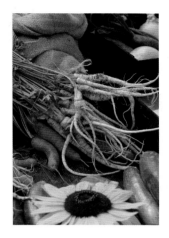

Nutrients in food and drinks

- *Good high-energy foods:* starches – wholemeal bread, pasta, potatoes, kūmara, taro, rice; fats – butter, cheese, full milk (all in moderation), cooking oils, salad oils.
- *Good high-protein foods:* milk (trim), butter, cheese, lean red meat, fish and other kaimoana, chicken (all freshly prepared), all types of beans (especially soya), nuts, lentils.
- *Foods rich in fibre:* wholegrain breads, cereals, vegetables, fruits, legumes.
- *Foods rich in iron:* lean red meat, fish and other kaimoana, chicken, eggs (all freshly prepared), wholegrain bread, legumes, dried nuts, parsley, spinach, silverbeet (you need large amounts of green vegetables to get significant iron from them). Vitamin C also helps iron absorption, so try to eat foods rich in vitamin C alongside iron-rich foods.
- *Foods rich in folic acid:* all green leafy vegetables (e.g. pūhā, cabbage, lettuce), eaten raw or lightly cooked.
- *Foods rich in vitamin B, especially B12:* meat, milk, fish, eggs, vitamin B12-fortified foods (some soy milks, textured vegetable protein).
- *Foods rich in calcium:* milk (trim), cheese, yogurt, canned fish with bones, dried fruit, wholegrain bread, cereals, nuts. Calcium metabolism is also helped by vitamin D (see box on p.137).
- *Fluids:* water and trim milk are best. Keep fruit juice, fizzy drinks and flavoured water to a minimum; they contain sugar but little else of value. Avoid drinking tea and coffee with meals as it reduces iron absorption. Avoid alcohol and energy drinks. Keep coffee consumption below one to two cups per day (see box on p.21).
- *Food preparation:* grill, boil, steam or microwave whenever possible. Avoid frying food. Vegetables should be lightly cooked to retain as many nutrients as possible, but meat, especially chicken, should be cooked thoroughly and eaten as soon as it is prepared.

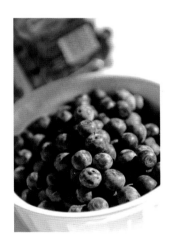

Dietary supplements

Iron

If your blood tests show that you need extra iron, it may be necessary to take iron tablets if you cannot get enough in your diet. Lack of iron can cause anaemia, excessive tiredness, slow healing of cuts and scratches, and poor health in your baby in the first months of life – especially if he is premature.

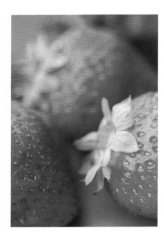

It takes a while to become iron deficient, and it takes a while (usually months) to build up your stores again. Although you may feel fine, if the tests show a need for iron, now is the time to take action. Getting enough iron-rich food is particularly important for Māori women, who seem to be at increased risk of iron deficiency, although exactly why is unclear.

Although you should first try to increase the amount of iron-rich food in your diet, several iron tablets are available in New Zealand. The usual dose is one tablet daily, but this can vary – stick to your recommended dose. Don't take iron tablets with antacids or tea, coffee or milk, as they interfere with iron absorption. Do take them with food rich in vitamin C to help absorption. Some women get nauseated and constipated with iron tablets, while others get diarrhoea. If either happens, check with your LMC about the best course of action.

Too much iron can also be a problem. Not everyone needs, or benefits from, iron supplements. Some research suggests that giving iron supplements to women who already have good iron stores in fact increases their chances of developing diabetes in pregnancy,[15] and decreases normal zinc levels in the body (this will not happen from iron in food, because of normal digestive processes). A few women have a condition called haemochromatosis, which results in excessive iron levels; if they take extra iron, they become ill.[16] Before you take iron supplements during pregnancy, have a blood test, and follow your LMC's advice.

Calcium

Your baby needs significant amounts of calcium for skeletal development. A healthy woman absorbs and retains more calcium during pregnancy, and transfers it to her baby, especially during the last trimester.

It is rare for New Zealand women to suffer from a calcium deficiency significant enough to affect pregnancy. Simply adjusting your diet should easily rectify any relative deficiencies. Any sort of milk is a good source of calcium. Supplements may be appropriate for women who find it difficult to eat any calcium-containing foods, as there is some evidence to suggest that good calcium levels help to reduce the risk of high blood pressure as pregnancy progresses.

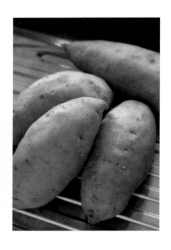

Trace elements

Zinc, selenium and magnesium are all required in pregnancy, but in very small amounts. A healthy diet containing foods from the four main food groups – with plenty of cereals, wholegrain breads, nuts and fish – will normally supply all you need.

Iodine

Iodine is an essential element for a healthy thyroid, especially in babies and children. (The thyroid gland in the neck maintains the body's steady metabolic rate, and a healthy thyroid is essential for normal brain development in babies and children.) However, New Zealand soils and New Zealand-grown foods tend to be low in naturally occurring iodine. For this reason, iodine has been added to salt for many years, and the incidence of thyroid disease in children has dropped to very low levels – although concern has been raised recently about declining use of iodised salt. Other iodine supplements can be toxic, so a much safer way to make sure you and your baby have normal levels of iodine is to use small amounts of iodised salt when cooking, and to eat fish regularly.

Vitamins

Unless there is good reason to think that you need additional vitamins, as in the special situations described in the box below, extra supplements are generally not necessary. It is nearly always better to get the vitamins and minerals you need from food, because the normal digestive processes will ensure you absorb only what you need. While most excess vitamins are simply passed out of the body in the urine, there are some that are stored in fat tissue and can build up to toxic levels if taken in large quantities.

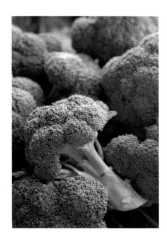

Vitamins

- *Vitamin A.* To ensure you get enough vitamin A, eat plenty of green leafy vegetables (e.g. spinach, pūhā), and yellow, orange and red fruits and vegetables (e.g. carrots, capsicums). Too much vitamin A, especially in the first trimester, can cause birth defects; avoid supplements containing vitamin A, any drugs associated with vitamin A metabolism such as the acne treatment drug isotretinoin (Isotane), and excessive amounts of liver and fish oil (which have relatively high concentrations of vitamin A).

- *Vitamin Bs.* There are several of these, all easily obtained through dietary sources. B6 (pyridoxine) supplements may be helpful for nausea (see p.86), but may be toxic above 200mg per day, so keep the dose as low as possible. Vitamin B12 is especially important for babies, as without good levels of it they will become deficient and seriously ill. If women are low in B12 during pregnancy and breastfeeding, their breast milk will also be low in B12. Vegan women often need to take extra B12 as supplements or from generous amounts of B12-fortified foods, because most natural sources of vitamin B12 are in animal products such as milk, meat, fish and eggs. For women who eat meat and/or dairy products, supplements are not generally needed.

- *Vitamin C.* This vitamin helps with iron absorption and skin health, and reduces the risk of pre-eclampsia (toxaemia – see p.139) in susceptible women. High levels of vitamin C are found in many fresh fruits and vegetables (e.g. citrus fruit, kiwifruit, capsicums, kūmara, potatoes). You will need extra vitamin C if you are a smoker or exposed to second-hand smoke (see also pp.23–24).

- *Vitamin D.* During pregnancy, this vitamin helps bone and skin health, and assists in calcium absorption for both women and their babies. Vitamin D deficiency in babies and young children causes abnormal softening of the bones (rickets), but does not occur if vitamin D levels are good during pregnancy and infancy. Vitamin D occurs in foods such as oily fish (e.g. sardines, tuna), but is also made in the skin when exposed to sunlight. Until recently, New Zealanders have assumed they have excellent levels of vitamin D because of good sunlight exposure, but this is not necessarily the case – especially in winter and in the more southern parts of the country. Women who spend a lot of time indoors, are dark-skinned (including Māori and Pacific Island women) or who do not expose their skin to the sun at all are particularly susceptible, and may well need a supplement.[17] However, for most other women, 20 minutes of sun exposure a day (before 11 a.m. and after 4 p.m. in the summer months) on their faces and arms, and a diet rich in foods containing vitamin D, will suffice.

- *Vitamin K.* This is essential for normal blood clotting, and is naturally low in newborn babies. Generous amounts of green leafy vegetables (e.g. spinach, pūhā) will boost vitamin K levels during pregnancy, making bleeding problems less likely in newborn babies. Even so, a single injection of vitamin K is usually recommended for babies immediately after birth, as this reduces the risk of brain haemorrhage. You should discuss this vitamin K recommendation with your LMC well before the birth (see pp.218 and 298).
- *Folic acid.* By the second three months of pregnancy, you no longer need to take folic acid in the form of tablets. However, good dietary levels of folic acid are still important, especially for multiple pregnancies. (See also pp.203–204.)

Heartburn

This is the name for a sudden sharp pain in the chest area after eating, sometimes accompanied by an acidic taste at the back of the throat. The problem is caused by the reflux of food and/or acid from the stomach up into the gullet (oesophagus). It can happen to anyone occasionally, but is more common in pregnancy as the growing uterus pushes on the stomach and intestines, and the smooth muscles of the stomach and oesophagus relax under the influence of pregnancy hormones. It tends to be worse in the second half of pregnancy.

You can minimise heartburn by eating small meals, eating the main meal earlier in the day, avoiding food in the evening, not going to bed straight after eating a full meal, and putting blocks or books under the bed legs at the head of your bed so that you're sleeping at a slight angle. Sometimes an antacid such as Quikeze, milk of magnesia or Gaviscon tablets (all available from a pharmacy) can help. These act to neutralise the stomach acid so that it doesn't burn as much, thus lessening the discomfort. However, don't take antacids with iron tablets (see p.136). Slippery elm-bark powder can be used for any digestive upsets but has been found particularly helpful for heartburn (it is available at any health food shop or via the Internet).

Sexual activity

A woman's interest in sex varies at different times in her life, and pregnancy is no exception. Many pregnant women find that they are more aware of their bodies and that sex can be especially pleasurable and fulfilling. Other women find that the increased awareness serves to make them feel less sexy. This whole range of emotions is very normal. Try to talk about your altered feelings with your partner. Changes in sexual response can be a source of frustration in any relationship, but you can't blame your partner for not understanding if you don't tell him (or her) about it.

Sexual activity is quite safe at this stage of pregnancy, unless (and this is rare) there is a threat of premature labour. But you do need to take things a little more slowly and gently than usual. Certain positions may be uncomfortable as pregnancy progresses. Orgasm may be dramatic, with the enlarged uterus contracting rhythmically. This is normal! Many couples find that pregnancy is a time of real joy and increased sexual fulfilment.

Practical tips for partners
(see also p.202)

- Find the right time, and create the right atmosphere, to talk about sex. Encourage your partner to express her feelings.
- Express your feelings and frustrations too, but do it gently.
- Talk about your partner's changing shape – is it a sexual turn-off (or turn-on) for either of you?
- Sometimes cuddles and kisses are more appropriate than intercourse.
- Allow more time for sex – be gentle and take things slowly, and use comfortable positions.

4. Complications

The middle three months of pregnancy are traditionally regarded as the 'good' months, and in many respects this is true. But while the chances of miscarriage are much lower, other problems can occasionally occur. All the following problems can also arise later in pregnancy, but are more fully dealt with here.

Hypertension of pregnancy and pre-eclampsia (toxaemia)

High blood pressure during pregnancy – especially if associated with protein in the urine or swelling of the feet, hands or face – can sometimes cause serious problems. These signs can herald the presence of a disorder known as pre-eclampsia.

Pre-eclampsia affects the placenta, reducing the blood supply and therefore the oxygen supply to the baby. Pre-eclampsia can also result in intra-uterine growth restriction (IUGR; see p.142).[18] It also affects the mother's health because the blood supply to her vital organs (brain, kidneys and liver) is compromised. In its most severe form (known as eclampsia), pre-eclampsia can lead to convulsions, premature labour, and the death of the mother and her baby. Fortunately, this is not common, and can be largely avoided by early detection and active treatment.

The causes of pre-eclampsia are still not clearly understood, despite much study of the problem over the past 50 years. It seems that a combination of genes, the immune system and the environment sets the scene for a woman to get pre-eclampsia. It is known to be more common with first pregnancies or first pregnancies with a different partner, with twins, and in women who have pre-existing high blood pressure.

Fortunately, not all women who have high blood pressure in pregnancy get pre-eclampsia. Mildly elevated blood pressure late in pregnancy often settles with rest, the placenta continues to function well until the baby is born, and there are no further problems. For other women, however, high blood pressure can continue and may be accompanied by protein in the urine and swelling of the legs. If the hands and face also become swollen, particularly on waking in the morning, this is likely to mean more serious problems. Severe headaches, visual disturbances or pain under the ribs on the right side may also be an indication that pre-eclampsia is developing. These symptoms can rapidly progress to seriously affect the mother and her baby. Take action early and contact your LMC if you are at all concerned.

At every antenatal visit, your blood pressure is recorded, your urine tested for protein, and any swelling is checked so that evidence of pre-eclampsia can be picked up as early as possible. There are also several blood tests that can help early detection. In women with some risk factors for pre-eclampsia, early warning signs can include changes in renal function tests (urea, creatinine and electrolytes), and rises in levels of uric acid and liver enzymes in the blood. These are sometimes tested for early in pregnancy to get a baseline and again later in pregnancy, particularly if the woman's blood pressure is starting to rise or she is feeling unwell for no other apparent reason.

Checking the blood pressure

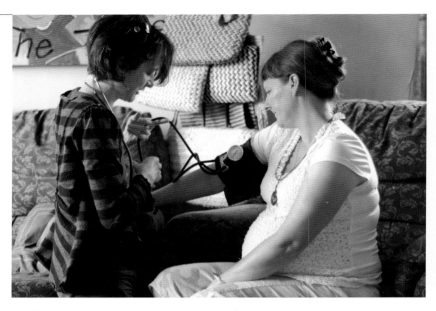

In general, the earlier in pregnancy that problems with pre-eclampsia arise, the more serious the potential complications. The best possible response is to be cared for in hospital, under a specialist obstetrician, as soon as a problem is suspected. This approach may seem overcautious at times, but because the condition can progress rapidly from mild symptoms to life-threatening disease, it makes sense.

Sugar diabetes (diabetes mellitus)

Diabetes is a condition where the supply of insulin (a hormone normally produced in the pancreas) is diminished or absent. Sometimes the body also becomes resistant to the effect of insulin, which can cause or worsen diabetes. The role of insulin is to remove sugar constantly from the blood and 'give' it to the cells in the body. If a person doesn't produce enough insulin, sugar levels in the blood will rise and they will be very unwell.

Nowadays, synthetic insulin is available in a wide variety of preparations, which are injected. Many diabetics keep their blood sugar under good control in this way, allowing them to live full and active lives.

Women who are already diabetic

Pregnancy presents particular problems for a diabetic woman, as her metabolism must change to meet the needs of her unborn baby. These problems are not insurmountable, but any diabetic woman contemplating pregnancy needs to be cared for by a medical and midwifery/nursing team skilled in managing diabetes. She must be prepared to have many tests done throughout her pregnancy, to put up with almost constant readjustment of her insulin dosage, and probably to have a more complicated labour than normal.

Ideally, special care should start well before pregnancy; it's wise for women who are already diabetic to plan their pregnancies and pregnancy care well before stopping contraception. Birth defects and early miscarriage are slightly more common with diabetic women, especially if their blood sugars are at all high. Because of this, it's important that pre-conception blood sugars are as normal as possible, and that diabetic women receive early folic acid (see pp.43 and 138).

If a diabetic woman's blood sugar goes much above the normal range during pregnancy, there are consequences for her baby. Because the baby is not diabetic, his metabolism has to try to adjust to the woman's higher blood sugar, often resulting in too much or too little weight gain, difficulties in labour, and a very unwell baby after birth. The risk of stillbirth is also increased. For these reasons, modern care for pregnant diabetic women involves complex regimes and different methods for keeping the blood sugar even lower than the levels acceptable for non-pregnant diabetic women, while at the same time avoiding low blood sugar symptoms. Diabetes in pregnancy is often also associated with high blood pressure and an increased risk of pre-eclampsia; frequent blood pressure monitoring and control is therefore also a necessary aspect of specialist care.[19]

Women who develop diabetes during pregnancy (gestational diabetes)

In all pregnancies, the placenta produces hormones to ensure the best nutrient supply to the baby. Some of these hormones can cause diabetes in susceptible women, even though they were not previously diabetic. This is known as gestational diabetes, and is likely to disappear after the birth of the baby. But the condition is likely to reappear with any subsequent pregnancies, and it also indicates that a woman is more at risk of developing long-term diabetes later in life.

Factors making gestational diabetes more likely

- family history of diabetes (especially immediate family)
- pre-pregnancy BMI over 30
- being over 25 years of age
- polycystic ovary syndrome (PCOS)
- sugar in the urine early in pregnancy
- high blood pressure (before or during pregnancy)
- woman's own birth weight was over 4kg
- having had a previous baby weighing over 4kg
- having had a previous unexplained stillbirth or baby with a birth defect
- Māori, Pacific Island, or South or East Asian ethnicity.

Gestational diabetes is the more common of the two forms. Routine testing of urine for sugar can help detect it before any symptoms appear and before the mother and baby become sick. In addition, a blood test is usually carried out at about 28 weeks to test for sugar (see p.213), because most pregnant women in New Zealand will in fact have one or more of the susceptibility factors. For particularly susceptible women, more complex blood testing over several hours may be recommended.

Possible signs and symptoms of diabetes

- no symptoms at all
- persistent thrush
- increased thirst
- urinary frequency
- dizziness
- vomiting
- sweating
- very fast breathing
- unconsciousness

IUGR – contributing factors

- smoking
- high blood pressure
- shape, size and blood supply of the placenta
- bleeding during pregnancy
- twins (or more)
- baby has a genetic or other abnormality
- mother is unwell or malnourished
- severe physical or psychological stress on the mother
- unknown

While mild cases of gestational diabetes can sometimes be managed solely by changing your diet, you may need insulin to keep your blood sugar under good control. The dose will change as pregnancy progresses.[20]

Regardless of whether your diabetes is pre-existing or develops during pregnancy, the aim is to maintain your blood sugar within a very narrow normal range to keep you and your baby in good health. This requires specialist team care. Sometimes, your blood sugar can be brought under control only in hospital, and you may have several hospital stays, especially towards the end of pregnancy. But this is well worth doing, as it may be the only way to keep your baby healthy and at a normal weight, and to avoid problems during birth – as well as having a well baby after birth.

Intra-uterine growth restriction (IUGR)

Also known as foetal growth restriction (FGR), IUGR is not a single illness – it is a label for a baby growing more slowly than normal.

Babies normally grow in the womb at a reasonably predictable rate. The range of normal growth has been determined by studies using ultrasound scans, and by closely observing many pregnant women of differing ages and ethnic backgrounds.

For a variety of reasons, some babies appear to grow too slowly. As a group, these 'small for dates' babies do seem to have more problems than their larger counterparts, although some will just be small because of family predisposition but are otherwise healthy.

In many instances, the function of the placenta is at fault. If the blood flow to the placenta is less than it should be, the baby gets less oxygen, less food and is smaller.[21]

The degree of IUGR varies widely: usually, it is relatively mild, but it may occasionally be severe. Less commonly, the baby may be very small because it is abnormal in some way. A chromosomal defect (see pp.90 and 147) could be responsible. In general, the earlier in pregnancy IUGR becomes apparent, the more serious it is likely to be.

By far the most common cause of IUGR is smoking. If you're still smoking, it's not too late to cut down or stop (see p.24), as the effect of smoking on IUGR is greatest in the second half of pregnancy.

At other times, no specific cause for IUGR can be identified and therefore no immediate action can be taken. But forewarned is forearmed, and potential problems, especially at birth, may be avoided if they can be anticipated.

Checking for IUGR

The simplest way to check for IUGR is to use a tape measure to measure the height of the uterus above the pubic bone (fundal height) regularly: your LMC will do this at each antenatal visit (see p.146). If it's suspected that your baby is growing too slowly, an ultrasound scan will normally be arranged to check this more accurately.

This ultrasound scan will usually be a special diagnostic one to check growth. Unless you have not yet had your routine anatomy scan between 18 and 20 weeks (in which case your LMC may be able to arrange for growth to be double-checked at the same time), this will be an extra scan. Because IUGR is more likely to become apparent in the second half of pregnancy, it may well not show up at your routine anatomy scan; a 'normal' 20-week scan does not rule out IUGR. The diagnostic scan may confirm your LMC's concern and show a 'small for dates' baby, but sometimes the result will be quite normal because fundal height is not that accurate in some women. However, if any suspicion of IUGR shows up, you will probably need to have more checks, more scans and more blood tests to monitor progress, because as pregnancy advances, any mild problems may become more significant. The placenta naturally 'ages' over the course of any pregnancy, and towards the end of pregnancy it does not function as well. In a poorly functioning placenta, this ageing process is often accelerated.

If the IUGR is getting worse, the baby may be better off being born early before the condition becomes severe, even if it means admission to a special baby unit. Babies with severe IUGR are likely to be adversely affected by the stress of labour, to breathe poorly, to suckle poorly, and to suffer from severe lack of oxygen in labour. Because they have little in the way of fat stores, they also have problems maintaining their blood sugar level, which is important for warmth, growth and brain functioning. There is also an increased risk of stillbirth.

Cervical incompetence/insufficiency

Very occasionally, the strong muscle of the cervix does not function properly, meaning it does not stay tightly closed as pregnancy advances, even though the baby seems to be normal and the placenta working well. The cervix softens and opens without the uterus contracting at all or very much, and the pregnancy sac is lost from the uterus, cutting off the blood supply to the placenta. The result is a miscarriage or stillbirth. If this happens once, it is likely to happen again with each successive pregnancy.

Management for cervical incompetence

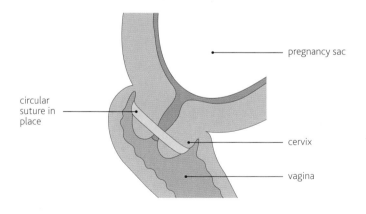

circular suture in place

pregnancy sac

cervix

vagina

Sometimes, medication such as progesterone can be used to stop the cervix softening. In other situations, a special encircling suture (stitch) can be inserted around the cervix to hold it closed until pregnancy is advanced enough for the baby to survive, even if born early. However, the suture has to be removed well before labour gets under way, or it will cause the uterus to contract against a closed cervix, obstructing labour and severely affecting the well-being of both mother and baby. To minimise this risk, a cervical suture is usually removed several weeks before the due date, and the baby is delivered early.

Cervical incompetence – possible risk factors [22]

- congenital variations in the shape of the uterus (e.g. bicornuate uterus)
- injury to the cervix during previous vaginal or Caesarean delivery
- previous surgery to the cervix (e.g. cone biopsy, cancer treatment)
- multiple pregnancy (especially triplets, quads)
- previous miscarriage in second trimester
- unknown

Very early premature labour and stillbirth

It's easy to assume that in a developed country like New Zealand, all babies are born alive and well, and that if they're not, obstetric and neonatal intensive care will be able to save them. Certainly, many more babies survive now than in the past, but there will always be some who are born too early to survive, and a small number who will die for a variety of reasons while still in the uterus or soon after birth.

Babies born extremely early, before 22–23 weeks of pregnancy, are just not ready to cope with life outside the uterus – even with expert neonatal help. Between 23 and 28 weeks, depending on their weight and constitution, some babies (but not all) have a reasonable chance of survival with the help of the latest technology in a special-care baby unit. Although advanced neonatal technology has become increasingly available in the last 30 years, many questions remain about whether such intense intervention is 'right' or 'wrong'. The risks of respiratory distress, apnoea (periodic cessation of breathing), gut problems, severe infection, kidney failure and brain damage are increased with these tiny babies, and some will have major persistent problems. Yet once past the first critical weeks, many grow up to become normal, healthy, intelligent children.

'I hadn't really thought about this lump too much before … and now that they were there, tiny but perfect, I desperately, desperately wanted them … longed for both my sons.'

The chance of a baby surviving without major problems rises significantly with every completed week of pregnancy between 23 and 28 weeks, but is still dependent on many factors. Beyond 28 weeks, a baby's chances of survival are much better. New Zealand neonatal unit survival figures are comparable with those of other developed countries. The chances of survival (without major long-term problems) are small under 24 weeks' gestation, but rise steadily to more than 90 per cent after 31 weeks' completed gestation.[23]

Premature labour in the second three months

Premature labour may occur in the second three months of pregnancy in these situations:

- uterine abnormality
- cervical incompetence
- bacterial vaginosis
- multiple pregnancy
- pre-eclampsia (toxaemia)
- diabetes
- IUGR
- some foetal abnormalities
- previous premature labour
- bleeding during pregnancy
- severe infection/illness in the mother.

Coping with the death of a baby (see also p.120)

Whatever the circumstances, the loss of a baby or babies at this stage of pregnancy is devastating. The birth will have been a 'real' labour and delivery, and the sense of loss is enormous.

Women in this situation have found great comfort in looking at, or holding, their dead baby or babies. You may want to name your baby, dress him, or take a photograph. Making an imprint of the baby's hands and/or feet also provides a tangible memory. Some women want to share this time with their partner, while others want to be left alone. Fathers and extended family/whānau grieve too, and it can be a time when relationships grow and strengthen.

There doesn't have to be a funeral if the baby is less than 28 weeks, but parents often choose to have one so they can 'say goodbye'. Making the arrangements can be very hard – yet parents frequently say afterwards that it was worth it.

The trauma of losing a baby takes time – sometimes many months or years – to come to terms with. It helps if you have someone you can talk to, cry with and be comforted by. Meeting and talking with other parents who have lost babies can also be a comfort. The Stillbirth and Neonatal Death Support Association can put you in touch with local people, including trained health professionals. (See Appendix: Stillbirth.) If things seem really hard, ask for help. Your LMC, obstetrician, GP and/or the hospital midwife who assisted at the birth may be especially helpful. They can also put you in touch with psychiatric services, grief counsellors and other forms of assistance.

'I was not coping at all, despite a very supportive partner and understanding friends. I sought psychiatric help, and I'm glad I did … I finally started the painful business of healing.'

5. Continuing health care

Continuing antenatal health care

By now, you will probably have had your first antenatal visit. You will have chosen and registered with your LMC (lead maternity carer) (see pp.94–99).

Over the next three months, your LMC will want to check you about once a month; if all is going well, these routine visits are often very short. If you have any questions, remember to ask them at the start of the visit. If you have trouble remembering what you want to ask, write it down beforehand and have your list ready.

All antenatal care aims to pick up problems with the woman's or the baby's health as early as possible, so that they can be dealt with promptly. At this stage in pregnancy, there are several potential problems that warrant early detection. Regularly checking your blood pressure, testing your urine for protein, examining your feet, hands and face for swelling, and checking weight gain will all help to detect pre-eclampsia early. Checking the blood for extra sugar will pick up diabetes.

Examining and measuring the uterus – and, later in pregnancy, feeling the baby's position and listening for a heartbeat – help determine whether he is growing at the expected rate. Small variations of plus or minus two weeks' estimated growth are not abnormal, but large variations (four weeks or more) are significant. The date of 'quickening' (when the first movements are felt) is a useful indicator to confirm dates. In first pregnancies this usually happens between 18 and 22 weeks, and in subsequent pregnancies from 16 to 18 weeks.

Antenatal visits in the second trimester

During these visits you will be asked about:

- how you're feeling
- the baby's movements
- any specific problems or concerns you may have.

The following will be tested or checked:

- your blood pressure
- your urine (for protein and sugar)
- your weight
- the size and height of your uterus
- the baby's heartbeat
- the position of the baby (after 24 weeks).

Position of top of uterus as pregnancy progresses

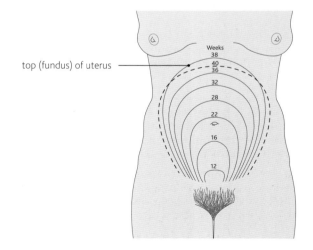

top (fundus) of uterus

Weeks
38
40
36
32
28
22
16
12

Smaller than expected

If the baby is smaller than expected, one of several things may be happening. He may simply be smaller than the norm for the population. This is more likely if you or your partner come from a family of small-sized people. Or the dates of your pregnancy may be incorrect. It is possible to be a month less pregnant than you thought you were, even if you were sure about your last period, because ovulation doesn't always occur on time.

Another explanation is that the baby may be growing too slowly (see 'Intra-uterine growth restriction', p.142).

Very rarely, the unborn baby may have died. If so, the uterus will no longer increase in size and some of the feelings of being pregnant will disappear. Sometimes, but not always, labour will start spontaneously after foetal death. If not, it will need to be induced. Either way, a woman in this situation needs support and love, both from her professional caregivers and those closest to her. Your LMC will consult with the specialist obstetrician to organise for you to go to hospital, as that is usually the most appropriate place for the delivery, where the obstetric, midwifery and nursing staff will have the experience and education to help women suffering the loss of an unborn baby (see 'Coping with the death of a baby', p.145).

Larger than expected

If the baby is larger than expected, he may simply be large compared to the normal range for the population, especially if you or your partner come from a family of big people. Once again, your dates may be incorrect, possibly because of an unusual period. A multiple pregnancy also makes a woman 'large for dates', as does a very large amount of amniotic fluid (a condition known as polyhydramnios, which sometimes, but not always, indicates a developmental problem in the baby).

Prenatal screening and diagnostic tests (see also p.105)

Maternal serum screening (possible from 14–15 weeks onwards)

This blood test for pregnant women is one of a number of tests that can be done to look for chromosomal and other abnormalities in unborn babies (for full details, see p.106). It is best done at the end of the 15th week of pregnancy, so is particularly useful if a woman has not had those earlier screening tests that can only be done before the end of the 13th week of pregnancy (see pp.105–106).

Amniocentesis (possible from 14–15 weeks onwards; see also p.106)

This test involves taking a sample of the amniotic fluid from the pregnancy sac. The earliest it can be done is at 14–15 weeks, as before then there is usually insufficient amniotic fluid. The fluid is then analysed to show the chromosomal make-up of the baby. Although a preliminary result may be available in a few days, the full analysis (which is the most accurate) can take up to two weeks. The procedure is done in conjunction with an ultrasound scan, as this helps to determine accurately the best place for taking the sample.

'The decision to have a younger sibling for Jay, who has Down syndrome, came after much discussion about whether we would have antenatal screens. In the end, we opted to go into it accepting what we were given, as I knew I couldn't terminate a pregnancy on the basis of the child having DS. To me, that would be saying that Jay isn't good enough, when he has as much – if not more – to offer us as parents than any other child. Having this test is a huge undertaking with risks for the baby; both parents need to be sure what they are prepared to do if the test is positive for an abnormality, before embarking on it. We just had a routine anatomy scan at about 16 weeks and everything was looking good for our next baby, a girl. She was born at 40 weeks, and does not have Down syndrome.'

Why have an amniocentesis?

This test is designed to detect chromosome abnormalities in the foetus. It also accurately shows the sex of the baby. Of all the tests to check for abnormalities, amniocentesis is the most accurate (about 99 per cent) for detecting abnormal chromosomes – not only those responsible for Down syndrome, but also other less common abnormalities.[24] However, the procedure does increase a woman's chances of having a miscarriage (a risk of about 1 in 200).[25]

For this reason, it should not be regarded as a routine test. It should be considered only when the benefit of having it outweighs the risk of miscarriage for any particular woman. The initial screening tests for abnormality now available (see p.105) are much safer and, for many women, results from those low-risk initial tests will mean they will neither want nor need to consider having an amniocentesis.

If you are thinking of having an amniocentesis, you need to weigh up the benefits and the risks carefully. You also need to remember that not all abnormalities can be picked up; very rarely, a baby with an abnormality will be born despite having a 'normal' amniocentesis result. Even though most women who have the test receive a 'normal' result, you also need to consider what you would do if the baby were found to be abnormal.

No woman should feel she has to proceed with an amniocentesis (or chorionic villus biopsy (CVS); see p.110) if she does not want to. If you would not consider having a termination under any circumstances, you may decide not to have the test at all. For most women in this situation, though, decisions about termination are complex, and very difficult to make until you're faced with the actual test result.

Amniocentesis

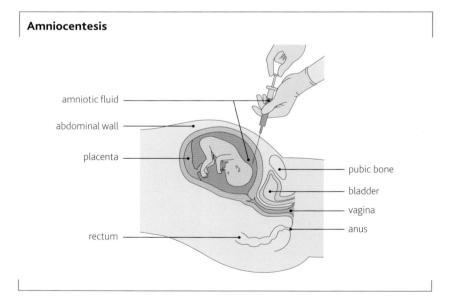

amniotic fluid

abdominal wall

placenta

pubic bone

bladder

vagina

anus

rectum

If the test does confirm that your baby has Down syndrome or another chromosomal abnormality, you then have to decide whether you want to continue with your pregnancy or have it terminated. Although the ultimate decision is yours, expert advice is on hand from the specialist obstetrician who performed your amniocentesis, from your local paediatric service, and (in the main centres) from multidisciplinary maternal-foetal medicine teams and/or specialist genetic counselling services.

Most women faced with this situation do elect to terminate their pregnancy. But for some, continuing with the pregnancy is a positive choice. Having the test allows these women and their families the opportunity to prepare for the rest of the pregnancy and birth (in which they are likely to need extra support), and for having a baby with a disability.

What happens when you have an amniocentesis?

Most amniocentesis procedures are carried out at dedicated hospital clinics, and you will normally be given an appointment to attend there, even if you have a private obstetrician as your LMC. Occasionally, specialist obstetricians will have facilities for amniocentesis at a private clinic.

First, you will be asked to lie down on a firm bed, and an ultrasound scan (see pp.107 and 150) will determine the position of the baby, the placenta, and the biggest pocket of amniotic fluid. The area selected for the insertion of the needle will be cleansed with a sterile swab.

Sometimes, you will have a tiny injection of local anaesthetic into the skin of your abdomen to make a small area of the skin numb. This is not always necessary, because the stretched skin of the pregnant abdomen is less sensitive than normal.

Then, the doctor doing the amniocentesis (a specialist obstetrician) inserts a long needle carefully through your abdominal wall until it reaches the amniotic fluid. Often this can be seen on the scan, which is being done at the same time. The scan equipment also has a special attachment that helps to guide the insertion of the needle. About 10–15ml of fluid is then slowly drawn up into the syringe over a period of about 30 seconds.[26] The amniotic fluid contains some of the baby's cells, which are naturally shed during development. These cells will be grown in the laboratory until the chromosomes can be clearly seen under a microscope.

Finally, the needle and syringe are taken out, and you will be asked to lie or sit quietly for 15–20 minutes before leaving the hospital or clinic. The whole procedure will have taken less than 15 minutes. You will be advised to take things easy for the next 48 hours, as you may have some mild cramping the next day.

Results

Before you leave, check how and when you are going to get the results. You should discuss whether or not a preliminary result (the fluorescent in-situ hybridisation test, or FISH, which gives a result in 48 hours) is going to be available, when to expect the final result, and who is responsible for getting this to you.

Although FISH analysis can be extremely useful if the results are positive (i.e. showing abnormal chromosomes), a negative (i.e. normal) result cannot be relied on. You will need to wait for the full chromosomal analysis result. In addition, FISH tests are expensive and often carry a patient charge. They are not routinely undertaken, but are reserved for specific urgent or unusual circumstances, such as where amniocentesis has been undertaken later in pregnancy. Even then, the full result will also be checked.

Most women need the full analysis and the most accurate result in order to make any decisions. You need to allow up to two to three weeks for this to come through. It can seem a very long time to wait, but at present it is the only way to get the best result.

Ultrasound anatomy (morphology) scan (best done at 18–20 weeks)

This type of ultrasound scan checks many details of the baby's anatomy, and is routinely available through your LMC. Although the procedure is very similar to that described for ultrasound scans in early pregnancy (see p.108), what can be seen is very different.

Taking an ultrasound scan

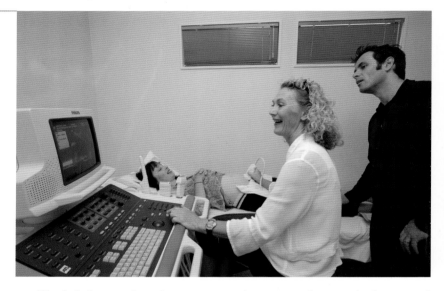

The baby's growth and maturity can be measured using the bi-parietal diameter (BPD), or distance across the head, and the length of the thigh bone (femur). The major organs are all observed, including the head, brain, spine, heart, lungs, kidneys, ureters and bladder, abdominal organs and limbs. The genital organs can often be seen, but accurate determination of the sex of the baby is sometimes difficult. One of the most important purposes of this scan is to check the spine and brain development, looking particularly for neural tube defects (NTDs), including spina bifida (see opposite). Close attention will also be paid to the heart, which is now big enough for a number of congenital heart defects to be evident (see p.329).

At the scan, the screen will usually be positioned so that you can see it yourself. Don't be disappointed with the image – to the unpractised eye, it looks like poor-quality black and white television. The ultrasonographer will often be able to explain what you are seeing.

Despite the picture quality, really 'seeing' your baby for the first time can be a very emotional experience. Try to take your partner or support person with you. (In most ultrasound scanning units, staff are happy for other people to be present, if you want them there.) Usually, the scan will show that everything is healthy and normal. If this is so, then you and your partner will really start to feel that your pregnancy is not just sickness, or a bulge, but a baby. And not just any baby – your baby.

If the news is not good (and very occasionally it will not be), having your partner or support person with you can be a great comfort. They will be better able to share your inevitable sense of loss about the possible abnormality or death of your baby.

Neural tube defects (NTDs)

When the baby is in the very early stages of development, the nerve tissue that will become the brain and the spinal cord 'folds together' along the length of the spine and the base of the brain. The resulting tube of tissue is known as the neural tube, and once formed, it develops rapidly into the future brain and spinal cord. This process is normally complete by the 12th week of pregnancy. Very occasionally, the neural tube does not form properly, resulting in incomplete closure, and normal development cannot proceed.

If neural tube development fails very early in the pregnancy, and to a major degree, this affects both the brain (causing anencephaly) and the spine (causing spina bifida). But if the failure occurs slightly later, it will affect only the spinal cord development, to varying degrees. Spina bifida can be minor, affecting only the skin and bones around the lower spinal cord; more significantly, it may leave the spinal cord exposed and non-functional from the lower back down. Bowel, bladder and lower limb function are all severely affected, creating significant and permanent disability.

These types of defect occur for a number of reasons. Genetic factors probably play a part, as certain families and certain populations have higher rates than others (people of Celtic origin seem particularly susceptible). But diet, and especially folic acid intake, is also important. The best protection against NTDs is good folic acid intake, using supplements both before and during the first three months of pregnancy (see p.43).

Major neural tube defects (where both brain and spine are affected) often result in miscarriage. Babies with spina bifida alone may continue to develop normally in every other respect, and pregnancy appears to progress as usual. The anatomy scan may provide the first and sometimes the only opportunity to detect this problem prior to birth, which is why it is so carefully looked for at this time.

If an NTD is detected at your scan, it is likely to come as a considerable shock and you will need time to adjust to this news. You may be offered another, more detailed scan and other tests. Prompt discussion with a specialised, multidisciplinary maternal-foetal medicine team (including an obstetrician, a paediatrician and a geneticist) can be very helpful. After reflection, most women faced with a significant NTD in their baby elect to terminate the pregnancy. But as with other major abnormalities, continuing with the pregnancy may be a positive choice. In these cases, the scan allows women and their families the opportunity to prepare for the rest of the pregnancy and birth (in which they are likely to need extra support), and for having a baby with a disability.

Dental health

Caring for your teeth and gums is just as important during pregnancy as at any other time. Gums may bleed more easily during pregnancy because the hormonal changes in pregnancy predispose women to gingivitis (where the gums become more soft and spongy than usual). If this becomes severe, it can lead to periodontal disease, which destroys the gums and bones around the teeth; it has also been linked to IUGR, pre-eclampsia and premature birth.[27] Brush your teeth daily and use dental floss regularly to minimise gingivitis and prevent periodontal disease.

A visit to the dentist during this second trimester is a good investment. Remember that it might be quite a while before you can easily get there again – unforeseen problems may arise towards the end of your pregnancy, and visiting the dentist when you have a tiny baby will not be particularly easy. At the visit, your teeth can be thoroughly cleaned, the gums examined and attended to, and fillings fixed if necessary. As long as the dentist knows you are pregnant, so that use of X-rays and other procedures is minimised, this type of care can be safely undertaken during the second and third trimesters of pregnancy.

Fresh fruit and vegetables, calcium and fluoride are necessary for your own good dental health, but there is no extra requirement during a healthy pregnancy if you are already meeting those needs. Calcium is efficiently transferred to your baby's bones and teeth during pregnancy (see p.136), and fluoride is also incorporated into the baby's developing deciduous teeth (the first, or 'milk', teeth) during pregnancy.

Fluoride

In New Zealand, only low levels of fluoride are found naturally in the soil, and therefore in our food. Many local authorities add fluoride to the water supply, but only up to the recommended levels that are found naturally in other parts of the world. Drinking fluoridated water is considered safe and helpful during pregnancy.[28]

However, not all water supplies have fluoride added. This is still a cause of controversy, as some communities do not wish to put additives in their water supply. To date, there is no evidence that fluoridated water is unsafe, and in fact the incidence of children with dental caries (holes in their teeth) is considerably lower in areas with fluoridated water.[29]

Fluoride is also present in some commercial toothpastes. If you live in an area with unfluoridated water, regular use of fluoridated toothpaste is recommended. Concerns have been previously raised that added fluoride might cause birth defects or miscarriage during pregnancy, but no evidence for this has been found.[30]

Education for parenthood

Pregnancy and parenting classes (see also p.128)

By now, you may be feeling overwhelmed by information. Is it interesting, or just plain confusing? Is it exciting, or do you just want it all to go away?

However you feel, attending some sort of pregnancy and parenting class will probably be helpful, especially if this is your first pregnancy. Attendance is not compulsory, but women in their first pregnancies (and their partners and support people) generally find them very helpful, as they give lots of practical information and help increase confidence. It's also a chance to get to know other people having a baby at about the same time as you; some enduring friendships are made in antenatal classes.

A variety of classes are available, depending on where you live and what stage of pregnancy you're at. There is often a charge for attending parenting classes. You generally need to book well in advance, by the fourth or fifth month of your pregnancy.

Most classes are organised so that you attend when you are well into the last trimester, between 30 and 38 weeks pregnant. But the timing of classes may mean you need to start earlier than this, or attend the end of one course and the beginning of the next to fit everything in before the end of your pregnancy. If in doubt, choose the earliest classes that are convenient; if you do have your baby early, or unexpected things happen, you will still have had the benefit of at least some of the classes. Different types of antenatal class suit different women – check all the available options in your area, and ask around to see which one is likely to work best for you. (See p.218 for what's covered in antenatal classes.)

Hospital pregnancy and parenting classes

A number of maternity hospitals run pregnancy and parenting classes. Some are offered free of charge, while there are fees for others. Some hospitals make their classes available to all pregnant women in the area, but at others, classes are restricted to women who are under hospital midwifery care.

The hospital midwives organise and run the classes, but will often get other people (for example, a doctor, a new mother, a physiotherapist) to come and talk to the class on a particular topic. Each hospital has its own special programme – some classes are especially designed for women on their own, some for those in their teens and some for couples.

Independent midwife classes

Often midwives who work together will offer pregnancy and parenting classes to their clients. These classes are often not widely advertised, but you will hear about them through the midwives concerned if you are going to them for your antenatal care.

Other organisations that provide classes

Parents Centre (NZ) is a nationwide organisation that has run antenatal classes for many years. You have to pay to attend classes, and normally get membership of the organisation as part of the cost. Parents Centre has over 50 centres and trains and supports over 100 certified childbirth educators across the country. (See Appendix: Parents Centre.)

Choosing an antenatal class – a checklist

- Is the cost reasonable?

- Is the venue convenient?

- Is the timing of the next series of classes right for you? (E.g. time of day – can your partner or support person also attend?)

- Is the type of class suitable? (E.g. is an exercise programme offered?)

- Is the standard satisfactory? (E.g. are the educators sufficiently trained?)

- Are you comfortable with the philosophy of the organisation?

- What sort of ongoing support is available after the birth if you want or need it?

Parents Centre has always encouraged partners to participate fully in preparing for the birth, and places great importance on the family as a unit. In addition to antenatal courses, the organisation offers parenting classes on wide-ranging topics that span the childhood years. Other services include a well-used website, post-natal telephone contact and neighbourhood support, easy access to (and discounts on) some items of baby equipment, online distance parenting education, and a parenting magazine.

Parents Centre also acts politically to promote parents' rights in the community. On many parenting issues, the organisation has been able to effect changes in attitudes towards parents in general and pregnancy in particular.

Home birth associations are committed to the practical and political promotion of home birth. Different associations exist in different areas of the country, but they are affiliated and easy to find through Home Birth Aotearoa (see Appendix). In some areas, local associations run their own classes. These are designed to help women make safe and responsible choices about home birth, to give all the practical information needed to have a baby at home, and to offer advice on all the other decisions that need to be made. In other areas, the local association liaises with groups such as Parents Centre to provide comprehensive courses on preparing for a home birth. Again, there is a modest fee to join the association.

Some iwi health agencies offer antenatal or parenting classes. These are often run by trained childbirth educators who invite midwives and other health practitioners to talk about specific topics. If your LMC does not usually access iwi services, they may not know the people to get in touch with; you may need to ask the Citizens Advice Bureau or another community information service to find out what iwi health agencies are available in the area. It is a misconception that iwi services are only for Māori. While the focus of their services is indeed to provide for Māori, they often welcome all women.

In some areas, Well Child health services such as Plunket run pregnancy and parenting classes, with their own experienced Well Child or Plunket nurses working in conjunction with local midwives and physiotherapists or qualified childbirth educators.

Pregnancy and parenting classes are also offered by a variety of other individuals and organisations. As there are no laws governing who can or can't offer these classes in New Zealand, it pays to check that whoever is running the class is reputable, and has had some training in childbirth education.

Pregnancy and parenting classes if you're expecting more than one baby
(see also p.203)

On average, about 850 sets of twins and 10 sets of triplets are born each year in New Zealand. Quads are much less common.[31] If you are expecting twins or triplets, the New Zealand Multiple Birth Association provides good practical information and support. They also hold an annual conference, hire out booklets and videos, give advice about publications written especially for parents of 'multiples', and have a well-used email correspondence column on their website. There is a modest fee to join up, but for many parents expecting twins or more, the cost is well worthwhile. Sharing experiences with others can be very helpful, as many valuable practical tips are common knowledge within the multiples community but not readily accessible elsewhere. (See Appendix: Multiple Birth Association.)

'I do tend to turn to other mothers with twins for advice because they really understand that it's about having two totally different babies. What works for one doesn't necessarily work for the other.'

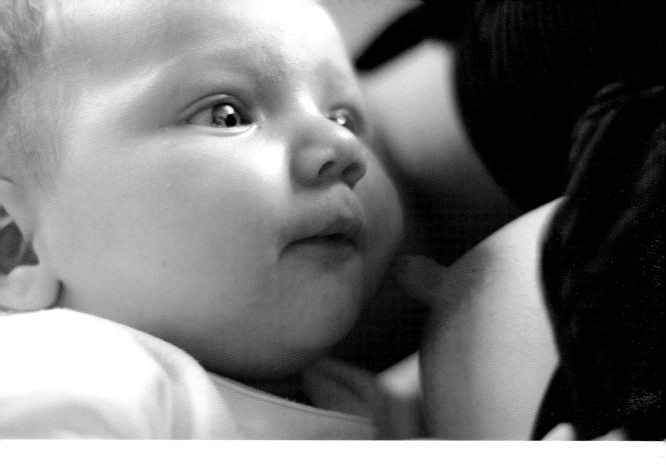

Education about feeding

Many women have found that standard pregnancy and parenting classes are not the best place to learn about feeding their baby, because they concentrate so much on preparing for birth. However, learning as much as you can now about feeding will help you to be well prepared when your baby arrives. It's a good idea to talk to your LMC about feeding at your regular antenatal visits.

Some women find it very helpful to visit a lactation consultant during their pregnancy, not only to gain detailed information about feeding, but also to have another expert on hand after the baby is born. If a lactation consultant is available in your area, you may really appreciate having another person to call on with your queries and concerns about feeding, especially if you don't stay in hospital after the birth. (See Appendix: Breastfeeding.)

The La Leche League (NZ) is part of a worldwide organisation that promotes breastfeeding. The League has over a hundred groups throughout New Zealand, and its members are available to help new mothers with practical aspects of breastfeeding. Their website provides details of local groups, useful books and leaflets, a telephone help service, and international contacts. You may find it very helpful to get in touch with the League before your baby is born to access information and find out who your local contact people are. (See Appendix: Breastfeeding.)

6. Planning for birth and beyond

Considering where you will give birth (see also p.94)

(see also p.94)

In choosing your LMC, you may have already considered where you will give birth. If you haven't, you should start thinking about the options now and discuss them with your LMC. There are three main possibilities:

- birth at home (planned home birth)
- birth in a small primary maternity hospital or independent birthing unit (these are said to offer 'primary maternity care')
- birth in a larger hospital with full facilities (these hospitals are able to provide 'secondary' and/or 'tertiary' care).

In New Zealand there are currently between about 58,000 and 62,000 births each year.[32] For example, in 2004 (the most recent year for which detailed and accurate figures were available at the time of writing), 57,591 women gave birth in New Zealand – nearly all (95 per cent) in hospital. Home births were planned by 2047 women (4.4 per cent), with just over half of these actually having their babies at home.[33] A small number of women who planned to give birth in hospital in fact had their babies at home following a rapid labour.

The choices available to you will depend, at least in part, on where you live. Home birth may not be an option in your area if there is no home birth midwife available. Giving birth in a small, intimate country hospital is not going to be possible if you live in a big city that has no such facility nearby. And an epidural will not be available anywhere except in a larger hospital.

Home birth

During the last decade or so, a small but increasing number of women have chosen to have their babies at home. Birth at home offers many different things to different women. It does not appeal to everyone, but it is a special way of giving birth that can be considered by any healthy woman who is enjoying a normal pregnancy.

Home birth is a choice that does involve taking responsibility for your own, and your baby's, health. It involves making decisions, and finding a qualified home birth midwife to be your LMC. Home Birth Aotearoa (see Appendix) can provide information and assistance, and put you in touch with your local Home Birth Association. Some local associations are very active, offering a wide range of support and resources, including pregnancy and parenting classes; others are small and rely on the larger associations for assistance.

As your LMC, a home birth midwife will undertake to look after you right through your pregnancy and labour, and continue to care for you after your baby is born. Home birth midwives must be experienced, competent and confident in assisting women who wish to give birth at home.

If you are considering a home birth, it is important to think about the twofold responsibilities involved. First, having a planned home birth means paying even more attention than usual to maintaining good health during pregnancy, and having good antenatal care. Second, planning for a home birth must always allow for the possibility of transfer to hospital if the need arises.

'My family is very important to me – to have my three older children present at Samuel's birth was a wonderful experience for us all.'

'Home birth has been an ecstatic, wonderful thing for me. I gave birth to Jessica beautifully, just beautifully — her eyes seemed to say thank you as soon as I held her.'

About a third of women having their first baby at home need more help during labour and delivery than their LMC can provide at home, and are transferred to hospital. This is usually because of slow progress in labour or the need for pharmacological pain relief. In comparison, women having their second or subsequent baby at home are more likely to enjoy trouble-free labours and births, and only a small number are transferred to hospital at any stage. These differing transfer rates for the two groups are not unusual or unexpected (see p.228 on planning for a first birth). Planned, responsible home birth can be a safe, private, relaxed and personal way of having your baby.

Birth in a small hospital/independent birthing unit

There are a number of primary maternity hospitals/birthing units providing primary maternity care in New Zealand. In 2004, nearly 9000 women (about 16 per cent) successfully gave birth at one of these facilities.[34] Most primary maternity hospitals are in less populated rural areas, where they offer an invaluable service. In many respects, having a baby in a primary maternity hospital is similar to giving birth at home. A very personal service can be offered, and most small hospitals have a relaxed atmosphere so that family and friends can come and go as you and they wish. There may be a staff of only three or four midwives, who will work with your LMC (midwife or GP) throughout your labour and birth, and in the hours or days after the birth; if you don't know them already, you can get to know them all before you go into labour.

Women giving birth in primary hospitals do sometimes need to be transferred to secondary hospitals to get more specialist care if their health or their baby's health is compromised during pregnancy or labour. Transfer rates are higher for first births than for all subsequent ones. Primary maternity hospitals do have more equipment than it is possible to provide at home, and this may avoid the need to transfer to a larger hospital, but epidural and other anaesthetic facilities are not available at primary hospitals.

Birth in a secondary hospital

In larger towns and cities, maternity services are available at secondary and/or tertiary level hospitals, and most women (about 80 per cent in 2004) give birth at a larger hospital.[35] These secondary and tertiary hospitals provide full obstetric services, including facilities for epidurals and Caesarean sections (see p.274), though only the tertiary hospitals in the main centres provide full intensive care for mothers and babies who need it (see p.331).

Because these hospitals have a large staff and look after women and babies from a whole region, the service can become rather impersonal, with different people caring for you in each area. Staff are more likely to be busy, and hospital midwives often have to care for several women in labour at once. However, some hospital midwives have arranged to offer a more personal service by working flexible hours. For example, some will have the facility to extend their normal shift and stay on with a woman in labour for a period of overtime. Independent LMC midwives also commonly care for women in larger hospitals. Even if your LMC has to transfer your care to the specialist obstetric team, they will often have contact with you, or with the staff caring for you, during your stay in hospital, depending on why you are there.

'My babies were all born at our district hospital ... and I enjoyed being there each time. After the first time, it was all a piece of cake. I knew everyone ... they knew me ... I just felt I was really well looked after, too. Lovely meals, better TV reception than at home, no cows to milk ... it was wonderful to sleep in as long as the baby slept.'

'I was very sure I wanted to have my baby in hospital. Because I came from a different country, I wouldn't ever consider having baby at home. In my country, it was the old-fashioned way. Personally I think it's a good idea to have baby at the hospital just in case something goes wrong – you always have back-up. You can still have a natural birth at the hospital.'

Each hospital is different. Not all larger hospitals are unfriendly places, and staff make every effort to ensure you are well looked after and comfortable, and that you have privacy and access to support and assistance when needed. Indeed, in most hospitals the staff work hard to ensure that women are given as personal a service as possible. Comfortable, private birthing rooms and spa baths are often available. Visiting hours may be limited – not because the staff don't want you to see your friends and family, but to ensure that there are quiet times when rest is possible.

However, the larger hospitals do specialise in active intervention. They have the sophisticated equipment, and specialist obstetricians, anaesthetists and paediatricians are on hand. So, if complex assistance is required during pregnancy, delivery or after the birth, then a larger hospital with competent staff and high-quality facilities is the right place to be.

Modern technology means that more healthy babies are born and fewer women die in childbirth than ever before (in 2004 there were only 6.8 maternal deaths per 100,000 births).[36] But modern technology has its dangers and its limitations. It may be used when it is not necessary; and it may cause more problems than it solves. Weighing up the potential risks and benefits is never easy. Women having their babies in hospital need to be just as responsible for their own health, and that of their baby, as those giving birth at home. It's only by knowing about pregnancy and childbirth, and knowing something about possible intervention, that women can weigh up the risks and benefits for themselves, and make informed decisions about their care.

Making your choice

'To be quite honest, I was dreading going to hospital. It had all looked very cold and clinical to me … but once I was in labour I was almost oblivious. Labour was hard, hard work … lots of sweating … Robert was the only important person at the time. No, in the end, the surroundings were totally unimportant …'

Just where you decide to give birth will depend on many factors. You may find it helpful to read the section on birth plans in Chapter 5, as well as running through the following checklist.

- What is your own personal/cultural/political philosophy on birth?
- Is this your first birth (see p.228)?
- Have there been any problems so far in this pregnancy, or in previous pregnancies?
- Where do you live? Does access or distance limit your choices? If what you want is not available, would you go and stay somewhere else?
- What support from others do you have for your choice of birthplace? And when the time comes, will your partner, family and other support people be there for you?

Considering breastfeeding (see also pp.308 and 342)

Around this time, you might start thinking about whether you will breastfeed or formula-feed your baby. 'Breast is best' is a phrase you will no doubt hear repeatedly at antenatal classes and when your LMC visits. You may wonder why there is so much emphasis on breastfeeding, when modern milk formulae and bottles are readily available.

With breastfeeding, nature has provided very well for babies' immediate needs. Breast milk is ideally suited to a small baby as it provides a complete, easily digested diet, with the right amounts of calories, protein, carbohydrates, fats and fluid. It contains vitamins, minerals and immunoglobulins – complex protein substances that help fight infection. In addition, whenever a baby sucks the milk from his mother's breast, he is held closely and warmly. He gazes at his mother's face, hears her voice, smells and touches her.

Breastfeeding ensures that a supply of warm, uncontaminated milk is available whenever a baby is hungry. The system is a natural one of supply and demand: the more milk a baby demands by feeding frequently, the more milk his mother will produce.

When breastfeeding works well, it is the ideal system for feeding a new baby, perfectly suited to his needs. It can also give a mother a wonderful sense of achievement as she supplies superb nourishment to her baby from her own breast. Many women find that they come to enjoy breastfeeding immensely; it can be a relaxing and pleasurable time. In addition, the weight gained in pregnancy tends to be lost more easily when you breastfeed.

Because breastfeeding is such a good method of feeding a baby, it is the method worth aiming for if at all possible. It's worth organising everything around breastfeeding for the first six months of your baby's life. Midwives, lactation consultants and the La Leche League can all provide more detailed information. (See Appendix: Breastfeeding.)

But there are some women who find that they cannot fully breastfeed their babies, or are unable to breastfeed at all. For women in these situations, modern milk formulae and sterilised bottles provide an acceptable alternative. Mastectomy, some other types of breast surgery, being on certain drugs or suffering severe illness may all preclude breastfeeding. Tiredness, frustration, and work and family pressures can all affect the let-down reflex and milk production (see Chapter 7). Some women elect to formula-feed after unsuccessful or unhappy breastfeeding experiences with previous babies. However, problems with breastfeeding one baby by no means preclude breastfeeding subsequent babies. Many women can successfully breastfeed second or third babies with good help and support from an LMC midwife (and/or a postnatal midwife, lactation consultant and family members).

With a first baby, it's difficult to know in advance just how it will be for you. The ultimate decision is yours. If for some reason breastfeeding simply does not work out, there is no need to feel guilty about this if you have considered things carefully. Breast is best, but formula can provide a good second choice.

Considering employment

Especially if you are pregnant for the first time, you may well be in full-time paid employment – possibly in a demanding and responsible job. Being pregnant raises two issues: first, will it be possible to continue to work throughout pregnancy, and if so, for how long? Second, what opportunities are there for paid work after your baby is born?

Working during pregnancy

Most women find that they can work at their usual job until at least 28 weeks into their pregnancy, and many continue happily until 36 weeks. It does depend on the nature of your job: heavy physical work, particularly stressful situations and some environmental hazards may preclude certain jobs during pregnancy (see box on p.160).

Breastfeeding benefits[37]

Breastfed babies are less likely to:

- have diarrhoea or vomiting
- get ear infections (otitis media)
- get coughs and colds
- develop bronchitis or pneumonia
- contract serious infectious diseases such as measles or meningitis
- die from cot death (SIDS; see p.381).

There is also some evidence that long-term breastfeeding (beyond six months) may reduce the severity of asthma, diabetes and obesity.

If everything seems to be going smoothly and you feel well, it's probably reasonable to plan to work until about 28 weeks. If things are fine then, you could choose to continue on a week-by-week basis (possibly part time) until around 36 weeks. Just be prepared to stop earlier if necessary. Increasing tiredness and rising blood pressure are the most common reasons for stopping work earlier than planned.

Remember that even when you're pregnant, you have a responsibility to your employer to perform the tasks expected of you. It makes for much better working relationships if you tell your boss about your pregnancy early on, so that you can both plan for you to have time off towards the end. It's reasonable to make a fairly firm commitment to the job until around 28 weeks, but make it clear that from then on you will be able to work only if you are well enough.

You cannot lose your job because you are pregnant, but you can be fired for the same reasons as any other worker – for example, for significant unexplained non-attendance. If you are dismissed when pregnant and believe this to be unfair, your union or the Human Rights Commission (see Appendix) may be able to help.

In general, pregnancy and paid work can mix very well, as long as you're realistic about what you can achieve in both areas. In the end, children are very precious – having embarked on pregnancy, it makes sense to maximise good health and happiness by treating pregnancy with the respect it deserves.

Parental leave[38]

If you are working, you may be entitled to paid parental leave. In general, you are eligible for parental leave if, during the six or 12 months immediately before the expected date of birth (EDB), you have worked:

- for the same employer for an average of ten hours per week or more *and*
- for at least one hour in every week, *or* 40 hours in every month.

There are different entitlements if you have been in work for more than six months, or more than 12 months, immediately prior to the EDB.

There are similar eligibility criteria for women who are self-employed; different types of self-employed work can be considered as one period of self-employment.

The primary entitlement for paid parental leave rests with the birth mother. In some cases, it may be possible to transfer some of the leave to a spouse or partner who will be the primary caregiver, including in cases of adoption. You can take parental leave several times, as long as six months elapse between the date you returned to work and the EDB for the next child.

Working out the exact proportion of paid and unpaid leave for any given situation can be complicated, so it pays to check what you are going to be entitled to well in advance. The Department of Labour can help with this; their website is a good place to look initially. (See Appendix: Parental leave; Financial support/advice for families.)

Some organisations offer additional benefits and arrangements, and there may be provision for more generous parental leave in some employment contracts. Government legislation (the Parental Leave and Employment Protection Act 1987 and subsequent amendments) goes a long way towards recognising the needs and rights of parents, although New Zealand's provisions are still not as wide-ranging as those in some other countries.

Examples of jobs not suitable when pregnant

- those involving environmental hazards or dangerous chemicals (e.g. firefighting, working with radioactive material)
- those where the oxygen supply is poor (e.g. diving, working in aircraft)
- those involving a big physical load (e.g. heavy warehouse work)

2008 paid and unpaid parental leave entitlements[39]

Where both parents meet the 'employed, 12 month' criteria, the mother is entitled to:

- 10 days' special leave

- 14 weeks' paid parental leave

- 52 weeks' unpaid extended parental leave (including the 14 weeks' paid leave)

The mother can transfer up to 14 weeks' paid parental leave to the father/partner. The father/partner is entitled to share remaining leave up to a total of 52 weeks (including 14 weeks' paid parental leave). The father/partner is also entitled to two weeks' additional unpaid paternity leave.

Applying for parental leave[40]

You should apply in writing by giving a letter to your employer, at least three months before your baby is due and preferably much earlier. Examples of suitable letters can be downloaded from the Department of Labour's website. (See Appendix: Parental leave.)

- Your letter should clearly state what type of leave you want, when you want the leave to start, and how long the period of leave will be.

- It will need to be accompanied by a certificate from your LMC stating when the baby is due.

- If you are sharing leave with your spouse/partner, the letter should also state the dates on which you and your spouse/partner plan to start and finish each period of leave, along with your spouse/partner's name, and the name and address of their employer.

- It will need to establish that both you and your spouse/partner are eligible for the leave you are applying for, and indicate that the total amount of leave you are taking jointly will not be more than 52 weeks (not counting any paternity leave taken).

Working after the baby is born

Caring for a small child, or children, brings a big change in lifestyle for parents. Pregnancy and breastfeeding are exclusively female functions, so women need to make the lifestyle adjustments to accommodate them. Traditionally, this has meant women being the primary caregiver, often temporarily (and sometimes permanently) giving up their place in the paid workforce in favour of home-based activities. The number of men who primarily look after children for several years remains small, although growing numbers are assuming prime domestic responsibility for shorter periods.

Every woman feels differently about what she expects and/or wants to do once she has a child. More women than ever before are choosing to return to paid work before their youngest child is a year old, often in a part-time capacity. Some women are under economic pressure to resume paid work. Many factors come into this decision about paid work, and each situation is different. If you have not had children before, the box on p.163 on the needs of a baby may be helpful.

'I'd always worked, and enjoyed it. It was a big part of my life, my career. I planned three months' leave, which I thought was ample... and do you know, once it was up I just couldn't bear to leave her. I took another three months off, then went back half-time, and we both felt much happier about that.'

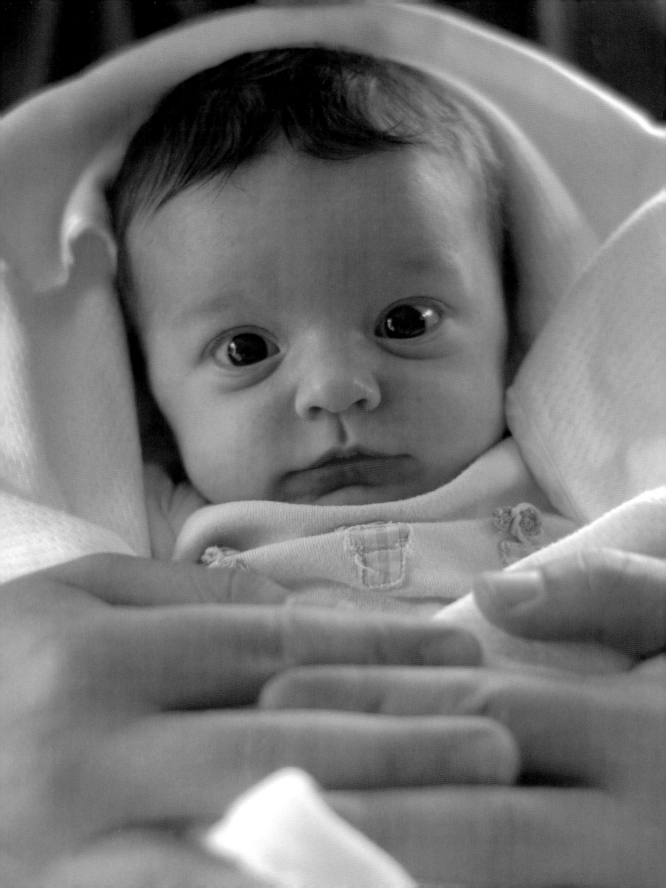

What do small babies really need?

Physical needs:

- *Food.* The advantages of breastfeeding, especially in the first six months of life, are discussed elsewhere (see 'Considering breastfeeding', above, and also the section on breastfeeding in Chapter 7). It's worth noting that breastfeeding is a learned art that requires time, patience and freedom from tight schedules.

- *Warmth and cleanliness.* Because babies are unable to clean themselves or adjust the air temperature, they need someone to do this for them. It sounds obvious, but having clean, dry clothes, frequent nappy-changes, and an environment that is neither too hot nor too cold are prerequisites for comfort.

Emotional needs:

Sometimes it's easy to forget that all babies, even the tiniest newborns, are human beings with emotional and social needs just like the rest of us. They need lots of people contact – cuddles for comfort as well as faces to look at and voices to listen to. They learn to identify with their main caregiver remarkably quickly, and can be very sensitive to mood changes or upsets.

Deciding whether/when to return to paid work

There are many benefits for a child who is cared for primarily by his mother for the first six months of his life. She is in a unique position to be able to supply him with breast milk (or, if that's not possible, expressed breast milk or formula milk), to pay attention to his other physical needs, and to get to know and love him. No matter what the circumstances, the relationship between a mother and her child is a very special bond that should be precious and rewarding. Early time spent together strengthens that relationship to become deep and resilient, ready for the challenges that will inevitably come with parenting. Other people – including fathers, partners, grandparents and other family members – may also be very important caregivers for this new baby. But if a mother and her baby are a close and happy unit, this is the best possible start in life for the baby, and everyone else in the family benefits as well.

If it is simply not possible for a new mother to be the primary caregiver for her baby – because of exhaustion, ill health or extraordinary work commitments – another person, or people, will need to be the loving and competent primary caregiver(s), perhaps temporarily or perhaps permanently. While this person, provided they are fully committed, will certainly be able to meet a small baby's physical and emotional needs, the relationship will be a little different from that between a mother and her baby (see p.302).

Working after your baby is six months old

Small children's needs are constantly changing, and around the six-month mark your working options tend to become wider. But it will depend on your child; he may be established on solid food and able to take a bottle, possibly of breast milk, or he may be steadfastly and solely breastfed. You will also have

'It's quite good to be studying rather than working. It means I can still be at home. Even though it's sometimes very stressful, I feel like I'm achieving something and still able to be a mother.'

Considering employment with a new baby – a practical checklist

- What are your ideas on your child's needs? Do you plan to breastfeed? Could/would you fit this in with your paid work? Will you work part time or full time?

- Can you leave your options open? Have you applied for parental leave? You may be unsure about when or whether to resume paid work; you may end up changing your mind either way.

- If you do return to paid work, who will look after your baby? Do you have relatives (e.g. parents, sisters) living close by? Could/would they be able to provide childcare? What sort of payment would they want/could you afford to give them?

- Would you employ someone to come to your home? Do you want to consider care at a child-care centre, if not immediately, then later on? What's available in your area and how long are the waiting lists? In some areas, especially in the larger cities, you may need to reserve a place right now, even before your baby is born.

- How much are you earning, as an individual and as a household? Could you afford the childcare you want?

- Is your paid work important to you? How committed are you to the type of paid work you're doing at present?

- Do you want to continue in your present job? Are you happy there? Or have you got into a bit of a rut? Could this be your opportunity to change direction and widen your horizons?

'I guess I've been lucky because I've always been able to work from home [as a graphic designer] — I worked from home before I had children, and just kept on ever since... While part of me resents not having that clear separation between work and family, the payoffs are really good too. I get to be at home with my kids every day. At the moment, I'm more interested in being a mum than in my work.

When Nadya was born, I was the only one earning an income so I had to work a lot more, and I guess I did feel a little bit resentful. Not of Jeremy, but just sad about the time I didn't get to spend with her. Now I have someone working with me, and it's great to be able to do more things with the baby — even silly little things, like hanging out the washing with Margot sitting on the grass beside me.'

a better idea of your own needs and priorities by now – it takes time to learn to become a mother.

Increasingly, women with very young children (under one year) are engaged in some form of paid work. Most of them choose to return to paid work sometime between six and 12 months, often in a part-time capacity. Other women decide that they do not want to leave their baby to go back to work. Many find that their priorities have changed, and that their mothering job has become far more important than any other. A significant number of women (about 40 per cent in 2003) still take variable amounts of time out from paid work when their children are small. The number of men taking time out from paid work to be full-time parents is much less.[41]

Combining paid work and parenting

When deciding whether to return to work, it may be helpful to talk to friends or colleagues who are already combining paid work and parenting small children. Ask them about childcare: what sort of choices did they have initially, and how long was the waiting list? How much paid work are they able to manage – and manage well?

A small but increasing number of women employ a full-time nanny to care for their children. While expensive, this arrangement may relieve them of some of the stress of doing two jobs – one at work and one at home. Ask friends and colleagues who have tried this option about the best way of finding a good nanny. Find out about the relevant qualifications, what agencies are available, and what they offer. Ask about the difficult times – what do parents do when children are sick or they have to stay late at work, or when the nanny is sick or unsatisfactory? What happens about pre-school education? Do they let the nanny drive the children to activities? In their car or in hers?

There are many such practical matters to consider once children are a bit older. Even though you don't need to deal with them all now, it does help to have some idea of the potential problems and challenges that lie ahead so that you can take them into account when planning for future employment.

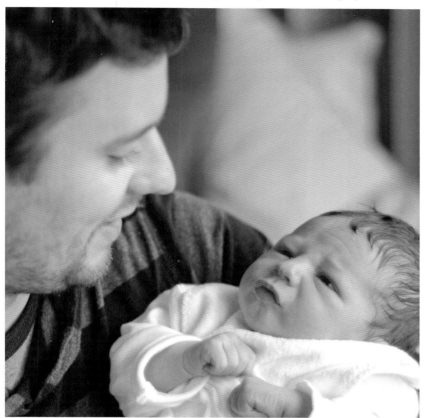

Income support

If you're not in paid employment when you become pregnant, or not earning a great deal, you will need financial support. Many women in permanent relationships are supported by their partners, particularly if they already have children. Others do not have this support, and need to draw the unemployment benefit or the domestic purposes benefit (DPB; see p.166). Benefit entitlements are subject to change, and are not always well advertised. Check with your local Work and Income office to find out what you are currently entitled to. Even if you have been on the DPB prior to this pregnancy, your entitlement is likely to change as your pregnancy progresses and once your baby is born. Check the Work and Income website for further information. (See Appendix: Financial support/advice for families.)

Sickness benefit

In New Zealand, if you are pregnant and have no financial support, have no other children and are not in paid work, you may be entitled to claim a sickness benefit and/or an independent youth benefit from Work and Income if you are 27 or more weeks pregnant – sometimes earlier if you have to give up paid work on the advice of your LMC. You will need a letter or certificate from your LMC to take to Work and Income. If you are under 18 years, your family circumstances will be taken into account.

Domestic purposes benefit (DPB)[42]

If this is your first pregnancy, and you have no other dependent children, you may be entitled to receive the DPB once your baby is born. You must be:

- a New Zealand citizen
- aged 18 or over (or have been legally married or in a civil union)
- not in paid employment
- living alone and without financial support.

If you will be under 18 when your baby is born, you may be entitled to an emergency maintenance allowance instead. For most benefits though, you will be required to name the father of the child, who will in turn be required to pay child support payments. There are exceptions, but this requirement is sometimes a barrier to would-be beneficiaries.

If you think you qualify (or will qualify) for any of these benefits, you need to go to Work and Income, where a staff member will ask you questions about your particular circumstances. You need to take some documents with you, so check what is required before you go (a checklist is shown on the Work and Income website). (See Appendix: Financial support/advice for families.) Take a knowledgeable support person with you if you feel at all unsure about your entitlements. Make sure you do all this well in advance, as payments take several weeks to start. They are usually paid directly into your bank account.

Working for Families

This tax credit scheme is administered by the Inland Revenue Department (IRD), and enables families who have dependent children to pay less tax. Greater financial support is now available for most families with dependent children; you need to check just what you are eligible for, as the rate depends on income and is recalculated to be more generous with each child. Depending on your circumstances, accommodation and childcare supplements may also be part of the package. Check the website to get an idea of the type of tax credit you are likely to qualify for. (Appendix: Financial support/advice for families.) Again, you should fill in application forms well in advance, as support may take weeks to filter through to your and/or your partner's pay packet. Application forms are available from the IRD, either in person or online.

Budgeting

Whatever your situation, it's likely that your finances will take a turn for the worse during the next year, even if you do qualify for paid parental leave. Many couples have to adjust to a single income, at least for a while. If you're on your own you may suffer a substantial drop in income.

Planning your finances for the year ahead can help ease the strain. If you need help, budgeting advice is available free of charge through the Citizens Advice Bureau. (See Appendix: Financial support/advice for families.) Find your local branch on the organisation's website or in the phone book.

If you are self-employed, check now whether you will be entitled to some paid parental leave, and consider how you will spread any income and ongoing expenses over the year. A good accountant can be of great assistance.

What to wear?

Depending on your size and shape, at some point between 14 and 24 weeks you'll find that your clothes are becoming tight around the waist. It's time to reassess what to wear.

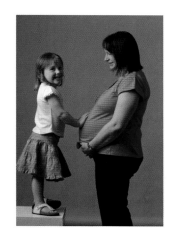

Stretchy tops, large T-shirts and singlets, low-cut jeans and loose-fitting pants are all popular in the middle months. If you want to wear tailored skirts or trousers, you may find that loose-fitting or longer tops, expandable inserts or an underlayer garment can help you get the most from your existing clothes. Not all pregnancy wear needs to be voluminous; many pregnant women see little point in trying to hide their pregnancy under shapeless clothes. Empire-line dresses and tops can show off an attractive bust line but cover the tummy area comfortably. Wear whatever feels comfortable; most women find anything that is too tight around the waist very annoying.

Once you're over 30 weeks pregnant, the range of ordinary clothes that still fit gets smaller, and some pregnancy wear will certainly make life easier in the last two or three months. If you are expecting your baby in late summer or early autumn, keep clothes cool and loose-fitting, as you will feel the heat much more than normal. Singlets and low-cut sleeveless tops in attractive stretch cottons can look stunning in hot weather, even when your pregnancy is well advanced.

Where to get suitable clothes

If you're planning to buy, there are an increasing number of good manufacturers and suppliers of smart, functional pregnancy wear in most parts of the country. New pregnancy wear tends to be rather expensive for what you get. It's a specialist market, so overheads tend to be high. But if good-quality clothes last for two or three pregnancies, they will be better value for money. You need to check more carefully than usual that the clothes are suitable for your particular figure and stage of pregnancy – it pays to check whether tops are easy to get on and off, whether trousers or jeans will stay up when you bend over, whether there's enough room around the bust, whether drawstrings are long enough, and whether the clothes might be suitable to wear after the baby is born and for breastfeeding.

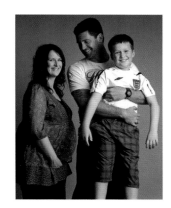

There are alternatives to buying new clothes that can be just as good, particularly if your budget is stretched. Most women can get away with just a small number of 'pregnancy' clothes, using larger sizes of ordinary clothing wherever possible. Home sewing, borrowing from friends, and checking out 'op' shops are all good alternatives. The Internet trading sites also have some excellent bargains, but it is difficult to try clothes on before you purchase.

Underwear

Cotton is more comfortable than synthetics, especially if vaginal thrush has been a problem (see p.87). Lower-cut briefs may be easier than pants that sit at the waist.

You may want to consider getting some nursing bras – from about 24 weeks, your bust size won't change much until 'the milk comes in'. Modern styles and fabrics have converted nursing bras from strictly utilitarian items to attractive lingerie, suitable to wear even after you stop breastfeeding. They are expensive, but are generally a good investment for the months ahead. A few women, particularly those with small breasts, find an ordinary bra (or no bra at all) quite satisfactory; but most women find that nursing bras are more comfortable and make breastfeeding easier. Try to find a firm-fitting, comfortable nursing bra, where the cup can easily be undone from the strap and done up again, preferably with one hand.

If you mainly wear trousers, then tights or stockings will probably be unnecessary in all but the coldest months. If you do need them, they will inevitably get tight around the middle, so it may be worth buying some with an expandable waistband from a pregnancy-wear shop. If you have varicose veins that are painful, and make your legs feel heavy and sore when standing, special support stockings are available that can minimise swelling and help your circulation. Some pharmacies stock these, and most can order them if you ask. They are quite expensive, but are much more durable than ordinary tights.

Clothes to wear in pregnancy

- Choose comfortable clothing: warm, but not too warm, in winter, and as cool and airy as possible in summer. Cardigans work well in winter, while singlets and sleeveless tops are good in summer.

- Big shirts, especially men's shirts, can be ideal.

- Wear a well-fitting, comfortable, supportive bra (perhaps a nursing bra), especially when doing any sort of exercise.

- Trousers tend to 'slip down over the bulge' – wearing braces is one solution, while a belt below the bulge is another.

- In the last month or so, everything gets rather uncomfortable – at this time, loose, very long tops or dresses are usually best.

- Flat shoes are best – high heels put extra strain on your already strained abdominal muscles and lower back. It's also easier to have footwear you can put on without having to bend down to do up laces or buckles.

- For walking any distance, or doing other exercise, wear sports shoes that will support your legs and feet better than scuffs, sandals or jandals.

- Don't wear any footwear that is too tight. Feet tend to get slightly bigger as pregnancy progresses; if you have any tendency to high blood pressure, this will often be accompanied by swollen feet. Or your feet may just swell at the end of the day or in the heat of summer.

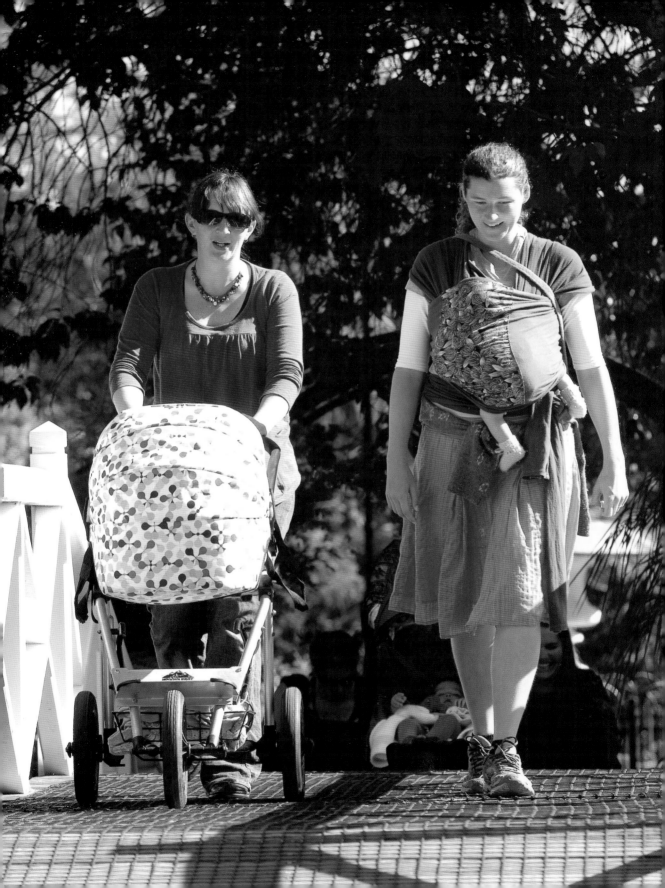

Household matters

Laundry facilities

Now is the time to assess your laundry equipment. Babies create more washing than you ever thought possible – how will your present facilities cope?

First, consider nappies. Do you plan to use reusable ones or disposables, or a combination? (See pp.172 and 358.)

Second, consider baby clothes. Small babies need frequent changes of clothing, and this continues when they are toddlers. Initially, dirty nappies are the norm rather than the exception, especially with breastfed babies. Even using really well-fitting nappies, the most expert nappy-changers are faced with frequent accidents and leaks in the first few months. In addition, many babies 'spill' a little milk after a feed, not just over themselves but over you too – you can't expect your own clothes to remain spotless either.

If you haven't already got one, a reliable, fully automatic washing machine is really worth investing in. Buy new if you can afford it, but if that's not possible, many whiteware retailers have good reconditioned trade-in models available with a short-term guarantee. If looking at Internet trading sites, check how old the machines really are before buying. The organisation Consumer NZ (see Appendix) can give you advice on different types of machine and what's best value for money.

A dryer may be a good investment too (or a combined washer-dryer), but it's an optional extra. It does save the time spent hanging out the washing, and can be a blessing in long periods of wet weather, but most areas of New Zealand enjoy good outside drying conditions for most of the year. A much cheaper and very useful alternative is two or three airing racks that can be moved around the house to make the most of warm and/or sunny rooms when outside drying is not possible. Even if you have a dryer, airing racks can give you substantially more inside drying capacity. Alternatively, if you have a garage or carport, a temporary clothes line can be a life-saver and reduce electricity costs, especially during the cold, wet winter months. You can purchase line from most hardware stores.

Heating

If your baby is due in the cooler months of the year, you will need to assess heating and its costs. Keeping at least one room in the house at a pleasant, even temperature (16–18°C) is a priority for a new baby and his mother. A thermostatically controlled unit may save on electricity or gas in the long run, and it's worth thinking ahead to systems that are safe for toddlers. Fire-guards and rails, child-proof switches and wall-mounted appliances are all safety features you will need to consider as soon as your baby is mobile.

Pets and other animals

If you already have pets, look at how they may affect your baby. If you are considering getting an animal, think about your baby's needs, as well as your own. Pets can be a wonderful addition to a family, bringing much pleasure as well as the chance for older children to learn caring and nurturing skills.

But they can bring disadvantages and dangers, many of which can be avoided with some common sense and forward planning. The following suggestions may be helpful:

- Have a room where your baby can sleep without animals. Cat and dog fur can easily cause allergic reactions and predispose children to coughs, runny noses, eczema and asthma. Cats may also carry toxoplasmosis (see p.80). Some dogs may be boisterous and unpredictable in their behaviour, especially in unusual situations. Kennel clubs can give advice about breeds of dog that are suitable for households with small children.
- When pets are inside in other rooms, ensure adequate ventilation and regular vacuuming, and keep cages and baskets clean. Keep any litter boxes outside, and avoid cleaning them when you are pregnant.
- Have an outdoor area fenced off so that children can play safely without animals. This is especially important on farms, where larger animals or working dogs can pose a frightening threat to babies or small children.
- When animals and small children are together, inside or outside, ensure that there is adequate adult supervision.
- Can you afford to get a pet just now? Consider the cost, especially if finances are going to be affected by your baby's arrival. Costs of keeping a pet include food, leads, collars, vaccination, veterinary care, medicines, flea prevention, cages, baskets, holiday care and contraception (usually a surgical operation).

House alterations

If you really think that some home improvements are necessary, now is the time to get on with them – not when the baby is nearly due.

A pregnancy in the household does seem to spur an extraordinary number of New Zealanders into action with additions and alterations. This is fine, and the end result will almost certainly be worth it, as long as you bear in mind a few salient points:

- Is the proposed alteration really necessary? Small babies don't have to have a room of their own – the need will be greater later. Perhaps a rearrangement rather than an alteration is all that's needed now.
- Will you get it finished well before the baby is due? More than one new mother has waited anxiously in hospital while the wall was hurriedly put back on the kitchen.
- Will the noise and inconvenience of the alteration make life difficult? Having to get up in the middle of the night to visit the hastily erected outdoor loo while the bathroom is being rebuilt is a stress new parents can do without.
- Can you afford it? Have you allowed for the cost of alterations and renovations, bearing in mind the financial constraints ahead? You may wish many times in the next year that you'd bought a new washing machine rather than repapered the hallway.

Baby clothes and equipment

It's worth starting to think about baby clothes and equipment, especially if you need to plan financially for big items. But don't feel you have to buy everything new. There's a strong tradition in New Zealand for baby gear to be given or lent long term to new parents. Small babies don't wear out their clothes, and there's a huge amount of beautiful clothing around – you may well be given some, and local fairs, 'op' shops and Internet trading sites often have good bargains. Some new items might be useful though, especially if you can afford to buy good quality that will last for another child.

Nappies (see also Chapter 8, pp.358–364)

There are two main choices: fully or partially reusable products; and/or disposable (single-use) nappies. A lot has changed in the last 30 years – in most developed countries, including New Zealand, traditional flat cloth nappies have largely been replaced by commercially made disposable nappies.

But although disposable nappies are convenient, they use up precious natural resources, contain a lot of plastic and chemical absorbents, and their safe and effective disposal is fast becoming a major environmental issue. Landfills are struggling to cope with thousands of used nappies – a potent mixture of non-recyclable plastics contaminated with faecal material which takes many years to break down, producing harmful leachates and methane gas in the process.[43] In response to this problem, enterprising parents, environmentally sympathetic businesses and even some local councils are now busy developing or supporting the use of excellent reusable products. These have features that make them superior to both traditional cloth nappies and disposable nappies.

For more on fitting and washing instructions, see pp.358–364.

Reusable nappies

- *All-in-one nappies.* These nappies are sewn and shaped to fit neatly around your baby's legs and fasten securely around the middle with Velcro tabs, snaps, hooks and loops, or buttons. A whole range of great colours and smart designs is available. If you want to sew your own, easy-to-follow patterns can also be found. Some brands come in different sizes, but there are also adjustable one-size-fits-all (OSFA) models. The waterproof cover forms the outside of the nappy, with the inner side being made of soft absorbent cloth materials. When changing, the whole nappy is removed, cleaned if necessary and then washed. A liner can be used to protect the inner fabric. Although the all-in-one models are fully machine-washable, drying times can be longer because of their thickness.

- *Pocket nappies.* As the name suggests, these nappies are made of a specially shaped cloth pocket, into which a reusable absorbent insert is placed. The nappy is then fastened securely with buttons, snaps or Velcro tabs for a snug fit. As with the all-in-ones, different sizes (including OSFA), colours and patterns make these nappies trim, attractive and fun to use. Sew-your-own patterns are also available. The outside material of the pocket is highly water-resistant to prevent leaks, but the inner stay-dry fleece material acts as a wick to transfer moisture to the insert. The insert is easily removed for cleaning and washing, but the pocket needs to be changed only if the

'With our first baby, we used cloth nappies just because it felt like a good thing to do. It felt so virtuous. But one of my enduring memories is of these mountains of nappies that had to be scrubbed, and we would always have to decide whose turn it was. Then with our second, we were completely over cloth nappies: we hardly used them at all, even though we'd occasionally feel guilty about it. Now with our third baby, we're using both disposables and pocket nappies, which are amazing, and also putting her on the potty – at nine months she does a wee nearly every time.'

nappy is soiled, especially if a liner is also used to protect the inner part of the pocket. All the components of the pocket nappies can be machine-washed, and because the layers are separated, they dry more quickly than the all-in-one models. Although a bit more fiddly to use – you need to 'insert the insert', and remove it afterwards – pocket nappies allow you to use different types of insert as your baby's requirements change.

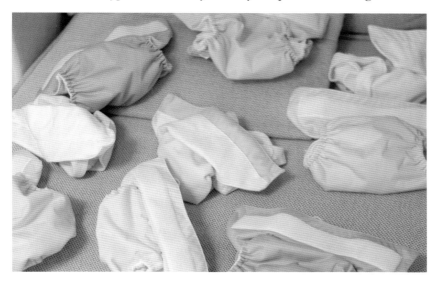

New-generation reusable nappies have several components, which affect washing methods (see p.363). The waterproof outer covering is generally made of a breathable plastic known as a PUL fabric, which lets through water vapour but not water droplets. Some brands use laminated cotton; although not quite as waterproof, these may be a good option for babies with very sensitive skin. Fabric technology is improving all the time as manufacturers strive for the perfect material that is soft and flexible, fully breathable, fully waterproof, non-allergenic, very durable, and environmentally sustainable. It doesn't exist yet, but some options come close.

The inner lining usually comprises a stay-dry fleece product. Its job is to move moisture rapidly through into the insert material, while staying dry and keeping the baby's skin dry too. In both the all-in-ones and the pocket styles, the lining is sewn at the edges to the waterproof outer cover, with the seam covered in a soft but robust border fabric so it fits snugly against the baby's legs and middle. To work efficiently, stay-dry material needs to be really clean and residue-free: all reusable nappies must be thoroughly washed and rinsed without the use of fabric softeners or bleach.

The absorbent insert consists of several layers of an environmentally friendly absorbent material that can be easily washed, dried and reused many times. It is sewn firmly between the outer and inner layers in the all-in-one models, so has to be washing-compatible with the outer covering and the inner lining. But with pocket nappies, several types of insert are available and two can be used together if necessary. Microfibre, cotton, hemp and bamboo-based materials are all in use. Microfibre is synthetic, absorbs about eight times its weight, and washes and dries very quickly. Cotton, hemp and bamboo products are made from natural fibres and are even more absorbent, but take slightly longer to dry. They may not last quite as long as microfibre inserts. It is also perfectly possible to use a traditional flat cloth nappy as an insert by folding it into several layers to fit the pocket.

Liners are optional, but they do help with nappy-changing, especially when babies are small. Reusable fabric liners (stretchy cotton or silk) are available, but more commonly, liners are made of disposable material. Most (but not all) are designed to be flushed down the toilet when soiled, and to degrade fairly quickly in reticulated sewerage systems. They are not suitable for septic tanks. Check the label before disposing of them. Some of the disposable types can be washed two or three times unless heavily soiled, thus extending their use to minimise waste. They help to protect the stay-dry fleece lining of reusable nappies, especially if your baby's skin needs barrier cream (which can otherwise damage the fleece material).

Traditional cloth nappies

Despite all the advantages of the modern, fitted reusable nappies, flat cloth nappies still have a useful place and are perfectly serviceable. They can be safely bleached, soaked, washed and dried for years. They need to be folded and pinned in place correctly to get the best fit and avoid leaks, and then are best covered with pilchers (soft overpants) or waterproof pants to protect outer clothing. Although this takes a bit of practice to get right, flat nappies can work well, and can be particularly useful at night for older babies. If you have been given a set of flat cloth nappies, you might use them in combination with a smaller number of reusable fitted nappies to save on cost. A reusable fitted nappy can be used over the top of a folded and pinned flat cloth nappy, and cloth nappies can also be folded and used as inserts for pocket nappies.

Disposable (single-use) nappies

Disposable nappies provide a useful alternative to cloth nappies. They are convenient, and save time on washing and drying. But for all the reasons mentioned on p.172, they are best reserved for use when travelling, if you are ill or exhausted, or if your washing and drying facilities are limited.

Some crèches and other child-care facilities require disposable nappies to be used, although parents are increasingly asking to be able to supply reusable nappies and take them home to be washed. Some babies with sensitive skins are unable to wear disposables, although better quality disposables are less likely to cause rashes. They can be used with the liners mentioned above if sensitivity is a problem. (For fitting and disposal, see Chapter 8, pp.361–362.)

Cost

By the time he is toilet-trained at the age of two or three years, your baby will have gone through somewhere between 5000 and 6000 nappies or nappy-changes: eight to ten changes a day when small, decreasing as he gets older. If you use disposable nappies, that's a tonne of landfill, over 300kg of plastic waste, and about $2500 a year (at 2007 prices).

Cloth nappies use only about a third of the energy that is required to manufacture and use the same number of disposable nappies, even if you take into account the energy used in manufacturing, washing and drying the cloth nappies by the most expensive methods. They are considerably cheaper to use than disposables over two to three years, taking the full costs of washing and drying into account, but they do have a higher up-front cost (especially if you have to buy a washing machine at the same time). Check with Consumer NZ if you need convincing. Most people find it costs between $400 and $500 to set themselves up with enough reusable nappies for their first baby, and less for the second, as often only inserts need replacing (flat nappies are cheaper: the initial cost of a new good-quality set is currently between $100 and $150).

To help with these costs, most reusable nappy companies will provide trial packs, starter packs and pay-by-instalment options. Look for cloth nappy hire schemes like the one run by Waitakere City Council (2007), or cash-back cloth nappy schemes such as that run by the Kaikoura District Council (2007); they will reimburse you for starter packs as long as you live in the area and are happy to provide feedback in six months' time. (See Appendix: Nappies.)

Shopping hints for nappies

Reusable and cloth nappies

1. How many? Assuming you use only one type:

- All-in-ones – somewhere between 15 and 20 will be plenty if you wash most days, more if you wash less frequently.
- Pocket nappies – 6–10 of the newborn size, then another 6–10 of the next size up (which are usually adjustable and last up to toddler stage) will be plenty if you wash most days. Inserts of various types can be used with all sizes; 18–20 is usually enough to get started.
- Flat cloth nappies – 25–30 will be usually be ample.

  Obviously, if you use a combination of types to give maximum flexibility, you can reduce the numbers accordingly.

2. Where to buy?

- In baby equipment shops – most shops carry a range of reusable and flat types, but may have to order some sizes and types for you.
- On the Internet – this is fast becoming the best way to buy new reusable nappies. Many excellent products are easily found by using keywords such as 'reusable nappies' (or 'diapers'), 'pocket nappies', 'pre-fold nappies' or 'twofold nappies'. You can usually order online. Suppliers range from small home-based New Zealand enterprises to much larger international suppliers. (See Appendix: Nappies.)

Disposable nappies

These are readily available in most supermarkets, and are cheaper if you buy in bulk. Several brands and many sizes are available. Costs can vary considerably between brands, so it pays to shop around. Some come in male and female designs. The more fitted designs are often more expensive, but minimise leaks and accidents. Reusable fastening tapes are useful.

Clothes

Your new baby's clothing needs will depend to some extent on the season and where you live. Very small babies sleep a lot, but within a few weeks they have wakeful periods and need clothes that minimise draughts and gaps. New fabric technology has resulted in excellent materials for baby clothes that are comfortable, smart, environmentally friendly, and easy to wash and care for. Some are synthetic/wool mixes; others are stretch cotton. Durability

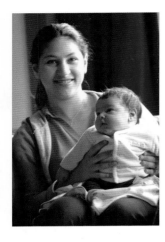

does vary, and while this is not a major problem for small baby clothes, it's a more important consideration when buying items that you want to last into the toddler stage. With all new products, check they are suitable for sensitive baby skin and that fabrics have low flammability. Wash well before use to get rid of any fabric dressings or odours.

With second-hand items, many will still be in excellent condition and will probably be well washed already, so virtually free of any fabric dressings. If you are offered good second-hand newborn baby clothes, make the most of them and save your money for the larger sizes you will need later. Older synthetic fabrics are easy to care for, but tend to be cold in winter and hot in summer. Natural fabrics such as plain cotton and wool are useful, as they 'breathe' and allow good temperature regulation. Plain, loose-fitting cotton garments are especially good in hot weather.

- *Nightgowns.* Useful in first few weeks. Easy for nappy-changes. Not especially warm if your baby is up in your arms. Three or four are usually sufficient. Easy to sew your own if you want.

- *Singlets.* Cotton is best next to the skin. Some come in stretch cotton so will last longer than plain cotton. Use a washable wool singlet over a cotton one if the weather is cold. A good number is three to six.

- *Sunhat.* Essential if your baby is born in the summer months. He needs to wear one whenever he's outside, even on cloudy days. One of each size is usually enough as babies' heads grow very quickly, and the size has to be right to get the hat to stay on. Ties or a stretchy band also help keep the hat in place.

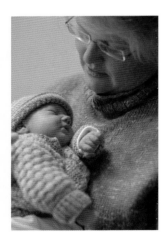

- *Bootees, socks and warm hats.* Necessary for the cooler months of the year. Knitting patterns for tiny bootees and woollen hats are available, but these will fit for only a few weeks. Some babies dislike ribbons – a knitted band attached to a hat may be better. Check that bootees have no loose threads inside or out, and that ribbons are tied properly – it's quite possible to catch a tiny toe in a loose thread and cut off the circulation. Small socks with an elasticised band to hold them on are safer, and easy to put on and take off. Small babies may need to wear socks or bootees in bed.

- *Warm tops, cardigans and jerseys.* Necessary in winter and for going out all year round. Warmer if they button all the way down the front. Safer if they have a fairly close knit – little fingers can catch in a lacy pattern. Jerseys can be tricky to get over the baby's head if the neck is too tight. Hand-me-down knitted garments can get matted and are prone to lose any stretch they once had; check before use. Partially synthetic stretch fabrics or machine knits are often easier to manage than tightly hand-knitted garments. Some babies get irritated skin under the chin if they dribble and the wool comes right up their neck. Garments made of pure wool may need to be hand-washed, despite the claims of the washing-machine manufacturer.

- *Shawls.* Useful for very small babies. One good-quality shawl that's fully machine-washable will often last for two or three children. Will keep babies warm while feeding or on outings. Again, watch out for lacy knits. Check that synthetic fabrics are flame-retardant.

- *Pilchers, or pants to go over nappies.* Not usually necessary with good-quality disposables or modern reusable nappies. Very useful to prevent (or at least reduce) leaks if you are using traditional flat cloth nappies. Will keep wet nappies warm, which helps prevent heat loss, and also help to keep the nappy on. Available in flannel, stay-dry fleece or PUL fabric (see p.173). Even if you're using traditional cloth nappies, two to three reusable nappies will make excellent, well-fitting pilchers.

- *Body suits, all-in-ones.* Very versatile and capable of some stretching as your baby grows. Important not to use any that are really too small; those with sewn-in feet can restrict foot growth, so most new ones are made without feet. Suits with domes, snaps or tabs right down the front are the easiest to put on. Worth getting some footless suits with long legs and some with short legs; the short-legged ones will last longer. Come in a wide variety of fabrics and colours, and look good even after lots of washes. Useful once your baby is up and about, helping to keep nappies on and minimising gaps around the tummy area. Most brands are fully machine-washable. Some are suitable for winter use; check the weight of the fabric if you are buying new. The summer-weight types will not be very warm by themselves and will need socks and an extra layer, worn either underneath or over the top, if the weather is at all cool.

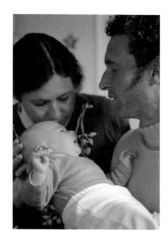

Bassinets and cots

Bassinets and baby baskets

These are useful for the first few months. They are usually portable, and bassinets will often lift off the stand to double as a carry-cot. They can often be borrowed, and some Plunket branches will hire them out. For those with stands, check that the basket is secure and cannot easily be pulled over.

Cots

Cots are very good once the baby is over five or six months. If no bassinet is available, cots can be used easily and safely from birth. They can often be bought second-hand – try the Internet trading sites. If you are faced with a choice between buying a bassinet or a cot, a cot is better value. Check that:

- the cot stands firmly on the floor
- the slats and bars are secure
- the gaps between both the slats and the bars are definitely too small for a baby's head to get through (no more than 9cm across)
- the drop side is well secured, yet easy to operate when you need to
- the base of the cot is in one secure piece (or if there are slats, they are very secure).

Portable cots

These are especially useful for travelling. Check that they cannot be collapsed inadvertently, and that the base cannot collapse with the weight of the baby. Most models are less than half a metre off the floor, so lifting children in and out can be difficult and bad for your back.

Sharing your bed with your baby

You may feel that your baby can simply sleep in your bed with you, and that a separate bassinet or cot is unnecessary. This may work well at times, but your baby will need to sleep when you don't, and it is not usually safe to leave a baby alone in an adult bed. Also, there is some evidence that bed-sharing under certain circumstances is linked to an increased risk of cot death (SIDS; see p.381).

Bedding (see also p.368)

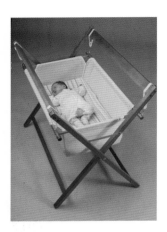

- *Cot/bassinet mattress.* Needs to be clean and well aired. Should fit into the cot well, with just enough room for tucking in the bedding. This is one item that is worth buying new if you possibly can – old mattresses tend to contain a lot of dust and other debris, including house dust mites, which may make your baby more prone to coughs, colds and sneezes. Recent research suggests that using old cot mattresses for babies may increase their risk of developing asthma.[44] There have been suggestions that cheap foam rubber mattresses may also give off formaldehyde gases, with a possible link to cot death (SIDS). Impermeable plastic coverings have been recommended to combat this problem. However, no link between foam mattresses and SIDS has been proven (see p.382).

- *Mattress protector.* A 'dry cot' blanket (absorbent, easily washable blanket made of synthetic or synthetic-wool mix) is easiest to use, but a plain cotton mattress protector or ordinary woollen blanket will work as well. Best placed across the middle section of the bed only. Needs to be removed frequently to air the mattress, otherwise mould may grow.

- *Sheets.* These go over the mattress protector. Cot sheets can be bought, or made out of half a single-bed sheet, and doubled over for use in a bassinet. Four to six are usually sufficient.

- *Duvets and blankets.* Cot-size duvets and covers are available in a wide range of colours and styles. Easy to wash and care for. They sometimes come in winter and summer weights, but a summer-weight duvet plus a good-quality blanket in winter will work just as well. (Full bed-size duvets are often too bulky to use easily in a cot, and run the risk of inadvertently covering a baby's head or making him too hot.) Blankets can be bought or made for a cot, and doubled for use in a bassinet. Cotton or washable wool is easiest. Shawls can double as blankets. The number and type required will vary depending on the time of year and the temperature of the room.

- *Padding for bassinets and cots.* Can be bought or made of cotton fabric and synthetic filling. Useful for stopping draughts. Once the baby is mobile, padding also prevents him from hitting his head on the side of the cot. Must be firmly attached so there is no danger of the baby's head getting caught under the padding. Must have some gaps to allow good ventilation. Plastic material is not recommended as it will reduce ventilation.

Nappy-changing equipment

Special tables and mats are useful but not essential. Any firm surface at bench height, with enough room to keep nappies, wipes and toiletries nearby, helps to avoid backache and makes changing quicker and easier. Check that a changing table is stable, has a safety strap, and has enough room to change the baby. Many have useful storage pockets or drawers underneath.

A portable alternative is a washable piece of heavy cloth and a prepared nappy bag. Foldable, washable plastic mats are also available. Check that there are no hard-to-clean crevices.

Nappy bags

Many well-designed, great-looking bags are available. If you can afford it, a quality bag is likely to be a good investment, especially if it lasts for two to three children. Nappy bags can be just as useful around the house as they are when you're out and about; wherever you take your baby, your nappy bag is likely to be your constant companion for the next two or three years.

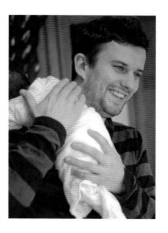

The more expensive bags tend to have insulated pockets and pouches to make everything easy to find and keep toiletries from overheating. Some buggy manufacturers make colour-coordinated nappy bags that fit in the back of, or underneath, the buggy.

But an ordinary day pack, a generous basket or kete, a reusable supermarket bag or even a sturdy plastic bag will all do the job of keeping everything you need together (see p.362 for what to put in the nappy bag). Whatever you use, make sure it cannot tip an older-model buggy or pram over when placed over the handles. Newer model buggies are less likely to tip over.

Bath equipment

- *Bath.* Plastic baby baths are convenient, but a small baby can quite easily be bathed in any tub or basin that is big enough (see p.365). You can also bath the baby with you in a normal bath, providing you have someone to help you undress and dress the baby. Otherwise, both of you can easily get cold and miserable. Babies may also enjoy showering with their mum or dad and being cuddled skin to skin.

- *Bath surround.* What's more important is to have a firm table or bench under the baby bath or next to the bath/shower, on which to undress and dress your baby. If this is not possible, put everything on the floor and kneel down. This may not seem important, but back strain really does need to be avoided; you need to be physically fit to care for your baby for many months to come.

- *Towels.* You'll need to keep a supply of bath towels exclusively for your baby's use (three to four should be sufficient).

- *Wash-cloths.* Any small, soft cloth will do. A piece of muslin, a disposable or reusable nappy liner, or a soft cotton wash-cloth will be softer than ordinary towelling ones.

Toiletries (see also p.365)

- *Soap/oil.* Several varieties of baby soap are available, which contain no perfume and only a minimum of hardening agent. Even the best soap dries the skin, so oil may be preferable. Various types of oil are suitable – some are available on prescription if your baby has sensitive skin. Products made from vegetable materials and without petrochemicals are better for skin and general health, as well as being better for the environment.
- *Powder.* Useful for areas such as under the arms to ensure dryness, but not essential. Special unperfumed baby powder is best. Must not be used on raw or broken skin.
- *Barrier creams.* A wide variety of creams are available; apply them to the nappy area to protect the skin from wetness. Not essential if you are prepared to be meticulous about changing dirty nappies immediately.
- *Wipes.* For cleaning the skin when changing nappies. Washable cloths made of towelling, soft cotton or muslin are good and should be kept only for this purpose. Disposable wipes in a special dispenser are convenient, especially for the nappy bag, but are more expensive. Like disposable nappies, they can create environmental problems.

Car seats

In New Zealand, every child under five years travelling in a motor vehicle is required by law to use an approved child restraint appropriate to their age. The law makes good sense; even in a low-speed accident, an unrestrained child is like a heavy bag of cement and impossible to hold on to. If children are securely buckled in, the driver (probably you) can concentrate on driving, not on trying to restrain them. Children secured in car seats are also less prone to travel sickness.

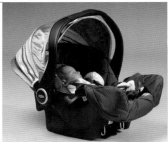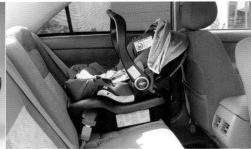

Car seat suitable for a newborn baby

Shown also in position – backwards facing on a rear seat

There are three main types of car seat:
- infant restraints for use from birth to when a baby weighs 9kg
- child restraints for use from 8kg to 18kg
- convertible models that can be switched from the infant style to the child style when the baby is about 8kg. When children reach 18kg, child booster seats are required.

Car-seat rental schemes

This is probably the cheapest way to get a car seat for a baby or small child. Plunket, iwi health agencies, and Māori and Pacific Island health providers operate car-seat rental schemes in most places throughout New Zealand. In some areas, charitable trusts further subsidise costs. Seats are usually hired out for as long as the baby or child requires them. Infant-size, child-size and booster seats are all available. There are long waiting lists in some areas, so get your name on the list several months before your baby's expected date of birth. If the seat is involved in an accident, take it back for replacement. (See Appendix: Plunket; Well Child/Tamariki Ora.)

If you are planning to buy a car seat, several models are available from baby-equipment retailers, including some excellent brands produced in New Zealand. Head cushions and weather protectors make for good baby comfort. Some retailers and car-rental firms hire out car seats on a short-term basis, which can be useful on holiday or when visiting grandparents etc.

If you are buying a car seat, check the following:

- Does the seat conform to a New Zealand or Australian safety standard? Any model that simply hooks over the adult seat is *not* safe, because in an accident it will act like an unrestrained piece of baggage.

- Will the seat fit in the car where you want it? Some models will go only in the back or in the front seat, not both.

- What method is used to secure the seat in the car? Some require a special fitting for a tether strap.

- How easy is it to carry the car seat with the baby in it? A handle that allows the car seat, with baby in place, to be picked up easily with one hand is invaluable.

- What harnesses and buckles are used to secure the baby? There should be shoulder, waist and crotch straps, all easily secured with childproof locks. Toddlers sitting beside babies in cars can undo insecure buckles.

- Is the seat in good condition, with no frayed straps or worn buckles?

- Has the seat been in an accident? The safety of most seats is no longer guaranteed once they have been involved in an accident.

Fitting and placing the car seat

All child-restraint seats must be fitted correctly according to the manufacturer's instructions. Safe2go is a training organisation set up by the Accident Compensation Corporation (ACC) and Land Transport New Zealand (LTSA) to promote the safe and effective use of child restraints in cars, and to train technicians to install child-restraint seats correctly. Advice about installing and using infant and child car seats, and a list of trained technicians, is available on their website. (See Appendix: Car seats.)

Safe2go recommendations for placing car seats[45]

- The back seat is the safest place for a child-restraint seat.
- Never place a rear-facing restraint on the front seat if an airbag is fitted.
- Babies are better protected in a rear-facing seat until they are one year old.
- If your child-restraint seat wobbles, try it in another place in the vehicle. A locking clip will help hold the restraint firmly.
- If there is a chest clip, ensure it is at chest level.
- The harness should be firm against your baby and go over his shoulders.
- Any blankets should be put over the baby once the harness is on, not under the harness.

Children, car seats and airbags[46]

Airbags in modern cars prevent injury to drivers and front-seat passengers in the event of an accident. The airbag 'explodes' on impact, rapidly filling with air to cushion the occupants. But for children in car seats, rapidly inflating airbags can hit them hard and envelop them – for a small baby this can lead to injury or even death. Front airbags on the passenger side are the biggest concern, but care must also be taken if there are side or roof airbags. The safest place for an infant or child seat is in the back, in the middle of the car. Some vehicles have a switch to turn airbags off; use this only if it's impossible to place the infant seat in the back.

Carrying equipment

- *Slings and front packs.* Several designs are available to hold a small baby snugly against your body. They are lightweight, and keep baby warm (and well protected if you wear a jacket over him). Very good for use on steps or uneven ground. Also useful to wear at home to comfort a grumpy baby, as they leave both your hands free. Ties, straps and buckles can be tricky to do up and undo by yourself. Will last only until baby is three to five months old. Some front packs will convert to a backpack for later use, but they can be very hard on your back once the baby is a bit bigger. Relatively cheap to buy, or make, especially if you simply make a sling with a large square of sturdy material that you can tie securely over one shoulder and around your middle.
- *Backpacks.* Useful for carrying older babies when out walking, especially on uneven ground. A variety of good lightweight models are now available, with cushioned backrests, neck supports, padded straps, sturdy frames, storage pockets and weather protection. Comfortable to wear. Limited use once the baby is too heavy to carry for long distances. More expensive than slings and front packs, but much better for your back. Babies need to be well wrapped to keep them warm enough. Models that can be set securely on the ground while loading or unloading, or even just having a rest, make life with a baby much easier.

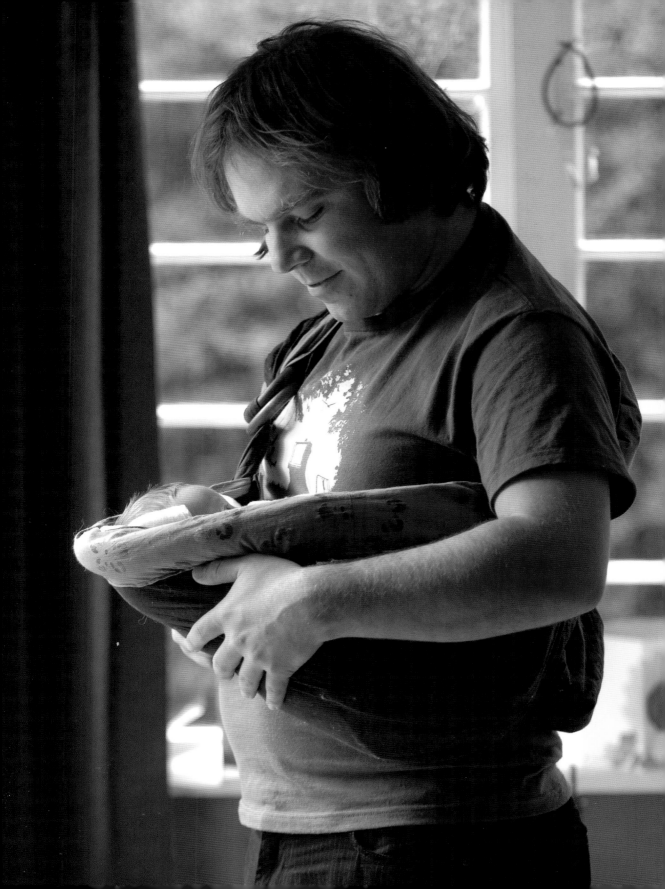

Buggies, strollers, pushchairs and prams

Modern, fully adjustable buggies can be used for very small babies right through to toddler stage. If you can afford one, they can be a good investment, especially if used for more than one child. But if the initial cost is simply too much, very serviceable good-quality older-style prams and buggies can be bought much more cheaply second-hand. Borrowing from friends or relatives whose children are now older is well worth looking into as well.

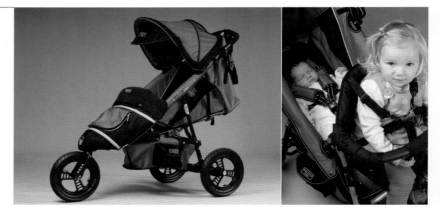

Modern all-terrain buggy

The toddler seat is in place, with the new baby behind.

- *Prams.* These can be useful for the first six months, and double as a bassinet. Babies can be taken outside without being disturbed, and prams provide good protection from rain and wind. They can be tricky on steps. Sturdy older-type prams will often accommodate a toddler seat, or twins. Some types will fold down to fit in a car, and some will convert to a buggy once the baby can hold his head up firmly (around six months).

- *Older-style pushchairs and lightweight strollers.* These are excellent for use with cars, buses and trains, but do tend to wear out with heavy use. Wheels tend to be small and hard to manoeuvre on uneven ground. Some have an attached shopping rack or bag. Not generally suitable for very small babies, unless fully adjustable to allow them to lie nearly flat. It's harder to protect the baby from rain and wind, although some are fitted with sun and rain shields. Double pushchairs for twins or two children close in age are available, as are clips to join two singles together.

- *Fully adjustable all-terrain buggies.* Several manufacturers, including some excellent New Zealand companies, are now producing high-quality, durable buggies designed to be taken 'off footpath' onto rough and/or soft ground. These give parents greater flexibility than the conventional pushchair, and are especially good to take running, around the farm or to the beach. Three-wheelers give maximum manoeuvrability. These can generally be used from birth, with a removable cocoon for when babies are small and need to be lying completely flat. Some have a fully supported seat that will convert to a certified car seat. Other models can also convert to an 'in-line model' where a second child can be seated, one behind the other. If necessary, the second child seat can be bought later, giving some saving on the initial cost. Twin versions (with babies side by side) usually come with four wheels to give the necessary stability to the wider base.

On the other hand, lightweight but fully adjustable two-wheelers (with a pop-out stand system) can be excellent if you frequently use public transport and/or have to negotiate steps and stairs. Most modern buggies come with good parcel trays, storm covers and sun-protection accessories, but check whether these are included in the initial price or whether you have to pay extra.

When buying any sort of buggy, pushchair or stroller, check the following points:[47]

- It is solid and sturdy, but light enough to be carried easily with one hand.
- It folds down and reassembles easily.
- It is stable when the child is on board (a gust of wind can blow over very light models).
- It has front wheels that swivel to make steering easier, but can also be locked if you are going to be travelling over rough terrain. Pneumatic (blow-up) tyres give a more comfortable ride, but need to be pumped up from time to time, and occasionally repaired.
- It has efficient brakes. Look for brakes on both rear wheels that are foot-operated and linked, so that left and right brakes are activated by a single lever. Check that your feet fit the brake easily, and that when you try to push the buggy with the brakes on, it will definitely not move.
- It has a secure harness, with adjustable shoulder, waist and crotch straps.
- It has handles that are either at a comfortable height or can be adjusted (an important consideration if people of different builds are going to be pushing the buggy).

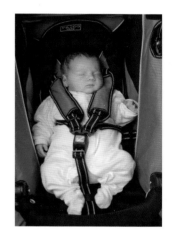

Five-point harness in a buggy

Buggy standards[48]

There are New Zealand and Australian standards for all new buggies made here and in Australia. Some international brands may also comply with US or European standards. Standards approval is not mandatory for sale, although it is highly recommended. If you cannot see a standards mark (the New Zealand 'S' mark or the red Australian 'tick' mark), then be sure to check that:

- There are no protruding parts that can hit your child's head.
- There are no small parts that could detach easily and pose a choking hazard.
- There are no gaps that could trap fingers – yours or your child's.
- There are no sharp edges or points.
- The stroller or buggy is stable enough not to tip easily.
- There is a child-resistant mechanism for locks.
- There is a five-point harness – two shoulder straps attached to the backrest, two waist straps attached to the frame, and a crotch strap.

Ngawari's story: A first birth at home

There are nine children in my family and I have four older sisters, three of whom have children. Most have been home births, including one I'd attended. So I was hugely confident about having a home birth, and in my ability to give birth naturally, even though it was my first pregnancy.

Even though my husband, Haymon, and I didn't go to formal antenatal classes, I talked to Mum, read books about birthing options, and made sure my support people understood what I wanted if we ended up having to go to hospital. But I was pretty sure that things would just go normally and naturally and without complications.

I was also very confident in my midwives, because I knew they had years of experience and supported home birth ideals. Because I trusted their ability to guide me, I knew taking their advice was my best option. Haymon was hugely supportive in all the decision-making. He said, 'Honey, it's up to you, you choose how you want to have baby.' So when I decided to have a natural home birth, there were no worries from him. He just said, 'If that's what you want, babe, I'll support you.'

I also knew from the start that I wanted my family there. When my sister had the first home birth in our family, she wondered later if it was a good idea to have Mum there because her own experience had been so different. Her nine children were all born in hospital, and everything was so medically oriented then — you were shaved, you lay on your back with your legs up, and the nurses would bring baby in and out when they wanted you to feed it. My sister remembers Mum being quite concerned about the whole home birth process. But since then, she's been at many births in our family and talks about how lovely it is to be in your own home, where the family, and not the doctors, are in control. She says, 'You girls are so lucky that these options are available to you now.' Because if she'd had the choice back then, she definitely would have chosen home births too.

Things got going on a Saturday morning. I started having these strange feelings — just very light contractions. I'd be walking around the supermarket, stop while I had a contraction, and carry on. Then we went for a walk, because I didn't want the contractions to stop — I wanted to get the ball rolling.

After that, the contractions got progressively stronger and we packed up ready to go to my sister's house. They'd offered their house for the birth because the birthing pool wouldn't fit in our little one-bedroom flat. I'd decided on a water birth because I love the water. I grew up in Tauranga with the beaches and coastal rivers all around. It was a natural choice for me.

Everyone had fun constructing the birthing pool and making it nice and cosy. We put a mattress and a bean bag under the bottom so I had a little ledge to lean on, and wrapped towels around the rim so it didn't hurt my arms. The other sisters who'd had water births gave us their tips. It was wonderful. The water helped with the pain so much — it almost felt like I wasn't having contractions when I was.

Through the evening, the contractions came and went. I'd get in the pool and the contractions seemed to level off, then I'd get out and they'd come on a bit stronger. I was getting incredibly tired. At one point, I was having doubts about whether I wanted something to help with the pain. But in the end, I just endured it. I tried to sleep in between contractions. Poor Haymon was rubbing my back, trying to stay awake. He'd have a bit of a doze, and I'd say 'Wake up, wake up, I'm having a contraction here!'

When Alena was finally born, there were just our two midwives, Haymon, my Mum and my two sisters. We're a very musical family: one of my sisters was singing and playing the guitar while I was having contractions, which helped take my mind off the pain. There were people massaging my back and shoulders, and wiping my forehead. I think I was holding on to Haymon's hand while I was pushing baby out — he said his hand was pretty sore afterwards!

The rest of the family came to visit soon after — my Dad and Haymon's dad first, then the other aunties, uncles, and tamariki. We ended up staying at my sister's house for a week after we had baby, which was such a blessing. They looked after us, cooked, cleaned and allowed us to have that much-needed recovery time.

After Alena was born, we kept the whenua (placenta) frozen for a while because we wanted to bury it at home, at my parents' place. Some of my nieces' and nephews' whenua are buried there too, each under their own tree. I made a clay ipu (container) to bury her whenua in. Making it was fun even though it didn't turn out like I thought it would. Alena was a few months old by then so we put her footprints and our handprints in it. It looked quite cool in the end.

So we took it up to my parents' garden, chose a tree, dug a hole and buried the ipu with the whenua inside. Alena was six months old by then. It was more of a casual thing than a ceremony, and we took lots of photos. We chose that particular place because Haymon's family don't live on whānau land and there's always the possibility they could move. So her whenua is buried in a place that will always be our whānau home, and a place she can return to and feel part of.

It's lovely for my parents to have this connection, to walk around at home and know that this tree is this grandchild's and this tree is another's. It's part of Māori tikanga, the continuity of the whānau, linking past generations to present and future ones. Having your whenua buried on whānau land ties you to the land and your iwi (people). That way, you'll always have somewhere you belong in the world.

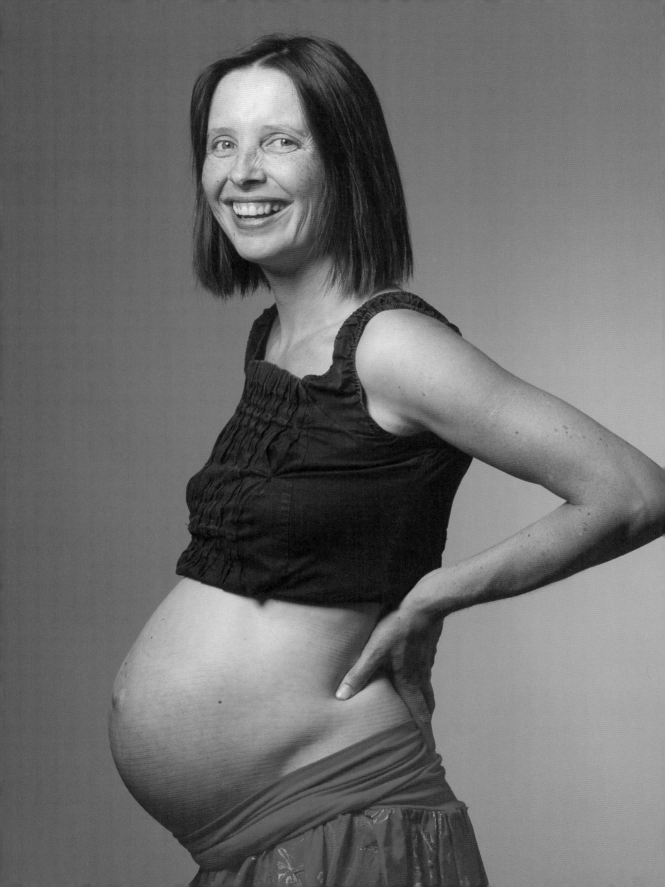

CHAPTER 5

The last three months

(Weeks 28–40+)

1. What's happening?

The baby

Pregnancy at 28 and 32 weeks

28 weeks pregnant

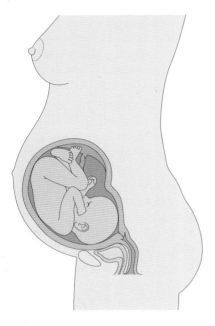

32 weeks pregnant

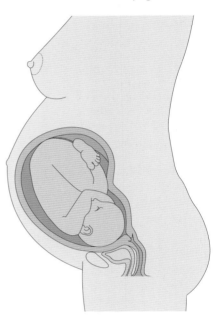

By 28 weeks, the baby measures about 35cm long and weighs about 1kg. She continues to grow a little in length, but she spends most of this last stage of pregnancy getting fatter, especially around her body. She is covered in a thick layer of white creamy material (vernix), which protects her skin from the amniotic fluid surrounding her. As pregnancy progresses, she gradually loses the hair on her body, and the vernix becomes thinner until, by 40 weeks, it is virtually gone.

The baby's heart continues to beat quite fast compared with that of an adult – normally between 110 and 160 beats a minute. During this time she also starts to make swallowing movements. Babies 'drink' some amniotic fluid in the last three months of pregnancy, and their kidneys start to work too, so they begin to pass urine into the bladder and out into the amniotic fluid. However, the waste products we normally associate with urine are removed from the baby's blood via the placenta.

'I'm now 28 weeks, and my baby is moving lots … at least, something is happening in there … it's still hard to believe it really is a baby, and that it's going to get even bigger before it comes out …'

Can the baby see or hear at this time? It is dark inside the uterus, but all the mechanism for vision is developed, and some women say their baby becomes more active if they sunbathe. Similarly, the baby's hearing is also well developed, and some women report increased or even rhythmic activity if they are exposed to loud noise or music.

Many babies develop noticeable patterns of restfulness and wakefulness. In some babies these patterns carry on after they're born, so that a baby who was very active in the mornings before birth is likely to be wide awake in the mornings after birth. Babies can get 'hiccups', too, which mothers feel and which can sometimes be heard when the midwife listens to the baby's heart at antenatal visits.

Lie of the baby within the uterus

The most usual 'lie', or position, for the baby from the 28th week onwards is with her head down (cephalic presentation). At 28 weeks, around 70 per cent of babies are head down; by 32 weeks, 85 per cent are. By 40 weeks only 3–4 per cent remain bottom down (breech presentation).[1]

Possible positions of the baby within the uterus

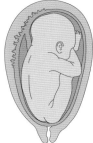 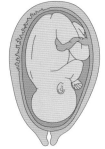 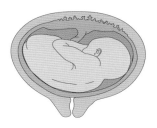

Breech (bottom down)   Cephalic (head down)   Transverse (back/shoulder down)

Breech presentations may sometimes occur for no particular reason, but are more likely if the shape of the uterus is altered or the baby is abnormal in some way. Babies can sometimes be born vaginally in a breech position, although complications may mean that a Caesarean section is required (see pp.225 and 278).

A few babies adopt a transverse lie, but this is very unusual after 37 weeks, especially in a first pregnancy. It generally occurs only if there is something obstructing the normal tendency to adopt an up-and-down position. A baby cannot be born vaginally in the transverse position, and this sometimes complicates premature births, because transverse lie is more common earlier in pregnancy. Caesarean section is necessary to avoid obstructed labour. In developing countries, where access to obstetric intervention is limited, transverse lie is still a major cause of death for mothers and babies during labour.[3]

Possible causes of a breech presentation near the end of pregnancy[2]

- no particular reason
- multiple pregnancy
- placenta praevia (see p.192)
- uterus is an unusual shape (e.g. bicornuate uterus, fibroids)
- too much or too little amniotic fluid
- mother's pelvis is misshapen

Note: these situations may occasionally lead to a transverse lie.

Maternal changes

Blood and body fluid

To supply all the extra blood required for the placenta, the total amount of blood circulating within the mother's body gradually increases. By the last phase of pregnancy, this increase is sizeable. To cope, the mother's heart must beat faster and her blood vessels carry more blood. In some women this increased blood flow enhances their appearance, giving them the classic 'bloom of pregnancy'. In others, varicose veins appear and ankles become swollen, due in part to the increased blood flow. Some women may also experience nasal congestion as a result of the increased blood flow, and may mistake it for a cold. The congestion disappears almost as soon as the baby is born. There is also increased pressure on the veins in the abdomen, which makes varicose veins and swollen ankles more obvious.

The uterus

The uterus continues to enlarge to accommodate the growing baby. At this stage, the lower part of the uterus expands more than the upper part, especially between 32 and 35 weeks. The muscles in its wall become very thin, stretched firmly around the bag of 'waters' containing the baby. In this last phase of pregnancy, the muscles start to contract from time to time in preparation for labour, although some women experience these mild contractions from as early as 24–26 weeks. Women notice these so-called 'Braxton-Hicks' contractions increasingly towards the end of the pregnancy.

The cervix (opening of the uterus) is also changing. It becomes softer and thicker, and small glands there become more active. There may be a noticeable increase in a white vaginal discharge, and/or a plug of mucous that fills the opening in the cervix.

Breast changes

Within the breasts, the milk-producing areas (alveoli) and drainage channels (ducts) are now becoming fully developed under the control of hormones – oestrogen, progesterone and prolactin.[4] Small amounts of milk, called colostrum, start being produced, and some women notice a few drops at the nipple, especially during sexual activity.

The placenta

By now this remarkable organ, which is still wholly responsible for the baby's health, has increased in size to weigh about 300g, and will continue to grow to about 500g. It is usually positioned high in the uterus, on either the front or the back wall, but occasionally it is positioned low down. If it is very low, over or near the cervix, it may cause a problem known as placenta praevia.

Placenta praevia

If the placenta is overlying the cervix, a major problem will occur during late pregnancy and then in labour. As the opening of the cervix starts to dilate, all or part of the placenta may separate and bright red bleeding will occur. In this situation the baby will die and the mother may haemorrhage to the point where her own life is at risk.

Because of the way the uterus enlarges, placenta praevia may not be evident at a 20-week anatomy scan (conversely, the placenta may appear to be very low-lying at 20 weeks, but as pregnancy progresses, the placenta naturally sits higher in the uterus). If the placenta is found to be low-lying at the 20-week scan, the radiologist will suggest to your LMC that a repeat ultrasound be undertaken at 30–32 weeks to determine its location at that stage. A true placenta praevia will often not be apparent until later in pregnancy, when the lower segment of the uterus stretches greatly (in comparison with the upper portion), causing the attached placenta to stretch and then bleed, a little at first, but then with increasing frequency.

As long as a placenta praevia is detected before labour begins, a planned Caesarean section can largely avoid the associated risks – that's one reason why any bleeding at all in later pregnancy, even a very slight amount, needs to be checked out urgently. Depending on the position of the placenta, not all cases of placenta praevia are life-threatening, but the situation needs to be urgently assessed by the woman's LMC and reviewed by a specialist obstetrician to ensure a safe delivery for both mother and baby. Placenta praevia is more common in women who have already had several pregnancies and/or Caesarean sections.[5]

Signs of a possible placenta praevia

- a little vaginal bleeding

- then, a few days later, a little more vaginal bleeding

- another painless bleed, which may be heavier than before

- an ultrasound scan late in pregnancy showing the placenta very near to, or over, the cervical opening (cervical os)

Placenta praevia

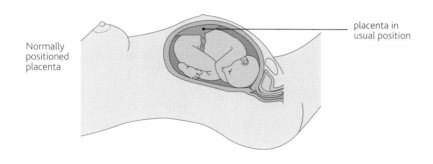

Normally positioned placenta

placenta in usual position

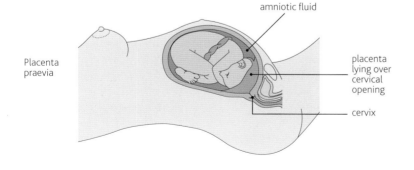

amniotic fluid

Placenta praevia

placenta lying over cervical opening

cervix

2. Feelings

Reaching the 28-week mark is a real milestone in any pregnancy. From now on, if your baby is born early she stands a reasonable chance of survival if good neonatal care is available. Does this knowledge make a difference to how you feel? For some women it does – they feel that only now can they start the practical planning for their baby, believing that it's all really going to happen. Other women start wondering just how big this 'bump' is going to get.

By now, most women certainly look pregnant. Reactions can be very different. Do you feel proud to be pregnant? Or are you conscious of discrimination at work because of your pregnancy? Do you want care and attention? Or do you want a bigger workload than ever because you feel so full of energy?

Feelings change tremendously over this last trimester. Energy levels tend to drop off until, by the last month, most pregnant women are feeling tired and often uncomfortable.

Practical problems

Having a large tummy makes for a number of problems, and even those women who manage pregnancy relatively easily find some adjustments are necessary.

- Sleeping is harder – you are really limited to sleeping on your side (see p.201). Lying on your front is impossible, and lying on your back can make you feel faint and sick towards the end of pregnancy. Cutting your toenails, and even putting on laced or buckled shoes, may be hard work.

- The enlarging uterus tends to press on the bladder, making frequent trips to the toilet a reality once again. Pressure on the bowel, as well as the continued effect of the hormones of pregnancy on the smooth muscle of the intestine, sometimes causes constipation as well.

- Heartburn (see p.138) may be a problem in these last three months. Some women find that the nausea and vomiting of early pregnancy return to plague them in the last month or so. This may occur particularly in the evenings when they feel tired after a day's work or activities.

- Bending and lifting become more difficult (see box on p.202), and your centre of gravity changes to put extra strain on your back. Swollen ankles and aching legs are common, particularly towards the end of the day.

Wrist pain from carpal tunnel syndrome

Occasionally, the extra fluid retention associated with pregnancy results in pain in one or both wrists, and/or the thumb and index finger. This is because the main nerve supplying that area of the hand naturally passes through a narrow tunnel of connective tissue (the carpal tunnel). Even a little fluid retention can cause pressure on the nerve at this point, resulting in pain and/or numbness or tingling. The problem can also occur when breastfeeding (see p.351).

Varicose veins and haemorrhoids (piles)

Both of these conditions occur when veins carrying blood back to the heart become congested, and their walls are a bit more relaxed under the influence of the hormones of pregnancy.

In the legs, the deep veins (which can't be seen) have valves that help the blood flow back up the legs, working against gravity. In some people these valves tend to break, forcing more blood than normal to travel back up the legs through the small veins on the surface. These small superficial veins become big and twisted under the extra strain, and can be seen in the legs.

The tendency to get varicose veins is largely a genetic one, but the condition is likely to be worse in people who are overweight or pregnant, because the blood flow back to the heart is restricted by extra pressure in the pelvis and abdomen. Exercise, and wearing support stockings, can help (see p.168).

Around the anus (back passage), the veins can also become congested. Constipation, straining to pass a bowel motion and pregnancy all put extra pressure on these veins, restricting the blood flow. Haemorrhoids, or piles, are lumps that form around the anus where the veins are congested, and can be painful. The treatment for haemorrhoids described in Chapter 7 (p.322) can also be used during pregnancy.

Symphysis pubis dysfunction (SPD)

As pregnancy progresses, there is a natural softening of the ligament that holds the two front bones of the pelvic ring (the symphysis pubis) together, making the pelvic ring more mobile in preparation for labour. For some women this softening of the ligaments causes considerable pain and discomfort low down in the abdomen, sometimes extending down the front of the legs. The ligaments in the two joints at the back of the pelvis (the sacro-iliac joints) also soften, so pain at one place may create pain in another.

The symphysis pubis joint

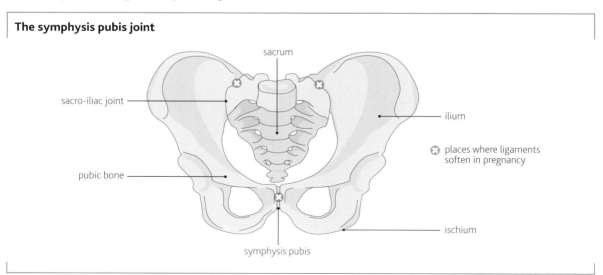

sacrum

sacro-iliac joint

ilium

places where ligaments soften in pregnancy

pubic bone

ischium

symphysis pubis

The problem most often becomes troublesome in the last month or two of pregnancy, but it can occur at any time, including suddenly during labour, during delivery or even after the birth. The pain tends to be made very much worse with movement, especially walking, going up and down stairs, going from sitting to standing, or turning in bed. It can also be hard to bear weight on one leg, making dressing difficult.

There are many things you can do yourself to help the pain (see box). A physiotherapist may also be very helpful – as well as advising you about activity, they can provide a belt for pelvic support, elbow crutches and pain-relief medication if required.[6]

For most women, the pain naturally improves once the pelvic ligaments tighten up again after birth – often this happens within days, but sometimes it takes several weeks.

Dealing with symphysis pubis pain[7]

- Reduce non-essential weight-bearing activities – e.g. climbing stairs, shopping, lifting and carrying.

- Rest when possible, but remain gently active at other times.

- Avoid leg-parting activities – e.g. when getting into a car, put your bottom in first and then bring your feet in, keeping your knees together; to get out, reverse the process. Avoid breaststroke if you go swimming.

- Avoid standing on one leg. Perch on a stool whenever possible and when putting on lower garments.

- Tell your LMC if you are getting this type of pain, so they can help you with appropriate positioning during labour.

Looking forward

All these problems can make pregnancy a real trial for some women, while others are much less troubled. But throughout, remember the end product of it all – your baby.

Sometimes, especially if you're pregnant for the first time, it's hard to look ahead and imagine what life with a baby is going to be like. But remember that pregnancy is only a means to an end, and focusing on the baby often makes it easier to put up with the tiredness and discomfort of being very pregnant.

One way of focusing on the baby is to get her clothes and room ready. Some women enjoy knitting and sewing tiny garments, while others attempt ambitious spring-cleaning programmes with varying degrees of success. Some will be trying to get things finished at work or completing other projects – this can be hard if you're tired and uncomfortable. Be realistic about what's possible in late pregnancy – you are better off working shorter hours and having more rest so that the work and activity you can manage is done well.

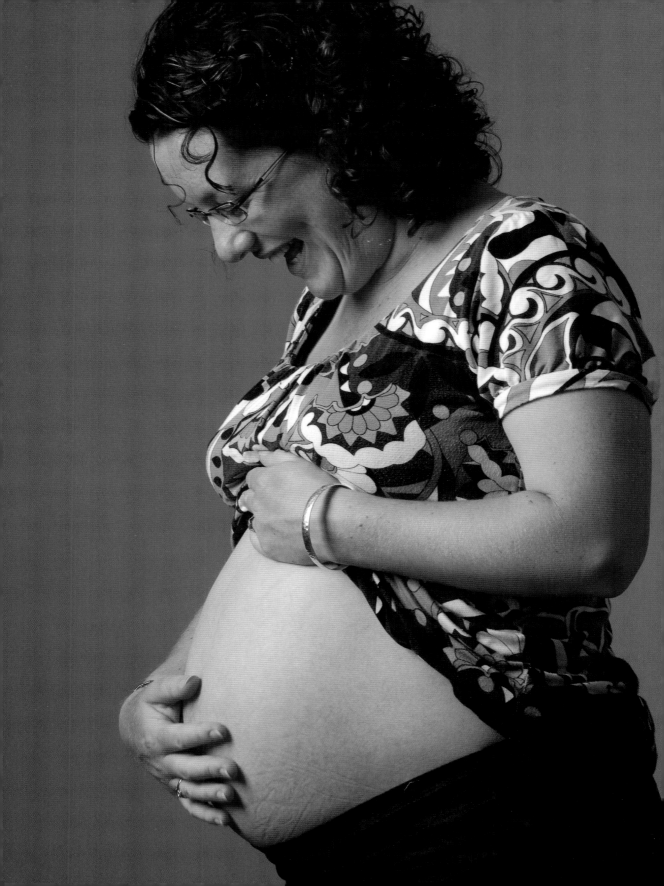

3. Helping yourself

A lot of the problems mentioned in the previous section continue to be helped by regular exercise (see p.124). Any sort of gentle exercise, especially swimming, will help to ease aching legs and varicose veins, reduce ankle swelling, and give you a better sleep at night.[8]

Looking after your pelvic floor

Keep up the pelvic floor exercises described in Chapter 4 (see p.126). The more you can do these exercises regularly, the more you avoid problems like urinary incontinence (leaking) both before and after the birth. Remember, too, that being able to control these muscles helps during the birth of the baby.

Perineal massage

The perineum is the area between the anus and the vagina, which stretches tremendously when your baby is born. The hormonal changes in pregnancy help to prepare the perineum for this stretching process, but some women find that massaging the area regularly during the last few months of pregnancy also helps. Certainly the massage will acquaint you with the type, although not the intensity, of sensation to be expected as the baby is born.

But with the best will in the world, not all perineums will stretch as much as they need to. Tears or splits in the perineal tissue may occur during birth, or an episiotomy (see p.265) may be necessary. It is more common to have a tear or episiotomy with a first birth; episiotomies are also more common with a vacuum (Ventouse) or forceps delivery (see p.280).[9]

If you want to do some perineal massage to improve the stretching of the tissue, try the exercise described in the box opposite during the last months of pregnancy. For women having their first vaginal birth, there is some evidence that regular perineal massage during the last 5–10 weeks of pregnancy reduces the chances of having an episiotomy, but it doesn't necessarily reduce the risk of tears or splits in the perineal tissue.[10] Many women try perineal massage with a second or subsequent baby, especially if they have a scar on the perineum from the first birth – they find it softens the scar tissue, making it more flexible.

The perineum

urethra —
vagina —
clitoris
vulva
perineum

Perineal massage – step-by-step guide

- Get a mirror, wash your hands, then sit in a semi-reclining position with your back supported and legs apart.
- Look at your perineum in the mirror. Find the midline. Touch the area gently, then more firmly.
- Put a little natural oil (e.g. wheatgerm oil) or vitamin E cream onto the fingers and thumbs of each hand.
- Place your thumbs or index fingers just inside the back 'rim' of the vagina, pressing towards the rectum, gently stretching the opening until you feel a slight burning or tingling. Maintain pressure for about two minutes or until the area feels a little numb. As you apply pressure, concentrate on relaxing your pelvic floor. If you have any previous episiotomy scars, concentrate on this area. (Some women prefer to omit putting the oil on their hands at this stage, as it may irritate the tender vaginal lining.)
- Then, on the outside, place two fingers of each hand in a V formation on either side of the midline and pull up and outwards, pressing lightly on the skin as you do so. If you have not already done so, apply a little oil or cream to your fingers at this stage. This area is surprisingly tender, so the pressure may be painful until you get used to it.
- Repeat until you can press quite firmly and still be comfortable.
- Now place your thumbs on either side of the midline near the back of the vagina and move them apart in opposite directions, pressing firmly. Repeat until you're pressing quite hard. Again, it may be uncomfortable until you're used to it.
- Lastly, place two fingers of each hand so they meet in the midline. Pull the fingers out towards your thighs.
- Repeat daily (or as often as you can), for about five minutes in total. Your partner can do this massage for you, but it's best to try the technique yourself first, and then guide him or her as to the amount of pressure you can tolerate. Avoid the urinary opening, and don't do the exercises if there is any infection or irritation in the area.

Perineal massage

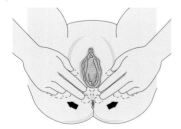

Press firmly and move fingers upwards and apart

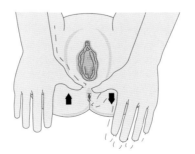

Move thumbs back and forth

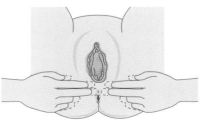

Press firmly and move fingers apart

Looking after your skin

The skin of the abdomen, nipples and surrounding area undergoes dramatic changes during pregnancy. Almost all pregnant women develop some increase in skin pigmentation, often most noticeable as a dark line running down the midline of the abdomen. As the abdominal skin stretches, it is often very itchy and 'stretch marks' (dark red wiggly lines around the abdomen) may appear. The itchiness can be helped by gently rubbing the abdomen with a bland oil, such as almond oil, or an anti-itch preparation containing tar derivatives (your pharmacist will be able to recommend suitable products). Try not to scratch, as this will make matters worse, and avoid soap if possible.

About a quarter of all pregnant women develop stretch marks. Whether you get them or not is largely genetically determined, so there is very little you can do about it. Some women have found that regular massage of the abdominal skin is helpful, but there is still no guarantee that stretch marks won't appear. The marks will gradually fade to a silvery colour and become less conspicuous after your baby is born.[11]

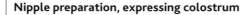

Nipple preparation, expressing colostrum

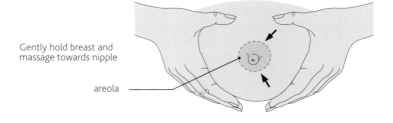

Gently hold breast and massage towards nipple

areola

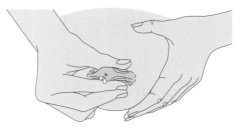

Hold behind the areola and gently apply pressure to express a few drops of colostrum

During pregnancy, the nipples tend to become more prominent and the areola (the pigmented area surrounding the nipple) becomes larger and darker. In the final three months, small amounts of thick yellow fluid (colostrum) may leak from the nipples in preparation for feeding.

For women with inverted or very flat nipples, some nipple preparation (expressing colostrum) may encourage the nipple to protrude (see diagram). However, most women breastfeed easily without doing any nipple preparation, and there is little evidence to suggest that it is really helpful.

Sleeping, bending and lifting

Sleeping on your side becomes increasingly necessary in these final weeks. One side may be better than the other, depending on the position of the baby. The baby may become quite vigorous as soon as you lie down – try to keep reasonably still, and she will gradually settle too.

A soft pillow that moulds under your tummy may help you (and your back) feel more comfortable. Sometimes it can be helpful to use a pillow to support your top leg when lying on your side. A tri-pillow works well (see photo below). Keep your ankle, knee and hip almost horizontal, and make sure your foot is not hanging over the end of the pillow. This can be especially helpful if you are experiencing pain in your lower back.

If heartburn is a problem, try putting one or two extra pillows under your head as well. If this causes back pain, it might be better to put some blocks or thick books under the legs at the head of the bed.

Getting in and out of bed may be a problem, especially if you're short and have a high bed. Getting a stool to stand on will make things easier. Some women have a tendency to faint in pregnancy; if so, avoid lying flat on your back, as this compresses the large blood vessels at the back of the abdomen. Get out of bed slowly (see pp.128–129).

If you are experiencing pain over the symphysis pubis (see p.195), when getting up from a lying position, or getting in or out of a car, make sure you keep your legs together; the relaxed ligaments around the pelvis may result in more pain if you open your legs wide.

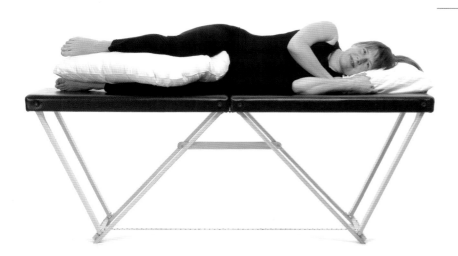

Sleeping position

> **Minimising bending and lifting**
>
> - Buy or borrow a laundry trolley for taking the washing out to the clothes-line, or put a table beside the line to rest the clothes-basket on.
> - Make sure the clothes-line is not too high – if it is, and cannot be adjusted, get a sturdy, wide platform to stand on.
> - Buy or borrow a high stool or find things that you can 'perch' on rather than standing or sitting.
> - Kneel down to do things at floor level, e.g. gardening, picking up toys, getting out files.
> - Absolutely minimise the lifting of toddlers and don't carry them on one hip. Make use of their strong urge to be independent – encourage them to climb into the high chair or cot using a small chair or step while you support them.
> - Remember, if you do have to lift, 'tummy tuck' first (see p.128), bend your knees and keep your back straight. Divide heavy loads into two lighter ones, one for each hand.

Sexual activity (see also p.138)

'I always get so incredibly tired in the last six weeks – sex just seems like too, too much effort.'

Do you still feel like sex? Some women find sex especially good in pregnancy. On the other hand, you may feel too tired, or have lost all interest. This is normal too. Try to talk with your partner about how you feel.

If you do both feel sexy, it's quite safe to have intercourse right up until labour begins, as long as the membranes around the pregnancy sac are intact and there's no threat of bleeding or premature labour. Intercourse and orgasm may set off runs of mild contractions, known as Braxton-Hicks (see p.192). This is quite normal, and may in fact help prepare the uterus for labour. In the last week or two of pregnancy, intercourse and orgasm may trigger the onset of labour if everything is 'ready to go'.

Some advice for partners

A pregnant woman's interest in sex may vary a lot, even from day to day. It's easy for partners to get a bit fed up with this – one minute it's all on, the next minute it's all off! The tiredness and hormonal changes of late pregnancy are largely responsible, so both of you need to be patient for these last few weeks. Remember that pregnancy doesn't last for ever, and it will be possible to enjoy sex again when things get back to normal after the birth.

If you are both in the mood for sex, take things slowly and as gently as you can. Avoid any activity that causes pain. Certain positions are better than others: side-by-side or sitting positions may work best. It's advisable to avoid really deep penetration.

4. When pregnancy becomes complicated

Multiple pregnancy (see also pp.78 and 154)

On average, about 850 sets of twins and ten sets of triplets are born each year in New Zealand.[12] Fraternal twins (who develop from two separate embryos) are becoming more common in developed countries as a result of increasing use of fertility treatments and the increasing age of mothers in general. The rate of identical twins (who have developed from a single embryo) is relatively constant.[13]

Twins (or even triplets) are generally accepted as a bonus in our society, so if you're expecting twins you're likely to be congratulated and considered 'lucky'. Two babies from one pregnancy is indeed a bonus, especially if pregnancy is not an easy time for you and you want more than one child. Twins can add a very special dimension to any family, and a very strong bond of support and friendship often develops between them.

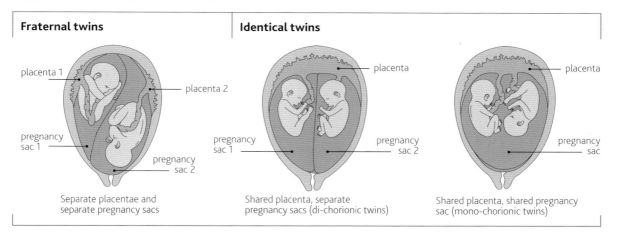

Fraternal twins

placenta 1
pregnancy sac 1
placenta 2
pregnancy sac 2

Separate placentae and separate pregnancy sacs

Identical twins

placenta
pregnancy sac 1
pregnancy sac 2

Shared placenta, separate pregnancy sacs (di-chorionic twins)

placenta
pregnancy sac

Shared placenta, shared pregnancy sac (mono-chorionic twins)

However, carrying more than one baby puts greater stress on both mother and babies, and problems are more likely as a result. Some women expecting twins may develop pre-eclampsia (toxaemia; see p.139) in the last three months of pregnancy, or earlier in some instances. This is thought to be related to the larger placental site in a multiple pregnancy. The possibility of premature labour is higher than normal at any stage after about 20 weeks, and about half of all twins are born prematurely before 37 weeks. In addition, the babies are smaller than normal because space is at a premium in the uterus, and intra-uterine growth restriction (IUGR; see p.142) is more likely. Twins (or triplets) may also be unequal in size, and this can be a disadvantage to both (or all) of the babies. There is a higher than normal risk of stillbirth, and sometimes only one baby will survive. The birth is often more complicated than with a single baby, as twins can get tangled up and obstruct labour. Quite often, one will be a breech, so it is common for twins to be born by Caesarean section. Some identical twins share the same placenta (mono-chorionic twins), and they have a much greater risk of problems than fraternal twins and identical twins who have separate placentas (di-chorionic twins).

Despite all this, plenty of twins have been born over the years without any problems; and today, twin pregnancies do better than ever before. Excellent nutrition, taking early supplements of folic acid, and avoiding smoking and alcohol are even more important than in a single pregnancy, so there is a lot you can do yourself to ensure that your pregnancy is as healthy as possible. In addition, expert obstetric care can help with many (but not all) of the problems mentioned above.

For all these reasons, the earlier a multiple pregnancy is detected, the earlier extra monitoring can be put in place – although this is most important from 20 weeks onwards. Twins are most often found on an ultrasound scan, although occasionally they will first be suspected at a routine antenatal visit. With twins (and even more so with triplets or quads), you just have to expect more antenatal visits, more tests and a closely monitored labour to give these babies optimal care.

Bleeding (antepartum haemorrhage)

In any pregnancy, vaginal bleeding is a sign that all is not well. It should be taken seriously at any time, but after 20 weeks the cause of the bleeding needs to be ascertained promptly. Contact your LMC immediately – if they are not readily available, go straight to the nearest delivery suite or hospital emergency department.

Why such concern?

The bleeding may well be from the placenta, and by late pregnancy the blood supply through the uterus to the placenta is about 600ml per minute. Sudden and very heavy bleeding is rare, but the danger is real – no one can survive blood loss like this for very long. Fortunately, most bleeding is initially slight – maybe only a few spots – but it is a warning not to be taken lightly.

Placental separation (abruption), where part of the placenta comes away from the inner wall of the uterus, can occur after a fall or a direct blow to the woman's abdomen. The force of a car accident can also occasionally cause some placental separation, which is why a check-up is advised, even if the accident seems minor (see p.122). More often there is no obvious cause. Usually, the affected area of the placenta is small and the bleeding light, and there may be some pain. In this situation things often settle down quickly, leaving mother and baby unaffected, although sometimes the baby's growth may slow down.

Occasionally, a larger area of the placenta separates, jeopardising the baby's blood supply and causing quite a lot of bleeding, and usually significant abdominal pain. The pain will sometimes occur before bleeding becomes obvious, as the initial bleeding may be trapped behind the placenta. If this happens, both baby and mother are at immediate risk. Fortunately, significant placental separation is rare.

Placenta praevia (see p.192) usually causes only a little painless bleeding initially. But if the placenta is right over the cervical opening, both mother and baby will be increasingly at risk of more bleeding as pregnancy progresses.

A clot may form between the placenta and the membranes, which sometimes causes the membranes to rupture early, making premature labour more likely. Sometimes a 'show' (a slightly blood-stained, mucousy vaginal discharge) may be the first sign of impending premature labour – another reason why prompt attention from your LMC or obstetric service is called for.

Occasionally, bleeding may come from the cervix or vaginal tissue. This is likely to be light and painless, and generally does not affect the baby. Its cause can be fully investigated after delivery.

So, not all vaginal bleeding in pregnancy is serious. But because the potential for catastrophic bleeding exists, it is important to determine the cause – and in the meantime to act as if it is serious. This usually means admission to hospital (to the antenatal ward if the hospital has one), and an ultrasound scan to determine the position and possible separation of the placenta.

Causes of bleeding in the last three months of pregnancy[14]

- a 'show' marking the onset of early labour (which will be considered premature if before 37 weeks)
- a 'show' associated with cervical incompetence
- a heavier, bloodier 'show', which may mean that this is not early labour, but that the cervix is already fully dilated and the baby is about to be born (especially if the 'show' is preceded by ongoing backache and abdominal cramps)
- placental separation (abruption)
- placenta praevia
- bleeding from the edge of the placenta
- bleeding from the cervix or vaginal tissue
- unknown

Blood clots (deep vein thrombosis, or DVT)

As if in response to this potential to bleed during pregnancy, hormonal changes alter the clotting ability of the blood. When a woman is pregnant, her blood clots more readily than usual, and this tendency persists and is even more likely for some weeks after her baby is born.

This is a normal physiological change which doesn't usually cause problems, unless there are other things going on that make clots in the blood vessels, especially in the legs, more likely. Immobility, for example in long-distance car or plane travel (see p.122), increases the risk of thrombosis during pregnancy. The risk is between three and ten times higher than for non-pregnant women, although the overall risk is still low.[16]

Clots in the legs are painful, and they also have the potential to break off within the vein in the leg and move to the lungs, interfering with or even stopping normal breathing. This life-threatening situation is known as a pulmonary embolus.

If you do suffer a clot in the leg, then rest is important initially, followed by a gradual increase in exercise. Anticoagulant drugs will prevent the clot

Factors making clots in the blood vessels more likely[15]

- a personal or family history of DVT
- partial obstruction of circulation, e.g. poor posture, being very overweight, significant dehydration, tight bands such as elastic around the legs, long periods of inactivity such as being in bed or travelling
- unusual anatomy, e.g. very narrow or twisted blood vessels to the brain or kidneys
- hardening of the arteries (atherosclerosis), making some blood vessels narrower than usual (very uncommon in women during their child-bearing years)
- no obvious cause

getting bigger, and prevent new clots forming. Several anticoagulant drugs are available; heparin is currently considered safest for the unborn baby, but it has to be given by frequent injection. You will probably be admitted to hospital initially until the risk of a pulmonary embolus has reduced. There, your situation can be monitored, and the pros and cons of heparin treatment carefully considered.

Severe abdominal pain in later pregnancy

This also needs to be checked out promptly, especially if it has come on suddenly, and does not come and go but steadily increases in intensity. Contact your LMC immediately – if they aren't readily available, go straight to the nearest delivery suite or hospital emergency department.

Concealed bleeding from placental separation could be the cause (see p.204); if so, urgent management in hospital is usually required. Other serious causes of ongoing pain in later pregnancy include appendicitis and pyelonephritis (see p.117). These also require hospital care, and may precipitate labour. Pain just below your ribs (from the liver capsule) may indicate severe pre-eclampsia (toxaemia; see p.139), especially if the pain is associated with high blood pressure, visual disturbances, headaches and irritability.

Very occasionally, significant abdominal pain will herald the onset of premature or abnormal labour, sometimes in association with one of the problems mentioned above. In any event, contact your LMC straight away. The pain of contractions in normal labour usually comes and goes in a recognisable pattern, and your LMC will be able to advise you on this.

The other problem that might cause significant abdominal pain is symphysis pubis dysfunction (pain from the softening of the ligaments in the pelvis; see p.195). However, this pain is usually distinctive, as it tends to come on gradually, and is more localised to the pelvic bones and lower back, rather than across the whole abdomen.

Important causes of severe abdominal pain in later pregnancy

- placental separation
- appendicitis
- severe pre-eclampsia
- twisted ovarian cyst
- pyelonephritis and/or other urinary tract infection
- bowel obstruction
- premature and/or abnormal labour
- symphysis pubis dysfunction

The Rhesus factor

All human beings have different antibodies in their blood, many of them genetically determined. There are two main blood group systems in each person's blood. One is the ABO group, in which individuals are either O, A, B or AB in type. 'O' implies lack of a particular protein or antigen, and 'A' or 'B' implies its presence. The other group is the Rhesus (Rh) group, in which individuals are either Rh-positive or Rh-negative. Of the total population, 85 per cent are Rh-positive and 15 per cent are Rh-negative. Thus the names of the common blood groups are a combination of the two systems:

- O-positive and O-negative
- A-positive and A-negative
- B-positive and B-negative
- AB-positive and AB-negative.

This means that people who are O-negative lack both the AB antigens and the Rhesus antigen.

A pregnant woman may have a different blood group from her unborn baby. Women who are Rh-negative have the potential to become sensitised (i.e. to develop antibodies) to the blood of their babies during delivery if their babies are Rh-positive. This can also happen during amniocentesis or miscarriage, or when there is bleeding during pregnancy for any reason. This means that the Rh-negative mother now carries antibodies that reject Rh-positive blood. This is not a problem immediately, but will cause a bad reaction if she has a blood transfusion or becomes pregnant with another baby who is Rh-positive. The latter situation can severely affect her baby: Rhesus antibodies cross the placenta and attack the baby's Rhesus positive red cells, causing the baby to become anaemic. If this is severe, the unborn baby develops heart failure. This sensitisation in the mother does not usually affect her first baby, but with each successive pregnancy the reaction becomes more marked.

It is possible to avoid this sensitising process by introducing a tiny amount of the Rhesus antibody into a pregnant woman's blood at or just after delivery (or at any other time where the mixing of the mother's and the baby's blood is possible – see p.208) in a process similar to vaccination. This antibody is known as anti-D, and is available to all Rh-negative women (although it is effective only in a woman who is not yet sensitised).[17] If used appropriately, anti-D will almost always prevent Rhesus disease.

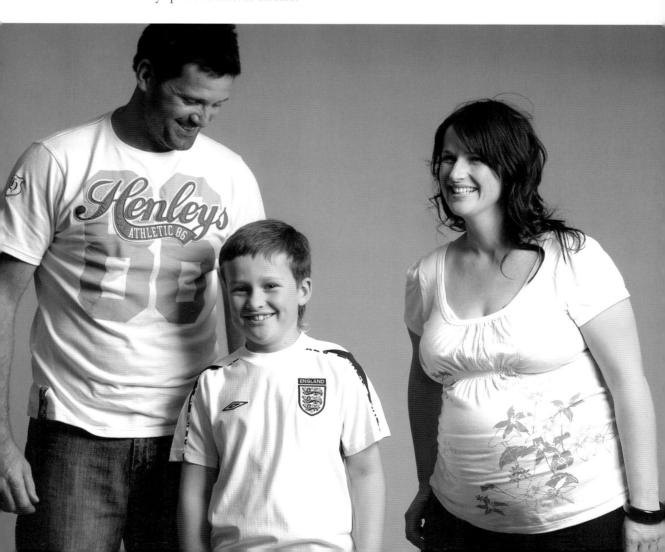

Avoiding Rhesus disease – current New Zealand recommendations[18]

- All pregnant women should have their blood tested and existing antibodies measured early in every pregnancy, to find those who are Rh-negative.
- All pregnant women should have antibody levels checked later in every pregnancy to detect any rise. This is usually done at 28 weeks and 36 weeks of pregnancy.
- All Rh-negative women are offered and should have anti-D at the time of any termination, miscarriage or amniocentesis (where the potential for the mixing of maternal and foetal blood exists).
- All babies of Rh-negative mothers should have their antibody levels and blood group checked (from the cord) at birth.
- If the mother's antibody level rises, either in pregnancy or at birth, the baby should be closely monitored. The baby can be given new, non-sensitised blood through an 'exchange transfusion'. This is usually done soon after birth, but in severe situations it is also possible to give the transfusion to the baby while still in the mother's uterus.
- All Rh-negative mothers with Rh-positive babies (identified from the cord blood) are offered an injection of anti-D. This tiny dose of Rhesus antibody needs to be given within 72 hours of the birth to prevent the woman becoming sensitised (developing antibodies) to her baby's blood. This means that her next pregnancy is very much less likely to be affected by Rhesus disease. (If the baby can be shown to be Rh-negative also, the injection can be omitted, but in any situation where doubt exists, it should be given.)
- After having anti-D, the woman's blood needs to be checked to ensure that the dose was sufficient. Sometimes a second dose is needed.
- The same regime needs to be followed with every pregnancy.

Heart disease in pregnancy

Because pregnancy puts extra strain on the heart and the circulatory system, women with significant heart disease need to consider the effects of pregnancy carefully. Until the last 40 years or so, women with heart disease (particularly congenital abnormalities of the valves or chambers of the heart) were either unable to become pregnant, or if they did, often miscarried or did not survive. However, with advances in cardiac surgery, women with congenital heart defects are increasingly able to conceive and successfully bear children. Even so, pregnancy for women who have undergone cardiac surgery is still a challenge; specialist obstetric and cardiology care is usually needed to keep both the woman and her baby well.

Depending on the circumstances, bed rest, rest in hospital and repeated adjustment of drugs may be necessary during the last three months of pregnancy. Premature birth is more likely, as it is the last weeks of pregnancy that place most strain on the heart, potentially compromising both the mother's and the baby's circulation. Once a baby is well able to survive in special care, premature birth may be less risky than the pregnancy continuing any longer.

Babies of women with congenital heart problems are also at increased risk of inheriting similar problems. Extra diagnostic scans to check on the baby's well-being mean that breathing or circulation problems at birth can be anticipated.[19]

Premature birth

Babies born before 37 weeks of pregnancy are not fully mature, and find the early weeks of life difficult. Generally, the more premature the baby, the tougher the fight for survival. But unless the baby has some serious abnormality, her chances of survival without major problems are good after 28–30 weeks, with expert neonatal care (see p.331).[20]

Premature labour may be unexpected, and often proceeds very rapidly. This makes it a very stressful experience. The following symptoms at any time in pregnancy should make you suspect premature labour, and act accordingly:

- a blood-stained vaginal discharge ('show') or bleeding
- runs of quite strong contractions, which get more frequent
- a lot of low abdominal pain or low backache
- suspected breaking of the waters.

If you think you are in premature labour, seek help immediately from your LMC, or at your nearest medical centre or hospital. Everyone (including you) will be relieved if it turns out to be a false alarm, but if it's not, it's wise to be where the best help is available.

If you are in premature labour, the best place to be is in a hospital that provides expert neonatal intensive care. Not all hospitals have this, but they will arrange for you (or you and your baby) to be transferred to a hospital where the required care is available.

A Caesarean section may be the best option if the baby is just too small to cope well with labour. A Caesarean section may also be quicker if the baby is in a life-threatening situation – for example, if there is heavy bleeding.

Premature labour is unusual. But it can happen in any pregnancy, so be alert to the warning signs and symptoms.

'I went to my doctor at 34 weeks for my routine check. I'd had a lot of low pain during the night, been going to the toilet a lot – I thought it was a urine infection. Well, the next thing I was in hospital and Timothy was born – feet first – two hours later!!'

Causes of premature labour in the last three months of pregnancy

- nothing obvious
- bacterial vaginosis (see p.87)
- multiple pregnancy
- pre-eclampsia (toxaemia)
- diabetes
- serious infection/illness in the mother (e.g. bladder infection, pyelonephritis, appendicitis)
- antepartum haemorrhage (see p.204)
- something wrong with the baby

Stillbirth (see also p.144)

All the factors that make premature labour more likely are also associated with a higher incidence of stillbirth. Modern obstetric and neonatal care is able to save more of these 'at risk' babies than ever before, but there are still a number of babies who die within the uterus in late pregnancy or during labour. Sometimes no cause is found, and this is especially hard to understand and cope with.

Women who lose a baby in this way need time to grieve, time to spend alone, and time to spend with their partners. Some parents gain much comfort from holding and dressing their baby, taking photographs and getting foot and hand prints, naming the baby, and blessing her before saying goodbye.

Post-mortem

If you are in this situation, you may be asked about a post-mortem. This is a thorough examination of a dead body, carried out by a doctor who has specialised in pathology. It is done to try to determine the cause of death where this is not clear.

The information gained may help you and your partner in planning future pregnancies, and may also help prevent future stillbirths for others. There are some situations where a post-mortem is required by law, but more often it is a request which you may refuse.

Burial

After 28 weeks of pregnancy, a formal burial or cremation is required by law and this may be accompanied by a funeral. Many bereaved parents gain much from a funeral service, and say that it helped them to come to terms with their loss.

It is usual to contact a funeral director to make the arrangements. Most funeral directors are happy to accommodate any requests you may have, and to arrange payment by instalment if necessary. It is also possible to arrange the funeral yourself.

You may find a meeting with one of the hospital chaplains especially helpful. They are available to everyone, not just those who have a nominated religion. If you prefer, your own minister or church elder, pakeke or kaumātua (tribal elder) can visit you in hospital – most hospitals have a very 'open door' policy in this situation, and are happy for you to have whoever you want to be with you in your grief.

You may want to leave hospital as soon as you can and, except in a few instances where your own health situation precludes it, you are free to do so within a few hours of the birth. Some women, though, feel they need more time in the 'neutral' hospital environment before facing going home. Either way, your LMC, hospital team and other hospital staff should respect your wishes.

Help and support

Your LMC can continue to care for you once you are home, and can then suggest other people to help you and your immediate family. Your GP, practice nurse and trained grief counsellors may all be appropriate people. The Stillbirth and Neonatal Death Support Association (SANDS) can also be a very helpful source of information and support. (See Appendix: Stillbirth.) Nearly every family in this sad situation benefits from expert help, so don't be afraid to ask.

'All the time I kept thinking – maybe they're wrong, maybe the baby's alive, just maybe the baby's alive … then she was born and I couldn't believe how beautiful she was. Very pale, but not really white – the most perfect beautiful doll I've ever seen. She wasn't alive – but somehow it helped to see how calm and beautiful she looked – untroubled by the trauma around her.'

5. Continuing health care

Antenatal visits

During the last three months of pregnancy, your LMC will want to see you more frequently – often every two weeks until the last month, and then every week until you go into labour.

Things change more rapidly towards the end of pregnancy, and there is more to check for. You will probably have more questions to ask on all manner of topics, and more frequent visits will give you the opportunity to voice your concerns. There is also a better chance that problems will be detected promptly.

Routine checks

All the routine checks mentioned in Chapter 4 (weight, blood pressure, urine, feeling the baby and listening for the heartbeat) are still done, and the same potential problems checked for. Pre-eclampsia (toxaemia), diabetes and unexpected changes in the size of the uterus can all develop at any time.

Checking the baby's position

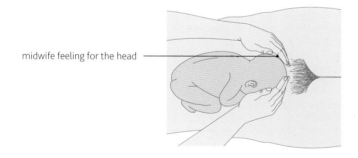

midwife feeling for the head

The baby's position

The position of the baby is determined at each visit. From 28 to 34 weeks, it can change from week to week. But beyond this time, the baby increasingly tends to assume the position she is going to be born in.

It is important to detect a breech presentation or a transverse lie early on (see p.191). During the last month, the position of the baby's head and its relation to the mother's pelvic ring are determined. To do this, your LMC will place their hands on your abdomen just above the pelvis and push quite firmly. It may be rather uncomfortable. You can minimise the discomfort by passing urine just beforehand so that your bladder is empty, and by trying to relax your tummy muscles as much as you can, as this makes your baby easier to feel. (See p.224.)

The baby's health

In these last few months, your LMC will focus as much on the baby's health as on yours. If serious problems are detected, it's increasingly possible to do something about them with appropriate intervention so that you will have a healthy baby.

It's possible for your LMC to check your baby's health in a number of ways. At your regular antenatal visits, the continued growth of your baby can be estimated by:

- checking that your weight gain is within the normal range
- checking the size of your uterus in comparison with the chart in Chapter 4 (see p.146)
- measuring the fundal height (distance from the pubic symphysis to the top of the uterus)
- measuring your abdominal girth (distance around your middle at waist level)
- listening for and counting your baby's heartbeat (normal range is 110–160 beats per minute); this is more accurate after 32 weeks, but is not always done if the baby's movements are good

Listening for the baby's heartbeat

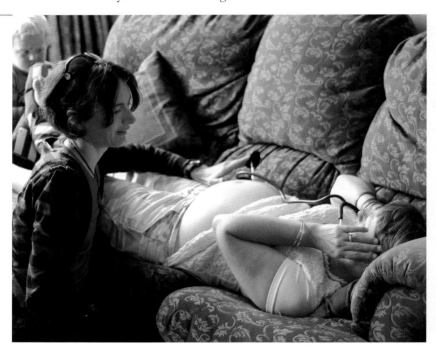

- asking you about the frequency of the baby's movements. Noting the frequency of movements in late pregnancy is quite an accurate way of checking an unborn baby's health. You may be asked to keep a 'kick chart' (see box opposite). You will probably become aware of some sort of pattern during the day – periods when the baby moves a lot, and periods when she is quiet and inactive.

Step-by-step guide to keeping a kick chart

- Keep the chart in a prominent place, e.g. on the fridge door.
- Start at 9 a.m. every day. Use an alarm clock or watch alarm if you forget.
- Each time you feel the baby move, count one movement. (Each separate movement counts as one – some are long, some are short, some are small and some are vigorous.)
- Continue until you have noted ten separate movements. Now place a cross on the chart for that day at the appropriate time, e.g. 10.30 a.m.
- There is nothing more to write now until the next day. If you notice long periods in which the baby is very quiet when she is normally active, contact your LMC.
- ACTION. If you have counted fewer than ten movements between 9 a.m. and 4 p.m., ring your LMC. A marked decrease in movements may indicate that your baby is not well. Ring the number you have been given promptly – don't wait until the next day. Your LMC will usually suggest that you have a CTG (cardiotocograph) reading done. Your local hospital will have a machine to do this (see p.214).

Possible tests in the last three months

Routine blood tests

- *Blood count.* Checks for any anaemia (including iron depletion).
- *Maternal antibodies.* Carried out to detect any changes from previous test (important in Rhesus disease).
- *Blood sugar test.* Checks for the development of gestational diabetes (see p.141). This may involve giving you a sugary drink, then taking several blood samples over about one to two hours. It is a much more accurate test for diabetes than a urine test. Some women have sugar in their urine but their blood sugar test result is normal; they are not diabetic.
- *Tests for early pre-eclampsia (toxaemia) and kidney and liver function.* Often done routinely in first pregnancies or first pregnancies with a new partner, but not necessarily in later pregnancies unless a woman has had pre-eclampsia in a previous pregnancy.

Urine tests

In addition to the routine test for protein and sugar, a mid-stream urine (MSU) test may be done at any time if infection is suspected (see p.104).

Vaginal swab tests

These are done if there is concern that a vaginal infection may be present. A persistent smelly greenish vaginal discharge, especially if you are also feeling unwell and have a temperature with no other apparent cause, may indicate a vaginal infection that could affect your baby after birth. A streptococcal infection (group B streptococcus, or GBS) is one such possibility; if this is confirmed, antibiotics may be advised to prevent your newborn baby being unwell with pneumonia or septicaemia. GBS can also cause urinary tract infections, and infection of the uterus in women after birth. Preventive treatment with antibiotics is much easier and more effective than trying to treat these serious conditions once they occur.[21]

Swabs may also be suggested if a herpes infection is suspected late in pregnancy, or for women who have a tendency to get recurrent herpes infections. Painful watery blisters with or without a vaginal discharge late in pregnancy may indicate a herpes infection. If this is so, the herpes virus can be transferred to the baby during birth. Because babies can become very unwell if infected, treatment with an anti-viral drug such as acyclovir, and/or a Caesarean section, may be advised to prevent this.[22]

Cardiotocograph (CTG)

This machine or monitor is designed to measure an unborn baby's heartbeat and the contractions of the uterus at the same time. It records both measurements on a long, continuous strip of paper.

CTG tracing

The uppermost line shows normal variation in the baby's heartbeat. The middle row of black bars shows the baby's movements. The lower line shows uterine contractions.

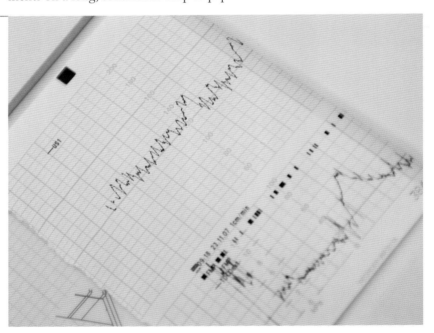

Changes in the rate at which the baby's heart is beating also indicate how well she is doing in the uterus. It is the pattern of change that is significant, and it takes considerable skill to interpret a CTG tracing. Your LMC will be able to tell you what the tracing means, and if in any doubt will seek a second opinion, even if no further action is required.

On a normal tracing, the heartbeat is 110–160 beats per minute, but this varies from beat to beat as the baby responds to her environment within the womb. The tracing will also show a change if the mother moves or has a mild contraction, or if there is a loud noise. The baby may then move, and her heartbeat will change, in response.

'The baby didn't move all day – I thought it was dead. Having the graph was wonderfully reassuring.'

The measurements are taken using two small, round, plastic or metal plates, which must lie in close contact with the mother's abdomen to get a reading. Contact is improved if a special jelly is used between the skin and the plate that detects the baby's heartbeat, and if each plate is held firmly in position by a strap that goes right around the woman's 'waist'. During pregnancy this is generally comfortable, but it can be uncomfortable during labour.

Pelvimetry

Sometimes there is concern that the mother's bony pelvic ring will not be big enough to allow her baby's head and/or shoulders to pass through unimpeded. If so, measuring the baby's head in relation to the mother's pelvic ring will give valuable information about the safest method of delivery. In some situations, a Caesarean section may be warranted.

The accurate measuring of the pelvic ring, both at the top (inlet) and at the bottom (outlet), is known as pelvimetry. It used to be done by taking several X-rays at different angles, and then calculating the measurements. Pelvimetry can now be done using computerised tomography (CT scan) or magnetic resonance imaging (MRI), involving a series of computerised X-ray pictures. The radiation used is less than that for normal X-rays, and the image created is much superior. Pelvimetry is rarely done – usually only when a woman has had a previous disease, fracture or surgery of the pelvis, has had previous proportion troubles in labour, or is of extremely small stature.

Cases where pelvimetry is sometimes advisable

- very small woman (e.g. shoe size 2 or less), with first baby
- very large baby
- breech position
- previous difficult delivery
- previous Caesarean because baby wouldn't fit through pelvic ring for some reason

The pelvic ring

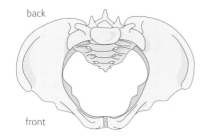

back   front

front   back

Looking down from above – pelvic inlet   Looking up from below – pelvic outlet

Antenatal admission to hospital

Most pregnancies are normal, needing only regular antenatal checks to ensure that all remains well.

A few women, though, have more complicated pregnancies that may best be cared for in hospital. Some women, for example those with diabetes, will have known from the start that hospital care would be necessary towards the end of pregnancy. For others, a problem may be found at a routine antenatal check or when a scan is done.

Having to go into hospital suddenly is never easy in these circumstances. Sometimes it's hard to believe that anything is wrong; sometimes, the reasons don't seem at all clear. If you are faced with admission to hospital before your baby is born, there are some things you can do beforehand to make it all a bit easier:

- Talk to your LMC as soon as possible. Get as much information about your condition as you can. Find out who will be looking after you in hospital. Sometimes the purpose of admission may be to find out more about what seems to be wrong, and your LMC may well be able to continue to care for you with specialist obstetric advice. You may be admitted only for the day, or overnight, as a precaution. In other circumstances, your care will need to be transferred to the hospital obstetric team or to a larger hospital some distance away from where you live.

- Ask how long you are likely to be in hospital. Make sure you're clear about what could happen if you're *not* in hospital.

- Ask for books and pamphlets about your condition.

- Find out whether you have time – a few hours, or a day – to get things organised at home.

- Contact your partner or support person as soon as you can. It may be helpful if they can be with you when you talk to your LMC, and it will almost certainly be helpful for them to go to hospital with you for the initial assessment.

- If you have other children, think who you can ask to look after them. If you are on your own, Child, Youth and Family (CYF) may be able to help (see Appendix). Talk to your children as soon as you can. Try to explain what's happening, in terms they will understand.

Day-stay unit/service

Several of the larger hospitals have a short-stay unit for pregnant women; if you are asked to go there, you can expect to be in hospital for just a few hours or perhaps overnight. This is a particularly useful service to check on potential problems. Quite often, you will be able to go home once tests such as repeat blood pressure readings, blood tests and/or CTGs have been done and found to be stable or satisfactory. Some women will end up visiting the day-stay service several times near the end of their pregnancy. These visits may seem disruptive and hugely inconvenient at the time, but they are an excellent way for your LMC to check out potential problems in a more thorough way than they are able to do at home or in a clinic. Often, the results of these further checks will turn out to be quite satisfactory, but occasionally a serious problem will be found that will be best managed in hospital.

In the antenatal ward

If you are admitted to hospital with an ongoing pregnancy problem, you will usually be transferred to the care of a specialist obstetrician and a charge midwife, and their team of doctors, midwives and nurses.

'The charge nurse was very understanding – I couldn't stop crying, I was so worried there was something dreadfully wrong with the baby.'

'I just needed to see my two other children every day. Then I was okay.'

Problems often warranting antenatal admission

- diabetes
- hypertension of pregnancy (pre-eclampsia/toxaemia)
- bleeding during pregnancy, usually after 20 weeks
- threatening premature labour
- multiple pregnancy (twins or more)
- intra-uterine growth restriction (IUGR), if moderate to severe
- where the baby has died in the uterus, or is found to be abnormal
- where the woman's health is at risk because of social circumstances

If you are asked whether a midwifery, nursing, medical or physiotherapy student may see you, think carefully about this. It is your right to refuse, but you can also help other women by ensuring that the students of today are the well-educated, sensitive health professionals of tomorrow. Students welcome feedback, and learn much from people who are prepared to talk to them. You will usually have plenty of time to do this.

There are usually some examinations and tests to be done on the antenatal ward (which in some hospitals may be combined with the post-natal ward), but most of the time you are left to your own devices. It can be frustrating and boring. But it helps to remember that pregnancy does come to an end, and that for most women, having a healthy baby to show for their patience makes it all worthwhile. Normally, partners or support people are not permitted to stay overnight, unless labour seems to be starting or there is some other unusual circumstance.

Staff in an antenatal ward (or general ward in smaller hospitals)

Midwives and nurses

- Charge midwife or nurse – takes overall responsibility for your midwifery and/or nursing care.
- Staff midwives and/or nurses – work in shifts to look after you and your baby.
- Enrolled nurses (no longer available in all hospitals) – have some basic nursing training, and also work in shifts to help look after you.
- Student midwives – work alongside experienced midwives as part of their education.

Care assistants

- Help with the routine maintenance of supplies etc., and carry out some patient care.

Clerical

- Ward clerk – handles all the day-to-day paperwork and answers the phone during office hours. Will bring you a cordless phone and post letters for you.

Cleaners

- They work rostered hours to keep the ward clean and tidy.

Doctors

- Specialist obstetrician(s) – in charge of the obstetric and medical care of their patients. Often there are several specialists attached to a ward.
- Registrar(s) – doctors who have already passed specialist exams and are in the last stages of training to be specialists. They work closely with the specialist and are responsible for your day-to-day obstetric and medical care.
- House surgeons – junior doctors who work closely with the registrar and specialist. They help with day-to-day care and paperwork.
- Trainee interns (final-year medical students) – work alongside the specialist team as part of their training. They have limited responsibility for patients.
- More junior medical students – work alongside the qualified doctors to learn about obstetric care.

Going to pregnancy and parenting classes

'We weren't enthusiastic. We
thought we'd be by far the
oldest couple there – so
we were amazed to find
that there were mostly
people about our age; a few
younger for sure, but quite a
few older, too …'

Most pregnancy and parenting classes are held once or twice a week for several weeks, and most cover similar material (see p.153).

Most classes are organised for women and their partners or support people to attend during the last few weeks of pregnancy, even though you usually need to book in and pay for classes when you're 4–5 months pregnant. But just in case you are unable to attend some or all of the classes for any reason, get hold of some information well in advance of the birth: online information, books, pamphlets and talking to other people can all be helpful. You may go into labour before you have completed, or even started, pregnancy and parenting classes – and you need just as much, if not more, information when having a premature baby.

Basic topics covered in pregnancy and parenting classes include:

- health during pregnancy
- exercises and relaxation techniques
- being a 'pregnant father' or 'pregnant partner'
- baby clothes and equipment
- information about the different stages of labour and the birth – what to expect
- the role of the partner and/or support person during labour
- after the birth, including life with a new baby, choices and decisions regarding vitamin K (immediately after birth, see p.298), and the recommended childhood immunisation programme (see p.396)
- breastfeeding
- sex after childbirth, contraception
- useful organisations.

The exercises are especially important even for second- and third-time mothers. It's hard to learn these from a book, although it can be done. Going to a class is much easier.

If you are planning a home birth, you will also want more information on preparing for a birth at home – contact Home Birth Aotearoa if you haven't already done so (see Appendix). Your local home-birth group can give you lots of practical advice online and sometimes in their own classes.

Pregnancy and parenting education for partners/support people

Most pregnancy and parenting education classes encourage partner participation and welcome support people – whether prospective fathers, partners, grandparents or other family members. In most areas, there is at least one set of classes held in the evenings or on Saturdays so that partners and other support people can attend more easily. Parents Centre (see Appendix) has always promoted this approach (see p.153).

Some organisations run special classes for grandparents, which can be especially helpful if they are likely to be involved in day-to-day care and support in the first weeks. Some same-sex couples recommend looking for same-sex-couple-oriented pregnancy and parenting education from a lesbian

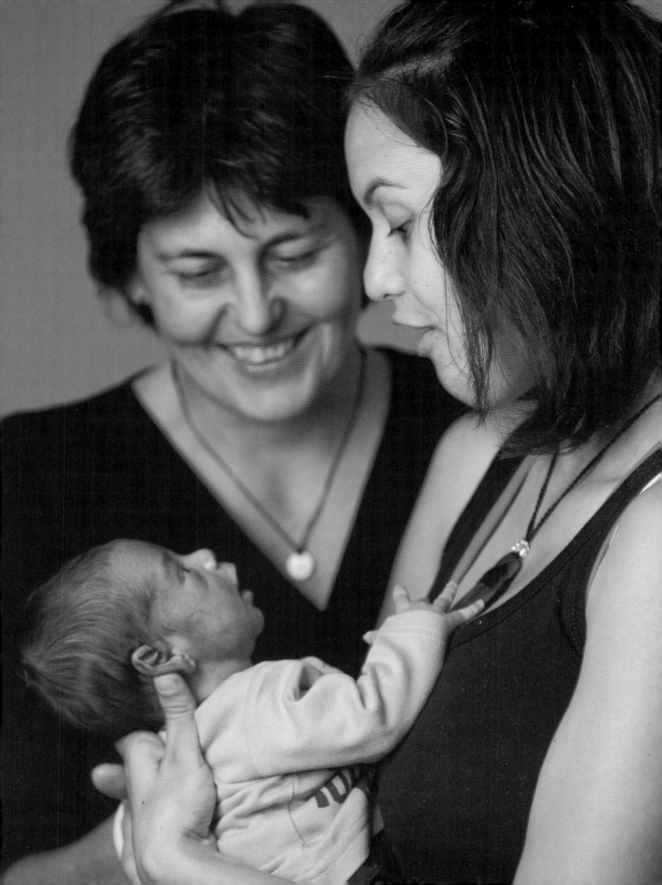

midwife, even if she is not your LMC, but other classes may also be suitable.[23] More general online courses are available too, but checking their credibility may be difficult. Ask your LMC for advice if you are not sure whether the particular course being offered is a reputable one. (See Appendix: Pregnancy and parenting classes.)

For men

If you are about to become a father, going along to pregnancy and parenting education classes will be really helpful. You may not relish the idea, and the thought of being present at the birth may fill you with apprehension. In the end, the decision on whether you will be your partner's 'mainstay' during her labour and delivery is yours.

But you can only make an informed decision if you have as much information as possible. So go along to some classes, read some books and pamphlets, and talk with your partner about her needs and expectations. Be reassured by other men's experiences – many men do attend the births of their children, usually in a very active, involved and fulfilling way (see pp.237 and 253).

But even more important than being at the birth itself is learning some basics about parenting, especially in the early weeks and months. Women having their first baby are not necessarily any better informed than you are, and unless you have the equivalent of a live-in grandmother, often it will be just the two of you who have to deal with an unsettled baby in the middle of the night.[24] Even if you decide in the end that you are not going to attend the birth itself, going to some pregnancy and parenting classes will still be really useful.

Breathing and relaxation for birth[25]

Breathing is something we all do every day without thinking about it. But it's quite possible to control your breathing consciously, and to make the most of every breath. Labour is a situation in which oxygen requirements are high, so it makes sense to take in as much air as possible. However, some types of breathing are very exhausting, so it pays to learn just what you can sustain and yet still breathe efficiently.

Breathing and relaxation go hand in hand with positioning as coping skills for labour. Women who learn good breathing control, combined with relaxation, find they are better able to cope with contractions in labour because they can breathe through them. It also gives them something to focus on and can help them relax. Think of breathing, relaxation and the use of positioning as your first means of pain relief.

Practising breathing for use during your contractions in labour

- To start, simply breathe in through your nose. As you do so, think of filling the base of your lungs so that as you breathe in, your tummy rises gently as your diaphragm (the flat sheet of muscle at the bottom of the chest) moves down. This is known as diaphragmatic breathing.
- Now breathe out through your mouth, slightly emphasising your outward breath; as you do so, think 'I must let go'. Let every bit of tension out of your body and think of opening up your body to give birth.

- Remember, breathe in through your nose, out through your mouth. Keep it slow and rhythmical, slightly exaggerating the outward breath. Literally 'sigh' it out.
- Practise until you can do this slow, deep breathing easily.
- In labour, this type of breathing can help you 'ride over' your contractions. Between contractions you can just breathe normally and rest. Going off to sleep at night is a good time to practise the breathing and relaxation together. Think about what other things help you to relax and make use of them – maybe a bath, shower, wheat pack, music, low lighting, special pillow or massage?

Positioning

Frequent position changes, movement, and use of the upright position will all help the progress of labour. If you choose to sit, use a forward-leaning position. This takes the weight of the heavy, contracting uterus off your spine and helps comfort levels.[26]

The more supported you are, the easier it is to relax. Have a look at the labour and birth photos with women using upright positions effectively (see pp.253 and 269) – this is 'active birth' in action.

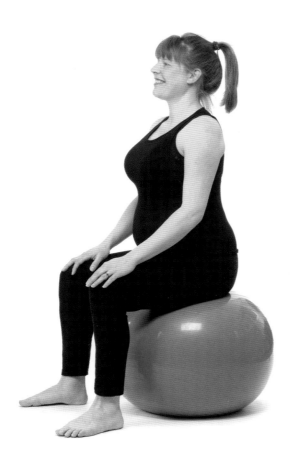

Sitting in the upright position, using a Swiss ball

Pushing

Pushing is really a reflex desire. It's all you want to do when you get to the second stage of labour, when the baby is moving down the birth canal from the cervix to the vaginal opening. While it's not something you need to practise, it's helpful to have some idea of positions that can be used. The best positions are going to be the ones that help your body to open up and make use of gravity. Squatting is ideal, but many women find this too difficult. A high sitting position, or kneeling and leaning forward over a support, or even on all fours, are possibilities. Your midwife will help guide you at this stage in labour, but you will know what is comfortable and helpful for you.

Practising birth positions and breathing

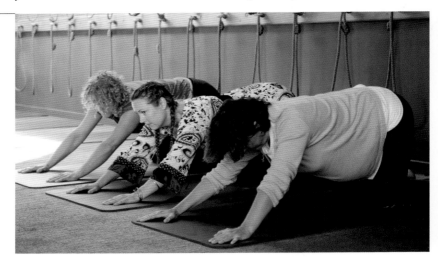

Breathing to stop pushing

There are certain times in labour when it is going to be necessary to stop pushing or to just push gently, even though you may have a very strong desire to do exactly the opposite. Be aware that at the end of the first stage (transition), it will be important not to push until the cervix is fully dilated (see p.263). At the end of the second stage, when the baby's head is emerging through the vaginal opening, everything should happen as slowly as possible to allow the perineum to stretch gently and naturally.

At both of these times, 'panting' will help. You can practise this by breathing in gently through your mouth with a very short breath, then emphasising your outward breath. This type of breathing is a lot lighter, just using the upper chest. As the baby's head is emerging, gentle pushes interspersed with panting can help slow things down and allow time for the tissues to stretch. You will be guided by your LMC, but it is helpful to be aware of what may be asked of you at this time.

6. Planning for birth

Changes at the very end of pregnancy

By 36 weeks, the baby weighs around 2.5kg (5½lb), or less if she is a twin. She has gained a lot of weight over the last six weeks, much of it as fat laid down under the skin. Some babies continue to gain a lot more weight between 36 and 40 weeks, while others slow down their growth as room within the uterus becomes limited. Their movements often become less vigorous because of this limited space, although they should not be any less frequent (see p.212).

During this last month, the baby's lungs become fully mature and ready to breathe air. The sucking and swallowing reflexes become stronger, the kidneys work more efficiently, and the liver functions better.

If the baby is born at 36 weeks or later, she has an excellent chance of surviving, although there may be some initial breathing and sucking problems, and jaundice is more likely (see p.333).

Pregnancy at 36 and 40 weeks

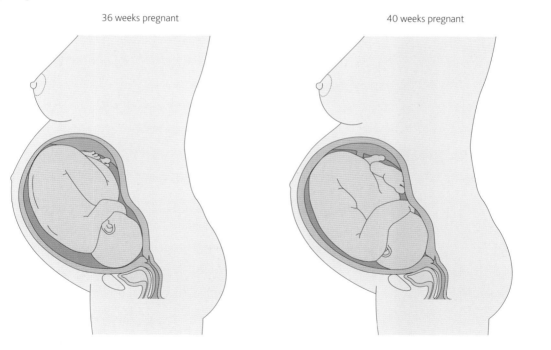

36 weeks pregnant

40 weeks pregnant

Positions of the head near the end of pregnancy

LOA – left occipito anterior

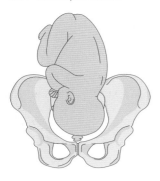

ROP – right occipito posterior

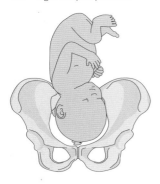

Position of the baby

During this last month, the baby also positions herself within the uterus ready for birth. The head, in nearly all cases, becomes 'engaged' in the pelvic ring and will stay in that position until labour begins. In first pregnancies, the head may engage somewhere between 36 and 38 weeks; in subsequent pregnancies, if may not engage until labour begins.

The clinical term describing the 'typical' position at this stage is left occipito anterior (LOA). This means that the back of the baby's head (occiput) is to the left within the mother's pelvis (and so, therefore, is the baby's back), and is angled slightly towards the front (anterior) of the mother. Other positions the baby may be in when the head is engaged are:

- right occipito anterior (ROA), meaning that the occiput is to the right within the mother's pelvis, and angled towards the front
- left occipito lateral (LOL), meaning that the occiput is to the left within the mother's pelvis, with the back on the left side of the mother
- right occipito lateral (ROL), meaning that the occiput is to the right within the mother's pelvis, with the back on the right side of the mother
- left occipito posterior (LOP), meaning that the occiput is to the left within the mother's pelvis, and angled towards the back
- right occipito posterior (ROP), meaning that the occiput is to the right within the mother's pelvis, and angled towards the back.

The LOA/LOL and ROA/ROL positions are the most favourable for labour, as they allow the head to descend firmly into the pelvis and press on the cervix, which encourages it to dilate. However, LOP and ROP positions often turn into LOA and ROA positions just before or during labour.

Problem positions

Occasionally the baby does not seem to engage in the pelvis, or the position she is lying in could cause problems if engagement does occur. If so, especially in a first pregnancy, certain conditions need to be looked for. Possible reasons for the baby not engaging include:

- wrong dates – the baby may be less mature than calculated
- occipito posterior position – the baby is facing forwards, not backwards
- transverse lie
- breech baby – the baby's bottom and/or legs, instead of the head, are in the pelvis
- the pelvic ring is very small or misshapen
- there is something in the pelvis (e.g. ovarian cyst)
- there is something in the uterus (e.g. low-lying placenta), there are unsuspected twins, or the baby's head is an unusual shape
- none of these! Occasionally, there seems to be no reason.

Helping yourself with a posterior baby

Labour is more difficult when the baby is in a posterior position (LOP, ROP), because the oval shapes of both the baby's head and the mother's pelvis are not well aligned. If room is tight, the head may then be effectively too large to come down through the pelvis, even though the same baby in an anterior position would have no problem.

During the antenatal period, work on keeping or getting your baby's back forward (i.e. anterior). You can help achieve this by:

- never slouching back on the sofa or on a chair while watching TV
- sitting upright while driving your car
- floating face down (with snorkel and goggles) in a pool, or while using a flotation board
- reading books or the newspaper on all fours on the floor, or adopting an all-fours position four to six times a day for 20 minutes each time and relaxing the abdominal muscles while doing so
- turning and sleeping on the opposite side if you consistently sleep on one side.[27]

Turning a breech baby[28] (see also pp.191 and 278)

If your LMC finds that your baby is (still) in the breech position when you are 36 or more weeks pregnant, they will consult a specialist obstetrician and discuss with you some options for delivery. Sometimes a breech baby can be turned around.

Moxibustion

Moxibustion is an acupuncture technique that involves burning herbal preparations to stimulate the acupoint by the fifth toe. There is some research evidence from relatively small studies that moxibustion can help to turn the baby from breech to a head-down position. Usually it is done between 32 and 36 weeks. As far as is known, this is not at all harmful, so it may be worth considering as a safe early option.

External cephalic version (ECV)

In some situations, it may be possible for an experienced obstetrician to turn a breech baby around between 37 and 40 weeks of pregnancy. This procedure is known as external cephalic version (ECV). It involves monitoring the baby's heart rate, then placing the hands firmly on the woman's abdomen and guiding the baby into the 'head-down' position. Sometimes a drug to relax the uterus can be used first; even so, ECV can be uncomfortable. Sometimes it will be successful, and as long as the baby's heart rate remains stable, normal vaginal delivery can proceed in due course. But sometimes the baby will simply revert to her breech position. Occasionally, ECV can damage the cord or placenta, immediately compromising the baby's well-being. For this reason, ECV should be attempted only by an obstetrician in supervised conditions where the baby's well-being can be closely monitored and facilities for an emergency Caesarean section are readily available. ECV is successful in just under half of first-time mothers and about two-thirds of women who have already had a child.

Other techniques

Traditional birth massage techniques, particularly those involving vigorous movements to turn the baby, are no longer recommended (although these would once have played an important role in reducing the high risks of unassisted breech birth on remote Pacific islands). Nowadays, the risk of damage to the baby and/or the placenta from traditional techniques greatly outweighs the very much smaller risks associated with expert ECV, assisted breech birth, and/or a Caesarean section, all of which are now relatively safe procedures.

Some other options that women have found helpful, although they have not been subject to specific research, include:

- *Positioning.* Some women have found that lying head down on a sloping board helps to turn the baby from breech to a head-down position.
- *Paying attention to the baby.* Some women believe that the baby has turned his head up near his mother's heart to get her attention. These women often admit to being fairly busy and not taking much notice of their baby. When encouraged to do so, they may find that by the next visit with their LMC the baby has turned to a head-down position.

The uterus

The uterus has now reached its maximum size, and the muscles and tissues within its walls are stretching very thinly and tautly over the pregnancy sac. It is now only about 0.5cm thick on the top, and even thinner in the lower part where there is less muscle. 'Runs' of contractions can occur quite frequently at this stage, and during the last two weeks or so they help prepare the cervix for birth. These runs of contractions, which may stop after a few hours, are known as pre-labour.

The cervix

The cervix at 36 weeks is about 2.5–3cm long, firm and tightly closed. By the time labour begins, it has become soft, slightly open and much shorter. This is known as the 'ripening' of the cervix. The mucous 'plug' at the opening sometimes comes away when the cervix is fully ripe, causing a slightly blood-stained, mucousy vaginal discharge, or 'show'. This may occur one or two days to a week before labour begins, or not until labour is well established. It may not be noticed at all by some women.

Cervix at 36 and 40 weeks

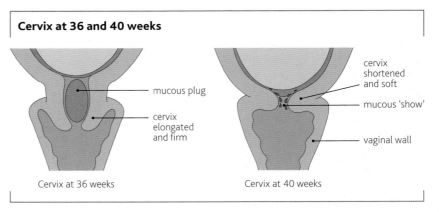

mucous plug

cervix elongated and firm

Cervix at 36 weeks

cervix shortened and soft

mucous 'show'

vaginal wall

Cervix at 40 weeks

The placenta

In this last month of pregnancy, the placenta starts to undergo a dramatic 'ageing' process. Towards 40 weeks it becomes less efficient as the blood vessels within it become narrower. Beyond 40 weeks (when the baby is past her due date) this process accelerates, to varying degrees in different pregnancies. If the 'ageing' is marked, the baby may suffer. When the placenta can no longer sustain the baby within the uterus, she will be better off outside it.

Considering the birthing of the placenta

Even though much of your discussion with your LMC about your preferences for labour and birth will obviously centre on the birth of the baby, you should also discuss the different methods of birthing the placenta. There will occasionally be times when, despite a straightforward birth, there is unexpected heavy bleeding, so you need to be well informed beforehand to be ready for any last-minute decisions that may need to be made.

There are two main approaches to managing this third stage of labour (see also p.271):

- *Expectant (physiological) management.* For some women, the natural production of the hormone oxytocin will be all that is needed to cause the uterus to contract and the placenta and membranes to separate. If a woman is not overly tired or dehydrated once her baby is born, there will often be an urge to push, the uterus will usually contract strongly, the placenta will be quickly expelled within a few minutes, and bleeding will be minimal.

- *Active management.* Sometimes (about one in every 20 births),[29] natural oxytocin alone is not enough to expel the placenta and contract the uterus efficiently. In these cases, a small dose of synthetic oxytocin, given to the mother by injection once the baby is born, can greatly aid the natural hormonal process and prevent subsequent haemorrhage. The placenta is then eased out of the uterus by gently pulling on the cord. This injection helps the uterus to contract down very firmly so that blood loss is kept to a minimum.

When considering your preferences for the delivery of the placenta, you need to be aware of the risks and benefits of each approach. Expectant management is the more natural approach, but it does increase the chances of needing later and much more aggressive intervention to stop bleeding or remove the placenta under anaesthetic.

On the other hand, active management involves a small preventive (and perhaps unnecessary) intervention early on to significantly reduce the risk of needing much more intervention later. The administration of oxytocin at birth or shortly afterwards is often recommended, and its routine use has meant that far fewer women suffer from post-partum haemorrhage (PPH; see p.282), and that if they do, it is likely to be less severe.

The potential for haemorrhage immediately after childbirth is very real. It was a common cause of women dying in childbirth before the twentieth century, and is still a major cause of maternal deaths in developing countries. Current available research shows that even in developed countries, post-partum haemorrhage is significantly more common when women do not routinely receive extra oxytocin, either as the baby is born or after delivery of the placenta.[30] Once rapid heavy blood loss occurs, a blood transfusion and manual removal of any remaining placenta are required extremely quickly (see p.282).

Other changes

In the last few days of pregnancy, many hormonal changes occur in preparation for labour. Often bowel movements become rather loose, the passing of urine becomes even more frequent, and the baby's head descends further into the pelvis. This can cause aching, a feeling of fullness in the vagina, pain in the top of the legs, and a low central backache, especially if the baby is in a 'posterior' position.

In addition, many women experience a sudden surge of energy over the day or two before labour begins. Most have a very strong desire to 'have the baby'. Pregnancy is, after all, just a means to an end, which has fulfilled its purpose by the time labour is ready to begin.

A plan for birth

During pregnancy, every woman has an idea in her mind of how she would like to give birth. Some women like the idea of avoiding pain and discomfort; others favour a totally natural approach. Your wishes and preferences for the birth should certainly be the subject of at least one discussion (and preferably more) between you and your LMC during your antenatal visits. Many women find that writing these things down helps to formalise and strengthen that discussion.

But a birth plan should be much more than simply a list of wishes and preferences. It should take account of your general health, your social and domestic situation, where you plan to give birth, any problems at conception or during pregnancy, possible problems detected during antenatal care, and whether this is your first birth or not. It is not until near the end of pregnancy that some of these things can be determined; even then, they may change at any stage. Birth plans are, at best, flexible plans with room for change.

Planning for a first birth

The majority of women having their first baby experience a normal, straightforward labour and birth. But as a group, women having their first baby are more likely to have longer labours, in both the first and second stages; are more likely to have a baby in a posterior position (p.277); and are more likely to require stitches in the perineum (for either an episiotomy or a tear). The obstetric terms 'primiparous' (referring to a woman who has given birth to her first baby) and 'multiparous' (referring to a woman who has given birth to her second or subsequent baby) acknowledge this difference. (The terms are sometimes shortened to 'primip' and 'multip'.)

There are several reasons for this difference. In a first labour, the muscles in the wall of the uterus are not as practised as in subsequent labours. So it takes more contractions, and more time, to dilate the cervix and push the baby down the birth canal. Moreover, the cervix has never previously opened, so it takes more force to dilate it. It also takes longer to stretch the skin of the perineum and the rest of the birth canal.

A longer labour does not necessarily cause a problem for either mother or baby. If labour is progressing steadily, and both mother and baby are well, there is generally no need for any intervention. But longer labours may, in some women, cause dehydration and exhaustion, a further slowing of labour, a need for pain relief, and abnormal stress on the baby.

So sensible planning for a first birth takes these possibilities into account. Your birth plan should include a discussion about pain relief and active intervention, should these be required.

Planning for a second or subsequent birth

Planning for a subsequent birth may well be different. Multiparous women, as a group, enjoy shorter, more efficient labours. In general, it is not until her fourth or fifth birth that the multiparous woman has once again an increased risk of complications.

There always has to be a contingency plan to cover problems that might arise, but most women can expect to have a shorter labour with their second baby, particularly in the second stage. However, if the first birth was by elective Caesarean section, a subsequent vaginal birth (VBAC, or vaginal birth after Caesarean) may be more like a first birth, because the cervix would not have dilated or the birth canal opened prior to the Caesarean. But if you did experience labour and then had a Caesarean section, the subsequent labour and birth may be as short and efficient as those experienced by someone who had a vaginal birth the first time around.

Preparation for birth

Gradually, as your developing baby gets bigger and demands more from your body, you will almost certainly slow down physically. Especially in the last six weeks, tiredness and lack of energy are likely to hamper your level of activity.

Different women are affected in different ways, depending on their constitution, the nature of that particular pregnancy, and the other demands placed upon them. Contrary to popular opinion, a woman expecting her first baby and continuing in full-time paid employment until 36 weeks may get far more opportunities for rest and relaxation than a mother at home expecting her fourth baby.

Stopping work can be difficult. You may be getting too tired to put in a full and productive day, and yet the first week at home may be rather boring and a real anti-climax. The waiting is not always easy, but make the most of it.

If you have other children, the situation is likely to be different. Often there are not enough hours in the day to get everything done, there seem to be endless toys over the floor, and lifting toddlers can be tiring.

Preparing for a hospital birth

In the last six weeks of pregnancy, it does help if you can be prepared to go to hospital at short notice. When babies decide to be born, they are no respecters of time and place.

After about 36 weeks, it's advisable to limit your travel to within an hour or two of the hospital you're booked into. If you absolutely and unavoidably have to go away, check the facilities at your destination and be prepared to use

'My three-year-old was getting rather disbelieving: "When is the baby going to come, when is the baby going to come?" he'd sing a hundred times a day.'

them if necessary. It's also wise to take a copy of your antenatal record and/or a letter from your LMC, plus your bag packed with the items you will need for you and your baby while in hospital.

Partner and/or support person

'I couldn't wait for 6 o'clock to come – I'd put the kids to bed and just climb in myself, leaving my long-suffering husband to get his dinner and clean up the kitchen.'

Know where you can contact your partner and/or support person if they're not at home with you. If they move around a lot in their work, a mobile phone or pager is an excellent way of keeping in contact.

Having a support person with you during labour is an invaluable asset, and helps most women a great deal. A support person need not be your partner: partners can be excellent, but for a variety of reasons they may not always be available. Even if they are, some families like to have another family member(s) present as well. For some women, a close friend or relative who has had a baby herself can be a very good support person.

If your main support person has to be away during the last few weeks of your pregnancy, you will want to arrange for someone else to be with you if you go into labour. In some areas, a paid support person may be available. Known sometimes as a 'doula', she is not an LMC but a person with special knowledge about pregnancy and childbirth who is there to support you during the labour and birth process, and as required after the birth. (See Appendix: Doulas.)

Contacting your LMC

Well before the end of your pregnancy, make sure you know how and when to contact your LMC if you think labour has started. They should discuss all this with you, and also give you clear instructions about contacting them if you are concerned about anything to do with your pregnancy in the last few weeks. Generally, they will want you to contact them before you leave for the hospital, unless you have planned to give birth at home. They will have a pager or a mobile phone number you can call. Make sure you have the relevant phone numbers in a prominent place at home and also in your wallet or bag, for easy reference – and check that the numbers are correct. Don't rely on texting your LMC or leaving a voicemail message if you are in labour or in need of urgent maternity care; phone directly or page them instead, as some texts and voicemail messages may have a delayed delivery.

Contacting the hospital

Your LMC will usually contact the hospital for you when you go into labour. But just in case you cannot get hold of your LMC, keep the phone number of the hospital in a prominent place for easy reference. Larger hospitals tend to have a direct line to the delivery suite, which avoids delays caused by going through the hospital switchboard.

Transport

Unless you're bleeding (in which case you should call your LMC, who may advise you to call an ambulance), transport to hospital is generally your responsibility.

If you're in established labour, you won't be able to drive yourself, so make sure you have someone on hand who can take you to the hospital. It's also a good idea to have several towels in the car to sit on in case the waters break on the way. Alternatively, take a taxi, but be warned – taxi-drivers don't like delivering babies, and will charge you several hundred dollars for cleaning their taxi if this becomes necessary.

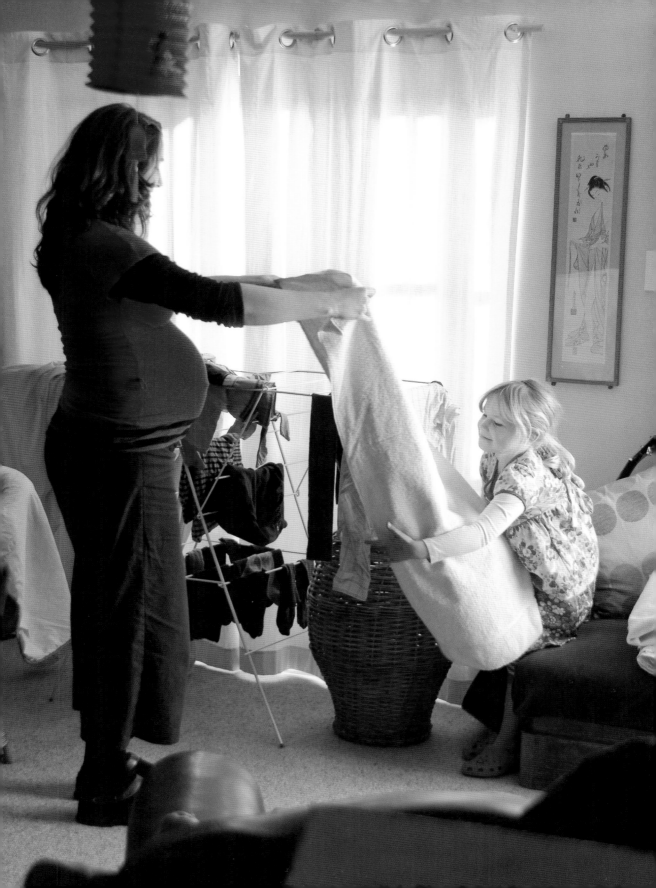

Expressing colostrum in advance

If you know in advance that your baby may be separated from you after birth because she is likely to be unwell or will need special care in some way (e.g. for a heart or lung problem), it is worth exploring the possibility of expressing colostrum before the birth and storing it in a sterile container in the freezer for use in the early hours after birth (see pp.332 and 346). Don't forget to take the stored colostrum with you when you go to the hospital and keep it frozen until it is needed.

Other children

Well in advance, organise the person or people who are going to look after your children when you go into hospital. Make sure they are going to be available when the time comes. If there's any doubt, make alternative plans, especially if the children have to be picked up from playcentre, kindergarten and so on.

If you are planning for the children to be present at the birth, you will still need someone to look after them and tend to their needs. Neither you nor your main support person will be able to take them to the toilet or get them a biscuit. If labour is longer than expected, or there are unexpected complications, the children will need adequate explanations and possibly some diversion tactics.

What to take to the hospital

This will vary from hospital to hospital, and most have lists available as a guide. Essentially, you need very little; even if you arrive without your bag, you will manage very well. Most items you take are not for your health but for your comfort, such as toiletries, pyjamas, underwear and reading material. A warm hat and booties for your baby are important, though, as these are generally not supplied by the hospital.

Hospital checklist

- nightgowns, with front opening for breastfeeding
- light dressing gown
- casual day wear – many women prefer to wear a light dress or tracksuit, but make sure it's suitable for breastfeeding
- toilet gear, e.g. toothbrush, hairbrush, chapstick, etc.
- slippers or slip-on sandals
- nursing bras
- nursing pads
- firm-fitting pants, but preferably not bikini pants that could interfere with a Caesarean wound
- juice, packets of biscuits, pre-packaged snacks, etc.
- books, magazines, pen, writing pad
- ear plugs
- mobile phone (although this will need to remain switched off in certain areas of the hospital)
- coins for pay phones, food and drink machines
- hot-water bottle
- baby clothes, especially a hat and socks/bootees
- nappies (either cloth or disposables), as these are not supplied
- jar of Vaseline to apply to baby's bottom to ease the cleaning of the first sticky bowel motion (see p.307)
- box of baby wipes
- flannels or small cloths (two to three) to help clean up the baby's first sticky bowel motion

Length of stay

How long you stay in hospital will depend on the type of labour and birth you have, your health and the baby's health, how well the baby is feeding, and how much support you have at home. The average stay in hospital after having either a first or subsequent baby is one to two days, although this will depend on your health and that of your baby, and how you are coping with feeding. Many women find that the most difficult time after birth is the second and third days, when the milk 'comes in'. Good post-natal support is essential at this time, ideally provided by the health professional you have come to know and trust, and preferably in your own home.

In some hospitals there is increasing pressure on new mothers to vacate beds, particularly if there is a shortage of staff or the maternity unit is very busy (which does happen from time to time). If you feel that you would benefit from staying longer, you should discuss this with your LMC, and if necessary ask to see the midwife in charge of post-natal services. If you still feel under pressure to go home before you are ready, you can ask to see the patient advocate. (This is a person experienced in hospital systems, who is appointed to protect patient rights in the hospital.) Make your decision about going home after considering your own circumstances carefully.

Planned early discharge

If things do go reasonably smoothly, you may opt to go home within a few hours or a day of delivery. Some women with their second or third baby find this suitable, while others need to stay in hospital for a rest.

Many women feel that their own home environment is preferable to hospital during the first week with a new baby, and a midwife (either your own LMC, a post-natal midwife working with your LMC, or a community midwife from the hospital) can give you good care at home. The midwife will visit daily, or as required, during the first two weeks to check on you and the baby and to help with problems. They should make at least five to seven home visits during the post-natal period (four to six weeks after the birth), and sometimes more.

Discuss planned early discharge with your LMC in the last few weeks of pregnancy. You can always change your mind if things don't go as expected.

Preparing for a home birth

By the last month of pregnancy, it helps if you can have everything you need for the birth ready and waiting. Discuss this with your LMC midwife, who will be your main caregiver during labour and birth. One of the advantages of home birth in New Zealand is that you get to know your midwife in your own home well before labour begins, so make the most of her visits towards the end of your pregnancy.

It's a really good idea if your midwife can meet and talk with your partner and/or support people too, so that all members of the home-birth team can get to know each other ahead of time.

Where will you give birth?

Choose a room in the house where you feel comfortable and there's enough space for everyone to move around. It helps if the toilet and/or bathroom are not too far away either. It is also a good idea to be flexible about this place, as you may change your mind when you are in labour and about to give birth.

'Jemima and I went home when she was four hours old; it worked really well … I was much more settled at home and wanted to be with my other children, too.'

'I loved my precious days in hospital. I knew it'd be the only time I'd have Matthew all to myself – before we had to cope with the demands of his three older brothers. I knew it was the only real rest I was going to get.'

What will you need?

Your LMC midwife will discuss preparations for a home birth. You are likely to need some sort of newspaper mattress, a waterproof cover, sheets, towels and wash-cloths. In some areas, midwives provide bags of hospital linen for you to use to cover areas where you may labour and give birth.

If you are planning a water birth at home, you will need either to hire a birthing pool and a califont to heat the water, or to buy a pool which can be used later as a paddling pool (after being thoroughly cleaned). You also need to consider whether your water supply is adequate and reliable, especially if you live in a rural area and it is summer.

You'll need a made-up cot or bassinet. Clothes for your baby should include a woollen singlet, cardigan, hat and booties, which can be warmed up either in the hot-water cupboard or in your oven (turn it on to a very low heat, to prevent the clothes from burning). You'll need a supply of comfortable clothes for yourself, including sanitary towels, to put on after your shower. Keep a warm dressing gown or blanket handy too, as many women feel cold after the birth – not only have they used up a lot of energy, but they also undergo rapid hormonal changes that cause their body's thermostat to readjust to a cooler temperature.

Temperature

Consider the time of year you'll be giving birth. If it's likely to be cold, you'll need the room at a warm, comfortable temperature. If it's going to be mid-summer, make sure you have plenty of ventilation – a fan may be really useful during labour too. But even in summer, a cool breeze may be too much for your newborn baby, who has not yet learned to regulate her temperature, so be sure to have a heater handy. Doors and windows will usually need to be closed and fans turned off as the baby is being born to ensure she does not get cold. Cold babies can experience breathing difficulties; avoid this by making sure the environment is really warm.

Equipment

Some midwives will leave a special delivery pack at their last visit before your due date. Others will bring it with them at the time. The pack contains basic sterile equipment for use when the baby is born, such as bowls, scissors, cord clamp and sterile drapes. The pack needs to be left intact until it's needed – if opened beforehand, it will be contaminated with bacteria from the air.

Cleanliness

Your midwife will discuss this with you. It makes good sense to have your birthing room clean, comfortable and dry, and the bathroom or washing facilities clean and tidy, with enough soap and towels for everyone to use. The kitchen will be used by a succession of people too, so have good supplies of tea, coffee and cups in obvious places, as well as a supply of nourishing food to keep you and your supporters going.

Contacting people

- *Partner/support people.* Know how to contact your partner and/or main support person, day and night, in the last weeks of pregnancy. A mobile phone or pager is a good idea (see p.230). The same goes for all your support people. If your partner or main support person is likely to be away, arrange a stand-in in case you go into labour unexpectedly.

- *Your midwife.* Make sure you know how to contact your midwife, and at what stage she wants to be called. If you live some distance away, get in touch as soon as you think labour has started. Have her phone number prominently displayed. In most cases midwives have pagers that should be used if you need them urgently; voicemail messages and texts sent by mobile phone may have delayed delivery. Get your midwife to explain how to use the pager, so that you know what to do when you need her urgently.

Other children

Are your other children going to be present at the birth? Discuss this with your partner and support people well beforehand, and with the children if they are old enough to understand. Whatever you decide, you will need to organise a support person specifically to look after them during the labour and birth. If the children are to be present at the birth, their support person can tend to their needs and explain what is happening. Contact your 'child support' person as soon as labour begins, so they can be present throughout the birth process and help your children to share it with you.

Some children find being present during labour and birth quite over-whelming or even frightening. They may need to go out for a while and do something different, or to come and go as they please, or to come in just for the actual birth or immediately afterwards. Make sure you and your 'child support' person have talked about roles and expectations. It is important that you are not anxious about your older children, as the anxiety may slow your labour.

A plan for transfer to hospital, if needed

Every home birth plan (and small birthing unit plan) needs to make provision for a transfer to hospital, if needed. The details of this will depend on where you live, the distance to the nearest hospital with full obstetric services, and the form of transport you would need to use. If you live in an urban area within 15 minutes' drive of the hospital, you have a lot more leeway than if you live in a rural area where the forms of transport available are limited. Air and sea travel can both be affected by bad weather, so if these are the only options for a quick transfer you may need to consider having your baby in a more accessible location. Your LMC will be able to advise you about your specific circumstances, so take advantage of their local knowledge and expertise when considering your plan for birth.

Who is going to help at the birth?

The process of giving birth involves a central person doing a job – a job of paramount importance. As a woman in labour, you need to be aided in your task by one or more assistants, who should be capable of participating actively and skilfully in the process, if required.

The Code of Consumers' Rights (see p.68) is relevant during labour and birth, whether in hospital or at home. It is important that your LMC, or other clinicians involved in your care, discuss all assessments with you. This will help give you confidence in those caring for you, and about your progress. In order to consent to any intervention in the natural course of events, you need to know what that natural course of events is likely to be, and the risks and

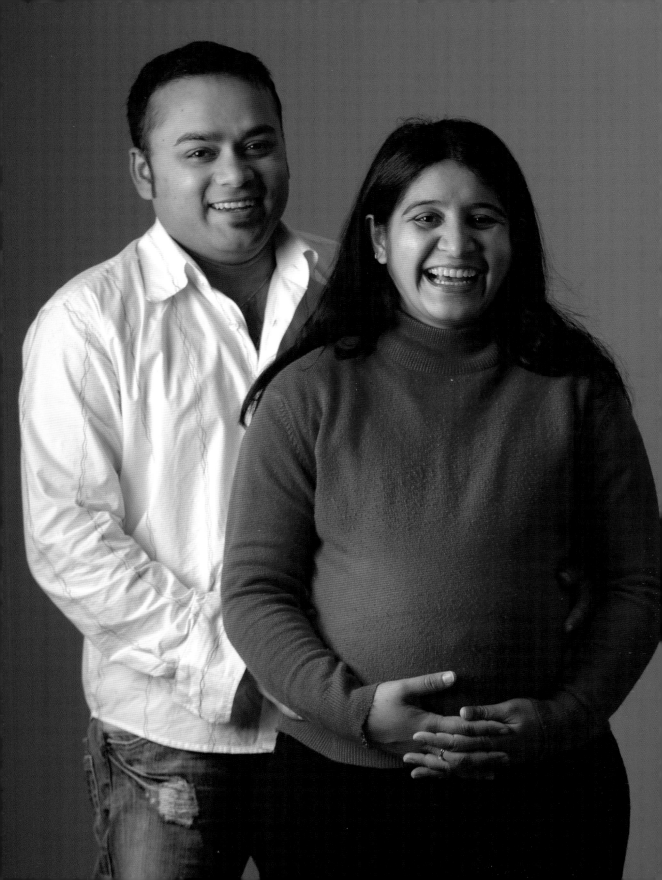

benefits of any intervention. You have the right to be consulted frequently about options and decisions, and to have your views respected at all times. You have the right to have procedures clearly explained, in language you understand, and the procedures cannot commence until you give your consent. This is known as 'informed consent'. Many hospitals now have interpreters and/or patient advocates available to help you if you need them.

The principal support person's role (see also pp.253, 301, 338 and 376)

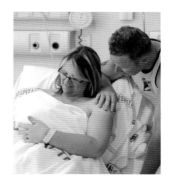

Contrary to what many people imagine, being present at the birth as a partner or principal support person is not just a matter of 'being there'. Being a support person means taking a very active and fulfilling part in the birth process. You are really doing two things: first, you are supporting and encouraging someone you love throughout her labour, both emotionally and physically; and second, you are there to welcome a very special person into the world. If you are the father or grandmother, the baby will indeed be 'your own flesh and blood'. Even if you are not a blood relation, that doesn't mean you are any less able to welcome this very newest member of the human family. Anyone who has had the privilege of being chosen by a pregnant woman to be her 'number one supporter' in the business of birth will always have a very special bond with her and her baby.

However, as in most jobs, some advance training and practice are necessary. At times you may need to be an advocate for the woman in labour, so you need to know her expectations and preferences beforehand, and to have agreed on priorities.

Communication

Can you talk easily with your partner/daughter/friend? Can you understand what she's on about even if she's not making much sense? Do you find all the technical words to do with birth confusing?

Towards the end of the pregnancy, you will both benefit from spending some time talking through what will happen, and what could happen. Try to become familiar with words such as 'cervix', 'transition' and 'perineum'. Talk about what she would like, and what you would like. Discuss possible complications, and how you each think you'd respond in these situations. Knowing what's likely to happen puts you in the best possible position to interpret what she needs and wants throughout her labour – and that may change with remarkable rapidity!

Continuity of care

One of the most important roles of a partner or principal support person is physically being with the labouring woman from 'before the start' to 'after the finish'. Other friends and relatives, midwives and doctors may come and go, change shifts or be away on holiday, but partners or main support people are there throughout. This means that you are a powerful source of emotional strength for the woman in labour. She cannot 'go away' either (even though at times she may very well feel like it!), and she will appreciate your constant presence.

You're also in a better position than she is to keep track of time. By keeping an eye on the clock, you'll be able to tell how long and how frequent her contractions are, when she needs to pass urine, and how long she's been in each stage of labour. Timekeeping also helps assess progress, both physically and mentally. However, some women may not want to be reminded of the time, but rather just encouraged to deal with each contraction as it comes. Labour is hard work; constant encouragement and ongoing support are vital.

Your own needs

In all the drama of labour and birth, it's easy to forget about your own needs as a support person. Throughout the labour, you'll need sustenance in the form of food and drink; and if labour is long, you'll want some rest, too. You also need freedom from worry – about other children, work, cars parked over driveways and so on.

A bit of forward planning goes a long way here – a couple of thermos flasks of coffee, some ready-made sandwiches, a comfortable chair, a clock, a mobile phone, some money (for drink machines, pay phones, etc.) and even an MP3 player can all help enormously. (Just remember that mobile phones and electronic devices may need to be switched off in certain areas of the hospital, as they may interfere with other equipment.)

Good forward planning for childcare, someone to cover for you at work, and a 'dummy run' to the hospital, including finding somewhere to park, all make things run more smoothly on the day (or night).

Role of the midwife

If you have chosen a self-employed midwife as your LMC, she will be responsible for your continuous care during labour and birth. Whether you are having your baby at home or in hospital, you will usually enjoy total continuity of care by the same midwife – before, during and after the birth. However, if there is a complication, she may need to call on extra help from another midwife or a doctor (possibly a GP if you live in a rural area; otherwise a specialist obstetrician, a paediatrician or an anaesthetist).

If you have chosen a GP or specialist obstetrician as your LMC, they will maintain overall responsibility for your care during labour and birth. However, they will not be present right throughout your labour. Instead, you will be cared for during labour and possibly delivery by a self-employed midwife who works with your doctor, or a hospital midwife or team of midwives, who will keep in contact with your doctor and report on your progress.

Hospital midwives usually work shifts of 8–12 hours in the antenatal clinic and delivery suite, and on the post-natal wards. During your labour, you may be looked after by several midwives, who undertake continuity of care as a group rather than as individuals. In spite of this, they can still provide very personalised care, and it is unlikely that you will have more than two midwives caring for you throughout your labour.

Increasingly, hospitals are providing a more personalised midwifery service. Doctors who are LMCs often work with a particular midwife or midwives to provide antenatal, labour and birth care. This means that you can meet your midwife well before you go into labour. She will undertake to attend you throughout your labour and birth, however long that may be.

So, whoever you have chosen as your LMC, and whether you are having your baby at home or in hospital, the midwife is the person who will be caring for you during labour, tending to your needs and monitoring your progress.

She will look after your health, but must also be very aware of the health of your unborn baby.

Your midwife is there to answer your questions, respond to your requests, listen to your worries, and keep you and your partner or support person fully informed about what's happening. She will keep a written record of your labour and check your progress from time to time, noting the frequency and intensity of contractions and occasionally examining you.

In a busy delivery suite, a hospital midwife may be looking after more than one woman at a time, and may come and go a lot during the first stage of labour. For this reason, it is very important to have your partner or support person there throughout.

However, once you're in the second stage of labour, your midwife will be with you continuously. She is well versed in the art of normal birth, but is also trained to detect potential problems, and will know when to call in specialist help.

After the birth, your midwife will make you comfortable so that you can start getting to know your baby. In the next few hours and days, her role will become even more important: she is there to help you get active again, to help you get breastfeeding established, and to teach you skills for looking after and enjoying your new baby.

Role of the doctor

If you have chosen a doctor as your LMC, they will be responsible for your overall care, but will not necessarily be present right throughout your labour. They will rely on your midwife to look after you, but they will expect to be contacted frequently about your progress – particularly if your midwife has any concerns.

During a normal labour and birth, the doctor may not play a major role, letting the midwife do most of the work. This is not an abdication of responsibility, but rather a recognition that normal labour and birth are physiological and not medical processes, and as such are best dealt with by someone who specialises in normal birth – a midwife.

If your labour is very quick and straightforward, you may not get to see your doctor at all until you're nearly ready to have your baby, or indeed until just after she is born. Most doctors, however, do visit at least once (and much more often if necessary) during labour, and are generally present for the birth. They are then immediately available and have the necessary skills to intervene if problems arise or if there are pre-existing complications.

Sometimes, specialist help is required, and your doctor may ask another doctor (for example, a specialist obstetrician, an anaesthetist or a paediatrician) to help give you the best chance of having a healthy baby and remaining in good health yourself. Sometimes decisions must be made in a hurry, and you may feel that you have not been adequately consulted. It is important to remember that your doctor and midwife have a duty to provide what they consider to be the best care *at the time*, and that occasionally time is at a premium. For these reasons, it is wise to have discussed the possibility of complications at one or more of your antenatal visits, well before you go into labour (see pp.146 and 228).

A couple's story: A first birth

Louise

My labour started a week early with a show, then gradually increasing contractions over the next day – just as my husband rushed around getting the last signatures to finally submit his thesis. Contractions became more regular as I helped him print out the final copy, and became painful walking back from dropping the thesis off to the photocopier's late at night.

Back at home, I was convinced things were happening rapidly as the contractions seemed strong and frequent. But when my midwife came to our home, I found I was only about 1.5cm dilated. This was a crashing disappointment and I remember thinking I couldn't do this for much longer. But time did pass and I lost all track of the outside world. I tried baths, different positions and going for a walk (surreal on a dark autumnal night, with frequent stops for contractions.) John was fantastic, although he wanted to do more: for those hours it seemed like just the two of us in our own world.

A few hours later I passed a bloody show: suddenly with a jolt I remembered there was a baby involved, and that bleeding might threaten the baby. My fantastic midwife came back and listened to the baby and thought the bleeding was within normal. Her presence helped ground me and everything felt better. I was about 3cm by this stage. More hours passed.

As it got light we headed for the hospital. I had one of the coveted natural birth rooms – welcoming and practical. I was about 6cm dilated then. Soon after arrival they monitored the baby. It was a routine short-term CTG. Suddenly my midwife told me to turn to my left side: I said I would after the contraction and she said firmly no, now. Again I was jolted back out of my pain and remembered with cold fear the baby. His heartbeat had dropped.

It soon returned to normal, but kept dropping with each contraction – variable decelerations, not the really dangerous type but potentially concerning. They called the obstetrician in; he was matter of fact, and moved me downstairs to 'High Risk'.

They wheeled me through subterranean corridors to 'High Risk' – lots of machines, more staff who introduced themselves but I never really grasped who they were. The CTG with my baby's heart rate kept beeping out, slowing to almost half the normal rate with each contraction then recovering, the trace showing all the dips as the paper spilled on to the floor. I was still having contractions – harder to deal with, as I was caught between the contractions – and listening to the heartbeat, watching the dips on the printout that was growing ever longer.

I was still only 6cm after one or two hours. I lost track of time and my main reaction was relief when the obstetrician recommended a Caesarean section as it meant an end to the beeps, my fears for the baby, and the contractions.

I was whisked into theatre. Forms were flicked before me, full of figures and complications – nerve damage, bleeding… And I signed, just wanting to get on with the Caesarean. The spinal was fantastic. Suddenly the pain of the contractions went and I could really focus on the baby's imminent arrival: thank goodness, I could be awake. Very soon, the obstetrician announced we had a son. I remember it took me a few moments in my exhausted state to work out that meant a boy. Just after, there was the magical sound of a baby's cry and I think everyone relaxed – I certainly did. My husband went to see the baby and soon arrived back with a bundle: small, wrinkled, wrapped, but utterly beautiful. I don't remember the rest of the operation; suddenly, it was back to just us again but now there were three. They said later the cord had been looped tightly around his neck, and this was why his heart rate had been dipping.

He was a lovely baby: calm and alert and a natural breastfeeder, and I had a very smooth recovery. My husband had finished his thesis and, despite the Caesarean, I had a strong feeling of completion and starting anew as I moved on from the birth to those magical exhausting days of early parenthood.

John

I found being a companion on the journey of pregnancy humbling. It challenged my far too ingrained (male?) sense of trying to control a situation and provide the answers.

There is so much you won't predict about the birth experience. But that (usually) one marvellous day is an experience that all carers are unlikely to forget. In this age of technology and professional support, you're there for the woman at your side who is even more amazing than ever during the ultimate journey of becoming.

What I feared most about the pregnancy process was the labour and the pain my partner would go through. Being focused on the growing baby, and talking a lot about things as they were and might be, helped me get that in perspective. It also helped to have a birth plan and to read about birth (and ohh, that birth video), but I still remember the nerves when labour began.

Then it was real. The contractions. The pain. The blood. Good grief, that birthing video was right! This is when you know you need to have read a book like this one, and to have made a birth plan. As labour progressed, we had a professional midwife at home to tell me it was normal. Before then it was scary, just my wife and I, living away from family. It was good to have built up a rapport with the midwife and to know something about the stages of labour. I rubbed Louise's back, helped her change positions, held her, got ice cubes, mixed energy drinks, applied cool flannels and remained on my toes.

All of us tired, we left for the hospital. We were renting and did not feel attached to our home or sure of a home birth. The streets were quiet, there were no traffic delays. We had the nice new birth room with a spa bath nearby, plenty of space and even windows: cool! Things seemed to be progressing, slowly but surely.

But it became clear the baby was in distress. My sense of stability wavered: so many monitoring machines, extra medics arriving, alarming changes in the baby's heart rate. We held each other's hands. Louise was shifted to the High Risk Unit, four floors below in a small basement operating theatre, and prepped for a Caesarean with me alongside. Then a nurse said, 'You're going to be a dad soon, have you got your camera?'! I zoomed back upstairs and grabbed it from our bag, running back through unfamiliar hospital corridors shouting 'where's High Risk, where's High Risk?'

I was directed through the maze to the place where everything important was happening. The team was great. The anaesthetist provided a (rather detailed!) commentary on Louise's Caesarean procedure; I was glad the wee screen was up. But I was lucky – I got to cut the umbilical cord.

Suddenly a person had arrived in the world, his imagined face here, right here, his breath coming in wails, his whole system shifting from living immersed in oceanic liquor to lung-inflating air, his cries carrying across the room and his eyes screwed shut at those too-bright lights. What a privilege to be passed this being, this person, and to move him to the arms of the beloved and lay him there for the first of many times. Flesh of our flesh, heart of our hearts, you live so suddenly and today you live on, so far removed from and so bound to that remarkable moment of your entry into our lives. And throughout your gestation, birth and growth, I am still learning, slowly, that both letting go and really being present are such important parts of birth and of parenting.

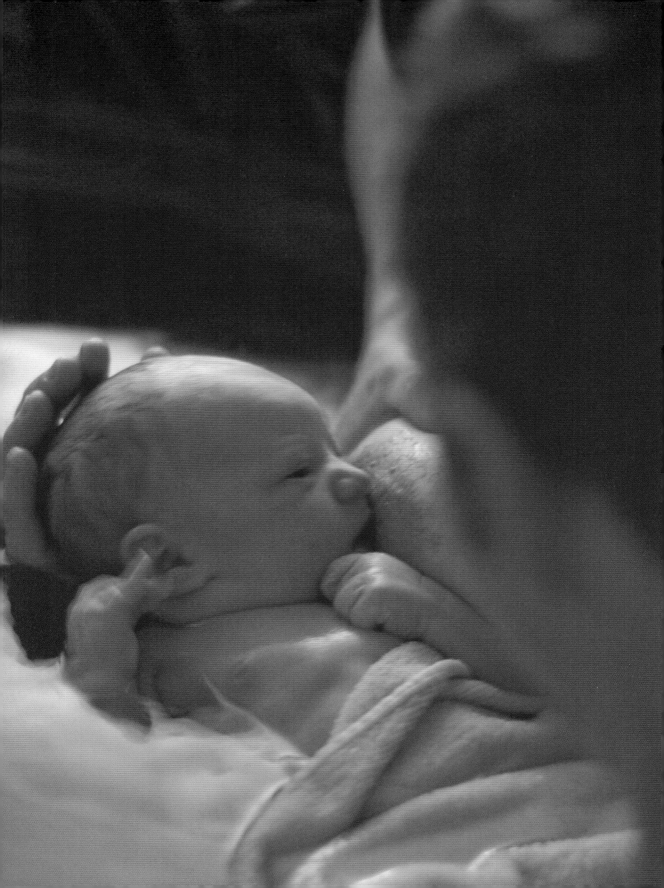

CHAPTER 6

Birth

1. The onset of labour

What's happening? Is this labour or not? Can you tell exactly why you feel you're in labour, or are you simply feeling uneasy or uncomfortable? Has this stage been a long, long time coming? Is it earlier than you expected; perhaps *much* earlier?

Labour starts in many different ways, and can be heralded by many signs and feelings. Some are more definite than others, and if several occur together, labour is likely to have started.

If you're not sure whether you're going into labour, it's worth waiting a while to see what else develops. If you feel nervous or uncertain, contact your partner or support person. Ask them to come and be with you if they're not already around. It can help to discuss the possibility that you're in labour, and then maybe do something else for a while.

If the signs continue or increase, but still nothing seems very definite, phone your LMC and tell them what's happening. They can help assess the situation from what you tell them, and advise appropriately.

Many women have 'false starts' to labour, often called 'pre-labour'. In the early stages, it can be very hard to tell whether this is really 'it'. For some women, early labour or pre-labour may last a day or two; for others, it may last up to several weeks. They may have frequent runs of contractions that come and go, sometimes over a period of six to eight hours. These are really 'practice' contractions, which are helping prepare the uterus for actual labour.

Definite signs of action

Contact your LMC if any of the following things happen:

- your waters break
- there is any bright red bleeding (see pp.192 and 204)
- the contractions are strong enough to take your breath away, or they stop you from interacting with people around you
- you are very worried about any aspect of your pregnancy or labour.

In any of these situations, your LMC will either make their way to you at home straight away, or arrange to meet you at the hospital.

Once your waters break, the potential exists for infection within the pregnancy sac. If labour has already started, it will usually speed up once the membranes have ruptured, and the contractions may become stronger and more frequent. If this is a second or subsequent baby, the birth may not be far off.

Even if there have been no contractions, labour nearly always starts within a few hours of the waters breaking. In this case, the baby is born before infection becomes a problem. However, if more than 24 hours elapse after the waters break, it may be advisable to induce labour, depending on the gestation of the pregnancy and the health of the mother and baby (see pp.260 and 275). It is common to get a blood-stained mucousy discharge, or 'show', just before labour starts, as the mucous plug in the cervix comes away. Contractions will usually start within 24 hours of the 'show', although occasionally several days

'I'd had so many runs of contractions over the last week that I'd stopped taking much notice. But this time, they didn't go away when I lay down ... I couldn't get comfortable.'

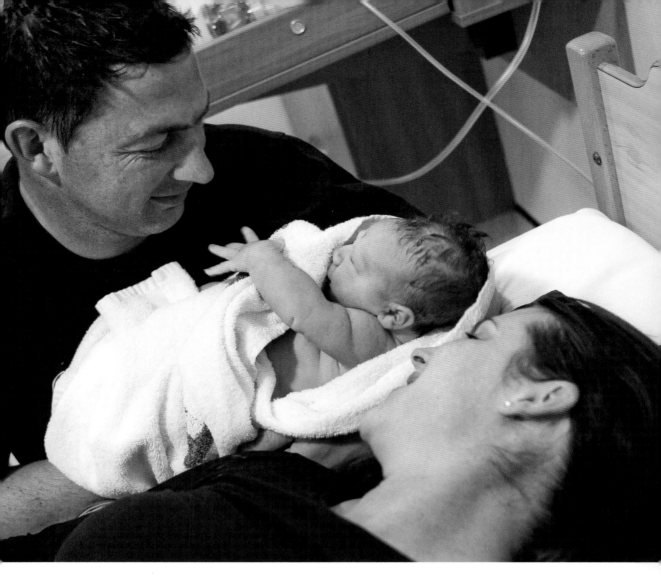

or weeks may elapse. However, any bright red bleeding, especially if it continues to trickle, should be checked straight away as there may be a problem with the placenta (see pp.192 and 204).

Helping yourself in early labour

The very early stages of labour, especially when you're not sure that it really is happening, can be very unsettling. It's hard to concentrate on anything, yet some women find it best to be active. This is especially the case at night, when you should be resting but may be too excited. As you do not know how long the early stages will last, it is best to try to sleep at night so as to conserve your energy for the later period of labour.

As the contractions become stronger and more frequent, you will no longer be able to lie down or sleep. As soon as you're reasonably sure, let your partner and/or support people and your LMC know (though if you are coping well and want to let them sleep until morning, then by all means do so). If you are anxious or becoming increasingly distressed, it is best to let others know that you think you are in labour.

Early labour can last several hours, or only a few minutes. Every woman and every pregnancy is different, although previous labours may be a guide. Some strategies that may help keep you comfortable:

- Walk around or keep upright as much as possible so that the contractions and gravity can help the baby to move down in the pelvis.
- Empty your bladder at least every hour, as a full bladder can get quite painful, even during mild contractions. It can also inhibit labour and prevent the baby's head moving down into the pelvis.
- Time the contractions – how long and how far apart are they? Once they're less than five minutes apart and getting stronger, you're likely to be in labour.
- Drink frequently, preferably water, but in small amounts. Alternatively, you can suck some ice. Isotonic drinks may also help.
- If you're really hungry and haven't eaten anything for some hours, have a light snack if you feel like it; otherwise eat nothing. You won't digest anything once you're in established labour, and eating may make you vomit. However, because labour is hard work, you will need to keep your energy levels up: try chewing some 'gummy' sweets or sucking on barley sugars. You'll also need reserves of energy immediately after the birth so that your uterus can contract effectively.
- Stay in your own home environment for as long as possible. You will usually feel more relaxed there, which will help your labour to progress.

If you are planning to have a home birth, make sure the place where you will give birth is warm enough for the baby but not too warm for your comfort while you're in labour.

If you're going to hospital, you will know when you need to go. Some women prefer to get there before they're really uncomfortable, especially if they have to travel for more than 10–15 minutes. If you have some distance to travel, especially an hour or more, it is best to head for the hospital at the earliest signs of confirmed labour. Any extended car travel can be extremely uncomfortable once labour is well under way. Despite occasional stories to the contrary, a car is not an ideal place to give birth.

Some signs that labour is starting

These signs are not necessarily in chronological order.

- a 'show' – slightly blood-stained mucousy vaginal discharge
- abdominal discomfort – often just a low, period-like pain at first
- backache – a low, central ache, gradually getting worse
- passing urine every few minutes
- definite contractions, or tightenings, in the abdomen
- contractions develop a regular pattern and become stronger, longer and more frequent
- the waters break – this may be a gush of clear fluid, or a little trickle at first. The liquid has a characteristic 'mousy' smell.

2. What's happening?
The normal pattern of labour

The birth process has three main stages. First, the uterus, which has firmly contained the baby within his sac of fluid for 40 weeks, must open up fully at the cervix. Second, the baby must pass down the birth canal from the cervical opening to the outside world. Third, the placenta must be expelled from the uterus, so that it can close right down, ready – in time – for the next pregnancy.

The first stage of labour

This is the longest stage, taking on average 8–16 hours for a first baby and 3–10 hours for a second or subsequent baby.

At the end of pregnancy, the cervix changes from its normal structure (with a narrow internal canal, about 2.5cm in length) to become softer, thinner and shorter. This is known as the 'ripening' of the cervix. In this state, regular contractions of the muscles within the uterus cause the cervix to become even thinner and shorter, until there is no length to the canal (a process known as 'effacing'). Then the cervix stretches and stretches – or 'dilates' – until it is fully open. The process of opening, or dilation, is estimated in centimetres. Labour is said to be 'established' once the cervix is 2–3cm dilated, and is said to be 'progressing' if the cervix continues to open. Full dilation is estimated to be 10cm across. Dilation of the cervix may not occur at a constant rate. The usual pattern is for the dilation from 1cm to 5cm to take much longer than that from 5cm to 10cm.

> **The stages of labour**
>
> - *First stage* – the cervix shortens, thins and completely opens up.
>
> - *Second stage* – the baby passes down the birth canal and is born.
>
> - *Third stage* – the placenta is expelled and the uterus contracts.

Cervical dilation during the first stage of labour – a typical pattern

As the diagram indicates, progress in early labour can be variable. But once labour is established, normal progress tends to be steady, until it slows down during the transition from first to second stage.

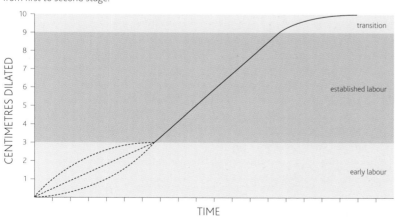

A contraction occurs when the muscles in the wall of the uterus contract in a coordinated way and the pressure within the uterus wall rises and then falls. During a contraction, the blood supply to the placenta (and thus to the baby) decreases, but it resumes rapidly once the contraction is over. Normal, healthy babies cope well with this stress during labour.

As a general rule, the stronger and longer the contractions, the more effective they are in dilating the cervix. Early in labour, the contractions tend to be infrequent and quite mild, and do not dilate the cervix very much. As labour progresses, the muscles of the uterus become more 'practised', and the contractions become more frequent, longer and stronger so that they dilate the cervix more quickly. Second or subsequent labours tend to be shorter and more efficient than first labours because the uterus has already had previous 'practice'.

Contractions are at their strongest near the very end of the first stage of labour, as the cervix nears its 'fully open' state. This is known as the 'transition' between the first and second stages. Once the cervix is fully dilated (i.e. 10cm), the first stage is complete.

Dilation of the cervix

head

cervix

5

10

vaginal wall

Cervix at 5cm dilated

Cervix at 10cm dilated

The second stage of labour

With the cervix fully dilated, the baby's head can now pass through it and down the vagina (birth canal) as the muscles of the uterus contract powerfully to expel the baby. These uterine contractions are helped along by the strong abdominal muscles, creating an urge to push that is very difficult to resist. The vagina has stretched remarkably during labour in order to accommodate the baby, but the bones of the pelvis are not capable of much stretching. So once the cervix is fully open, the next obstacle the baby's head must pass through is the bony 'pelvic outlet' (see p.215). To do this, the head must twist to a sideways position and then to a backwards-facing position again (see opposite).

At that point, the baby's head is visible at the vaginal opening and the skin of the perineum starts stretching to allow it to pass through. As the head presses against the perineum, the skin stretches and stretches until the widest part of the baby's head is born, usually facing his mother's back. Next the shoulders come through the vaginal opening, the baby once again rotating to the side to allow first one shoulder and then the other to emerge. The baby is born and takes his first breath. The second stage is complete.

The baby passing down the birth canal

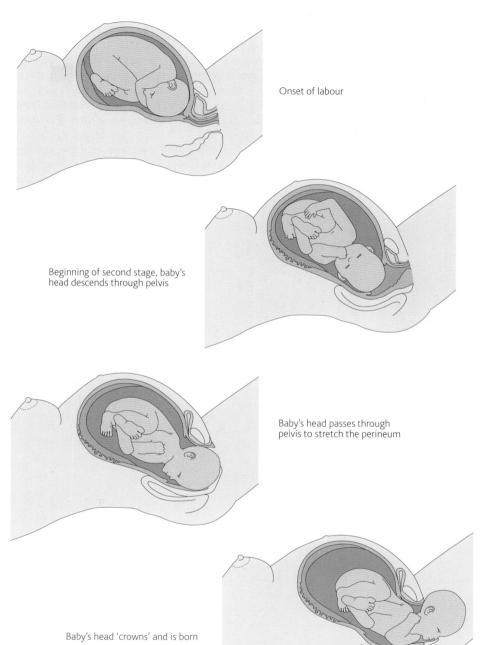

Onset of labour

Beginning of second stage, baby's head descends through pelvis

Baby's head passes through pelvis to stretch the perineum

Baby's head 'crowns' and is born

The third stage of labour

All that now remains within the uterus is the placenta with the attached cord, and remnants of the pregnancy sac. After the baby has been born, the uterus continues to contract, allowing the placenta to separate from the wall of the uterus. This process starts as the baby is emerging through the vaginal opening, and is usually complete within a few minutes. Then the uterus must contract again to expel the placenta through the cervix. Sometimes the uterus goes through a brief resting phase before this happens, but the placenta is usually expelled within 10–15 minutes of birth, and passes out of the vagina along with the cord and membranes.

Now the uterus can contract and stay contracted, preventing all the open blood vessels that previously supplied the placenta from bleeding. Immediately after birth the uterus becomes hard and much smaller, the cervix closes up, and the vaginal walls and perineum all start to shrink back to their normal size and shape. Labour is complete.

The delivery of the placenta

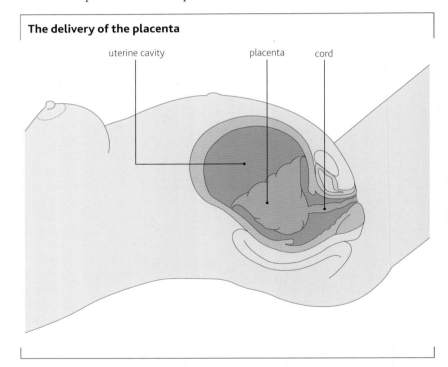

uterine cavity   placenta   cord

3. Working as a team during labour

First stage of labour

By now, you've met up with your LMC midwife, either at home or at the hospital. You've told her what's happening and how you're feeling. She can help confirm that you are indeed in labour, both from what you tell her and by being with you during contractions. To assess just 'how far on' you are, she needs to do a vaginal examination (VE) to determine how much the cervix has dilated (see box below). Dilation is an important sign that labour is progressing. In addition, your LMC can determine the thickness of the cervix, the part of the baby that is presenting first, the position of the baby, and the relationship of the baby to your pelvis.

If you are having regular contractions, the cervix is thin and more than 3cm dilated, and the baby's head is well down in the pelvis, you're in established labour and well on your way. Now, it's a matter of concentrating on the contractions, breathing through each one as it comes along.

Sometimes, however, labour can slow and stop, even though the cervix may be well dilated. This can be disappointing, but there are a number of possible reasons, and possible responses (see p.276).

Signs that help to confirm you are in labour

- Contractions increase in strength, length and frequency.
- Contractions take your breath away.
- VE shows that your cervix is shorter and thinner (effaced), and is opening up (dilating).

Having a vaginal examination (VE) during labour

Because of the discomfort and the risk of infection once the membranes have ruptured, it is wise to keep VEs to a minimum during labour. They should be done only if there is a real need to assess progress, about once every three to four hours. To ensure a successful VE:

- Go to the toilet and empty your bladder if you haven't done so within the last half-hour.
- Lie down on your back, preferably with a couple of pillows to keep you slightly propped up. It's best not to lie flat on your back, as this may cause the heavy uterus to press on the big blood vessels that supply your uterus.
- Bend your knees up, put your ankles together and let your knees flop apart.
- Your LMC will put on sterile disposable gloves, and apply some lubricating cream to their fingers.
- Between contractions, your LMC will gently insert two fingers into the vagina and feel for the baby's head and the cervix covering it. To get an accurate estimate of how dilated the cervix is, they need to feel right around the edge of the cervix. It is also important that they can feel for the fontanelles (gaps) of the baby's skull to estimate the position of the baby's head (i.e. anterior or posterior) and how far down in your pelvis the head is.

This examination should take only a minute or two, but it can be uncomfortable. You can minimise the discomfort by relaxing as much as possible, and concentrating on your breathing. You can also ask your LMC to stop and wait if another contraction starts.

Different positions

Many women find they are much more comfortable moving around than lying down during the first stage of labour. Any position in which gravity can help the baby get as low as possible helps labour to progress:

- walking around between contractions
- getting into a kneeling position, leaning on a chair or bed
- sitting astride a chair
- squatting in front of a chair or bed
- standing against a wall
- sitting in a bath or standing in a shower (for as long as you like)
- squatting or sitting in bed, leaning forward on pillows
- lying propped up in bed on your side or back.

You may want to try all of these, or only some – certain positions will work better than others for each woman.

Handling labour – some options

- Some women like the feeling of solitude as they concentrate on breathing through painful contractions; they may wish to be alone in a room for a time. In hospital, the sense of solitude can be created by lowering noise levels as much as possible, e.g. by shutting the door and asking other people present to keep silent during contractions.
- Other women may prefer being surrounded by their whānau/family/loved ones and they may enjoy hearty company, laughter and chatting.
- Some women like to hear soft music in the background. Some women may want to sing or be sung to.
- Some women like the aroma of a cake baking, or meat roasting, or the smell of pine, kawakawa or the sea air; other women are completely averse to any such things. In a large hospital, there is less ability to control the environment, but a little creative thinking can go a long way.
- What actually happens in labour may be spontaneous and totally unplanned. Support people need to be 'in tune' (attentive) to the woman and recognise that what she wants can change over the course of labour.

Hope Tupara

Relaxing between contractions

It's hard to imagine, but there is often quite a lot of time between contractions. It helps to use this time to recover as fully as possible from the previous contraction, so that you are well prepared for the next. Try to relax completely – loosen your arms, hands, face, neck, legs and feet. Think consciously about relaxing each area of your body, and get your support person to remind you. Or you might want to move around, have a sip of water, suck on a piece of ice, or wipe your face and neck with a cool, damp wash-cloth. Don't forget to empty your bladder – the normal sensations of bladder fullness are often altered during labour.

Positions of uterus while mother is in different positions

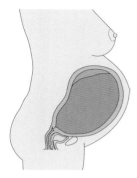 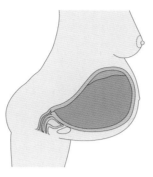 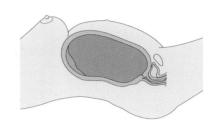

Standing – gravity
helps contractions a lot

Leaning forward – gravity
helps contractions a lot

Lying down – gravity
helps contractions a little

Helping a woman in labour (for partners and support people)

- See if a back-rub during and/or between contractions will help. A firm, circular motion over the small of the back, using the heel of your hand with a little oil or talcum powder, works well, but any massage that gives relief is fine. Some women prefer a lighter touch higher on the back, so check what is most helpful.

- Encourage her to sip a little water or suck some ice between contractions if she is thirsty. Lip salve may be good, too.

- Check that she empties her bladder at least every hour and preferably more often. Help her to the toilet if you can; otherwise get assistance from your midwife or another support person.

- Encourage her to move around as much as she can. Help her to get into different positions, but don't be surprised if she doesn't like that position and wants to change again!

- Help her to concentrate on breathing through the contractions once they start getting stronger. Do the breathing with her, so she can follow your pace. Remind her of what you've practised, and slow her down if she starts to breathe too fast (see p.220).

- Don't be offended if she gets irritated and impatient with you. Labour can be extremely intense and overwhelming; you may be the only person to whom she can express this intensity, knowing that you will continue to love her just the same.

Relief from pain

If the contractions seem to be getting much more painful, and are becoming unbearable despite your best efforts, it's worth considering some other ways of getting relief. Your partner or support person and midwife can help you make an appropriate choice.

Having another VE at this point can be a good idea, unless you've recently had one. It may well be that you're nearing the end of the first stage (transition), and that the contractions are much stronger and more frequent because of this. Knowing that you're nearly fully dilated, and that it won't be much longer now, may give you the encouragement you need to get through this phase. If this is not the case, several alternative forms of pain relief are available.

What pain will I feel in labour?

Every woman's experience of pain in labour will be different, but it does help to have some idea of what it could feel like at different stages. Below, three women talk about their own experiences:

- [1] At home, I used Rescue Remedy to relax me, and I sat in the bath for quite a while. That helped me to deal with contractions. Towards the end, my husband didn't know what to do, how to help me. He was going mad. In the end, I got a bit annoyed. I didn't want anyone to help me: I knew I just had to deal with the pain myself. I didn't want anyone else to see me in pain other than my mum and my midwife. I didn't want people to see me struggling – if you are a strong person, you don't want people to see that side of you.

  Once I went to hospital, I used a Swiss ball – I had used one throughout my pregnancy. Deep breaths, using Rescue Remedy with every third or fourth contraction, different positions with the Swiss ball – that was all I actually used. And I managed to handle four hours of intense labour, real bad labour.

  There was one point where I said to my midwife, 'I don't think I can handle this any more.' She said, 'Yes you can. He's coming, he's going to be born – don't you want to see your son? Well, just a few more minutes and you'll meet him.'

  I enjoyed pushing, because I felt under control and working towards something. That was the most enjoyable part.

  Friends who are pregnant have asked me to describe the pain, but I can't. It's a lot of pain, but it's a pain you can live with.

- [2] First stage: cramps across my lower stomach felt like period pains, and then a ring of pain at the cervix. A bit of backache as the head turned. I felt early on that the pain was becoming unbearable – then as I relaxed and breathed through the contractions, I realised that the contractions were much stronger, but that the pain had remained at a level I would call uncomfortable but bearable. No pain between contractions, so time to rest.

  Transition: this was fighting the urge to push, and if I did push the pain told me that wasn't what I should be doing. I found it took all my concentration to keep going … it was nice to know that the gas was available, but it would have broken my concentration to ask for it.

  Second stage: suddenly my baby's head moved from the uterus to the vagina, and I could feel it with the vaginal nerves so I could now feel exactly what was going on, rather than pain … everything stretched apart … then, as the head crowned and the perineum stretched, there was some intense pain – but this only lasted for five seconds. By the time I drew breath to complain, the pain was over and everything was numb. And feeling the baby slither out was a delightful sensation.

- [3] I found actively relaxing through contractions was the most important technique to cope with pain.

Mirimiri

Mirimiri is a Māori therapeutic practice that is often equated with massage, though it is not the same. It can be used in pregnancy, during labour and after the birth (for mother and baby). The tactile application of mirimiri is just one aspect, because there are other equally important dimensions.

Mirimiri services may be offered in your area, so it is worth making enquiries to local Māori health providers as a starting point. To find out who the Māori health providers are in your area, contact either the local iwi organisation, the primary health organisation or local hospital, or search the Ministry of Health website. (See Appendix: Māori health providers.)

Hope Tupara

Bathing

Some women find that having a warm bath is a good way to relieve pain, as long as the bath is big enough to move around in. Most women naturally find the best position to relieve pain by moving around quite a lot, and taking a spa bath (without using the jets) can be ideal for this. Some hospitals have spa baths installed in the delivery suite, where there is privacy but also plenty of room for the midwife and your partner or support person to help you.

Using water in labour and birth

Advantages

- The buoyancy of the water enables you to move more easily.
- Immersion in warm water is a good form of pain relief in labour; some women find that even a warm shower is helpful.
- Being in water reduces the use of narcotics for pain relief in labour; in fact, narcotic drugs such as pethidine are not recommended for women who are labouring in water.
- You will not have to get out of the water for VEs – or to deliver the placenta, as long as this happens promptly and without the need for assistance.
- Babies can be born safely in the water, providing they remain fully submerged during the birth and there are no medical problems that preclude a water birth (see p.270).
- Newborn babies can remain in the water to keep warm, unless their condition makes this impossible.

Disadvantages

- You cannot labour in water if you have had any form of narcotic pain relief, or if you or your baby are not well.
- You cannot labour in water if your baby's condition needs continuous electronic monitoring and the transducers are not water-resistant.
- You may have to get out of the water if your temperature rises more than 1°C above your baseline temperature (i.e. your temperature before you got into the pool).
- Contractions may slow down if you enter the water before you are in established labour.
- You will have to get out of the water if the birth of the placenta needs to be actively managed, you are bleeding excessively or require suturing.

Transcutaneous electrical nerve stimulation (TENS)

This technique helps to lessen the pain of contractions by temporarily blocking the nerve pathways that carry pain messages to the brain. Four sticky pads are applied to your lower back. They are attached to a control box that sends tiny electrical pulses to block the nerve pathways, and help to stimulate the production of endorphins (naturally produced hormones that help to reduce pain sensations).[1]

It can take a while to get used to the sensations TENS produces, and trying it out in advance can be helpful. TENS can be used successfully at any stage, but has been found to be most effective when used from early labour. While some women find it extremely helpful, others don't. (Note that it is not available in all hospitals.)

Pethidine

An injection of this narcotic painkiller into a muscle (usually in your bottom) or directly into a vein helps take the worst of the pain out of the contractions. It takes about 15 minutes to work, and lasts two to three hours. Because pethidine tends to make you very sleepy between contractions, you will probably need to be in bed, although you can still be propped up in various positions. Be aware that narcotic injections can make you vomit, although sometimes an anti-nausea drug such as metaclopromide (Maxolon) will be given with the pethidine. It is important to realise that no narcotic drug takes away the pain completely, but it is likely to change your perception of the pain from intensely unbearable to a duller sensation.

Rarely, babies born soon after a pethidine injection can be slow to breathe, although drugs to reverse the narcotic action can be given to the baby straight after birth. But it's best to avoid this type of pain relief towards the end of the first stage of labour or during the second stage, when the baby is moving down the birth canal. You will usually have a VE to check the baby's progress before a decision is made to give you an injection for pain relief.

Fentanyl

This is a more potent narcotic analgesic drug than pethidine. Small doses are given either into a large muscle, or into a vein if you have a drip (IV line). Although fentanyl can be very effective, it must be used with caution. High doses of fentanyl have recently been associated with impaired reflex responses in newborn babies. While the long-term significance of this is uncertain, it makes sense to avoid this potential complication by restricting the use of fentanyl to the smallest doses.[2]

Entonox

This anaesthetic gas is a 50:50 mixture of nitrous oxide and oxygen, and is also known as 'laughing gas'. You breathe it in through a mask or a mouthpiece when you need to take the worst of the pain out of each contraction. If you are offered a mask and you find it claustrophobic, ask for a mouthpiece.

This gas mixture is very fast-acting, but because the effect wears off equally quickly it is recommended that you start breathing in the gas as soon as you begin to feel a contraction. It works only for as long as you are breathing deeply, in and out, with the mouthpiece between your teeth or with the mask over your mouth and nose. You can continue with your controlled breathing patterns when you do this. A 'click-click' noise tells you that you are breathing deeply enough to activate the valve to release the gas.

It's also very important that you hold the mask/mouthpiece yourself. Too much gas will make you so drowsy that you will drop the mask/mouthpiece and breathe air again, regaining your normal level of consciousness within a few seconds. On the other hand, if someone else holds the mask/mouthpiece, you could drift into unconsciousness.

It's hard to use the mask/mouthpiece for any length of time as it gets very claustrophobic, so it's best reserved for use near the end of labour. The gas will not affect the baby unless you have enough gas to make you unconscious.

Epidural and combined spinal epidural (CSE)

An epidural/CSE is a type of anaesthetic that affects just the lower half of the body. It is the most effective form of pain relief, making even the strongest contractions barely noticeable. A Caesarean section can be done using an epidural/CSE.

Epidurals (where an anaesthetic drug is placed in the space around the spinal cord) have been used for women in labour for the last 35–40 years, and there is no doubt that for long and difficult labours they are invaluable. A CSE is a more recent approach to this type of pain relief, where some anaesthetic drug is also placed into the spinal cord, theoretically speeding up the onset of pain relief, but with lower drug doses. However, from a practical point of view, the differences between the two approaches are not often noticeable. Instead, many anaesthetists suggest using the lowest possible epidural drug dose that will give reasonable pain relief, but still allow you good movement and some sensation.[3]

Epidurals must be given by highly trained people, using impeccable techniques and instruments. Epidurals also need to be carefully monitored, from both the mother's and the baby's point of view. This makes them quite unsuitable for use at a home birth, and you will have to transfer from a small hospital to a larger one if the need for an epidural arises. Epidurals/CSE are very safe in the expert hands of a properly trained anaesthetist, but the decision to have one must never be taken without realising that they do carry a small risk of potential complications (see box on p.258).

Advantages of an epidural

- It allows virtually pain-free labour.
- It doesn't affect your level of consciousness, so you are mentally alert throughout labour.
- Only a tiny amount of anaesthetic passes through the placenta, so the effect on your baby is minuscule compared with that of a general anaesthetic.
- It allows you to relax, and often means that labour will progress faster.
- It usually causes your blood pressure to drop, which is helpful if it has been too high. However, it is important that it does not drop too low.
- If a forceps or vacuum delivery is necessary, this can be done comfortably.
- If a Caesarean section is necessary, this can be done without any other anaesthetic and you can be awake to see your baby being born,
- The cannula can stay in place for as long as you need pain relief.

Disadvantages of an epidural

- It may confine you to bed (although 'walking' epidurals are now available in some larger centres).
- It must be given by a fully trained health professional, and such people are available only in larger centres.
- It usually involves having an intravenous line (drip) inserted into your arm to give you extra fluid.
- If given before labour is established, it may stop labour proceeding.
- You need to wear a monitor continuously, or at least at frequent intervals.
- The assessment of progress is more difficult, so there will be more VEs.
- It may be harder to push your baby out at the end of the second stage, because of decreased sensation. There is a higher rate of forceps or ventouse (vacuum) delivery with epidurals (see p.280).
- An epidural may not be possible if your blood pressure is already too low and/or there is bleeding or a risk of bleeding, or if you have any skin infection on your back.
- Rarely, it may be difficult to insert the epidural correctly, so that there is too little anaesthetic given (i.e. it is ineffective) or too much (i.e. there is complete loss of sensation or movement). The latter is a serious situation, and this is why full emergency equipment and trained staff must be on hand in any hospital where epidurals are given
- Very rarely, the epidural cannot be inserted because of small anatomical variations of the spine. It is not usually possible to predict this situation, so every woman should be aware that there is a very small possibility of epidural failure.

Insertion of an epidural

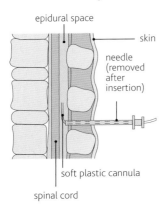

epidural space

skin

needle (removed after insertion)

soft plastic cannula

spinal cord

Inserting an epidural

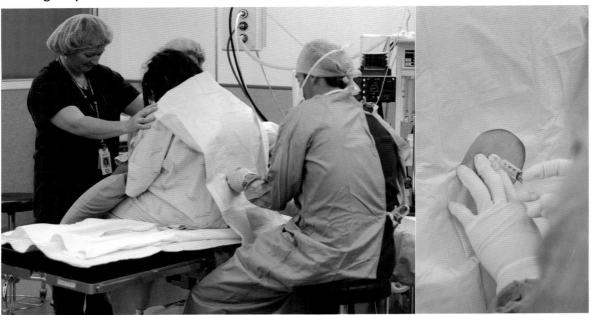

Having an epidural

- Before the epidural is inserted, you will usually have an intravenous line (drip) inserted into a vein in your arm or hand so that you can be given some extra fluids. This will prevent your blood pressure dropping too rapidly once the epidural takes effect.

- You will usually be asked to sit up with your body straight and your feet on a chair or stool, and to lean over a pillow so that the spaces between the bones of your spine (vertebrae) can open up. You will need to keep very still and tell the anaesthetist when a contraction starts, especially if they are about to insert the larger needle.

- A small amount of local anaesthetic is injected into the skin in the middle of your back, using a tiny needle.

- A larger needle is then inserted between two vertebrae into the epidural space around, and not in, the spinal cord. Next, a fine hollow plastic tube (cannula) is threaded through the needle into the epidural space and the needle is removed, leaving the cannula in place. This is then secured with sticky tape.

- A small amount of long-acting anaesthetic is inserted into the cannula, via a tiny tap with a filter, to surround the spinal cord. Sometimes, a little pump is used to give a small but continuous supply of anaesthetic.

- Within a few minutes, you will lose sensation in the lower half of your body. Your ability to move is usually reduced, though not completely; this means that you may be confined to bed. The anaesthetic lasts between one and three hours, and then gradually wears off. If necessary, further doses, or 'top-ups', can be given through the cannula. Sometimes the analgesic drug is administered as a continuous infusion, so that it flows in at a steady rate. The rate of flow can be reduced once you are ready to give birth, enabling you to feel the urge to push and the sensation of moving your baby through the birth canal.

- Your midwife will monitor your blood pressure regularly after the epidural is inserted and will also check the level of the anaesthetised area to ensure it does not go too high and affect your breathing.

- Once your baby is born, the cannula is simply pulled out. You will need to lie quietly for a while afterwards.

- The insertion is nearly always done by an anaesthetist. Top-ups can often be done by your midwife, if she has had the extra training required to look after a woman with an epidural anaesthetic.

Acupuncture[4]

This Chinese technique is becoming popular in New Zealand, with some midwives being trained in its use to deal with specific issues in pregnancy and labour. It involves having tiny needles inserted into particular pressure points to relieve pain. Not everyone is suited to acupuncture, and some women find it ineffective.

If you wish to consider this method of pain relief in labour, you will need to find a skilled acupuncturist who is willing to do it for you. You will need to discuss with them your expectations, and what they can offer, before you go into labour. You will also need to discuss it with your LMC, unless they also practise acupuncture. (This is becoming more common as the technique gains acceptance within Western health systems.)

In skilled hands, acupuncture can be a very effective form of pain relief in labour which allows you and your baby to remain alert throughout.

Rupture of the membranes (RM)

This is also known as 'the breaking of the waters'. It often occurs spontaneously during labour (an event known as SRM), but may sometimes occur before labour begins. Once the membranes rupture, labour is inevitable (except sometimes in a premature situation, when it may take up to one or two weeks for spontaneous labour to start). Contractions often become stronger, more frequent and more painful. Labour nearly always speeds up, and the cervix dilates quite quickly.

When the waters break, there may be just a trickle of clear fluid from the vagina, which is easy to confuse with a little leaking from the bladder. Or it may be a dramatic explosion, at which time most women hear a 'popping' sound – so be prepared! The fluid (liquor) is normally quite clear; if it is cloudy, green or brown, or contains bright red blood, this can indicate problems – alert your LMC straight away.

If the membranes do not rupture spontaneously, and providing the cervix is sufficiently dilated for them to be reached, they can be artificially ruptured (a process known as ARM). This is a simple procedure carried out by a midwife using a little hook-like device during a VE, and takes only a minute or two (see also p.275).

However, an ARM should not be done without good reason: the waters provide protection for the baby from the stress of labour, because the pressure from the contractions is spread throughout the liquid rather than being directly on the baby. If a baby is more than a week overdue, the membranes are often ruptured so that the colour of the liquor can be assessed. Babies under stress usually pass meconium (their first bowel motion), which makes the liquor cloudy. There are other situations where ARM may be indicated, especially in a long labour when progress is slow. Both you and your support person should be part of any decision about whether ARM should proceed, as in most situations the membranes rupture spontaneously towards the end of labour.

Rupture of the membranes without labour

If labour does not start within 24 hours of the membranes rupturing, you and your LMC will need to make a decision about what happens next. This will depend on both the duration of your pregnancy and the health of you and your baby.

If you are within two to three weeks of your due date, then your baby is probably mature enough to be born. Because the risk of serious infection is likely to outweigh the risk of immature lungs and breathing problems, it is advisable to plan to induce labour within the next day or so. It is quite common in this situation for women to go into labour suddenly anyway, and induction becomes unnecessary.

However, if your membranes rupture before you reach the 37th week of pregnancy, the baby is still premature. More time in the womb will give a pre-term baby just a little bit longer to mature – even a few days can make quite a difference to a baby's lungs and his ability to breathe after birth. But because of the risk of infection, you will need to be on high doses of antibiotics and under the care of a specialist obstetric team in hospital. However, there is research which indicates that women can sometimes be safely managed and monitored at home if their membranes rupture early and there are no contractions,[5] although this does depend on the reason for the waters breaking.[6] Either way, both mother and baby will need close monitoring for any early signs of infection, and the baby's growth must also be checked.[7] If there is any doubt at all about the continued well-being of either mother or baby, it is advisable to induce labour as soon as possible (see p.275).

Intravenous (IV) lines, or drips

IV lines are a way to give fluids, and sometimes drugs, directly into a vein in the arm. They are not required or recommended in a normal labour, but they do have an important role if progress is slow or labour complicated. Sometimes an IV line may be needed to supply fluids to rehydrate your body and to give you a little bit of extra energy for your uterus to work effectively.[8]

A special needle with an outer plastic covering is inserted into a vein in your arm, using a little local anaesthetic. The needle is then removed, leaving only the flexible plastic cannula, which is held firmly in place with sticky tape. IV lines are a bit restricting, but certainly don't have to keep you in bed.

Situations where different fluids need to be given via an IV line

- woman dehydrated and/or vomiting (a special salt and sugar solution)
- labour slow, sometimes owing to the woman's lack of energy (salt solution)
- labour slow or induced (salt solution plus syntocinon – the synthetic form of the hormone oxytocin)
- when an epidural anaesthetic is used (very weak salt solution, which helps to keep the blood pressure normal)
- if there is bleeding, or a danger of bleeding (salt solution and/or blood transfusion and/or blood products)

Checking on your baby

Throughout labour, your health and that of your baby are of paramount importance. Labour is not just hard work for you; it's hard work for your unborn baby, too. Normal, healthy babies take the stresses and strains of a normal, straightforward labour in their stride (in fact, it is thought that they initiate labour when hormones are released from their adrenal glands). Many of those stresses and strains prepare your baby for life outside the womb, when a dramatic change in his whole physiology must take place within a few minutes of birth.

Labour seems to become a problem for a baby only when the normal course of events falters, putting extra strain on the environment within the womb. Whenever this seems likely to occur, it's wise to keep checking on his well-being. This can be done in several ways:

- Listening frequently and regularly to the baby's heartbeat with an ear trumpet or sonicaid. The normal range is 110–160 beats per minute, and a slow or a fast heartbeat can indicate stress.

- Observing the colour of the liquor (waters) once the membranes have ruptured. If there is concern about the baby's welfare, the membranes can be artificially ruptured (see p.275). Cloudy, green or brown liquor indicates that the baby is or has been under stress.

- Using a CTG (cardiotocograph) or monitor (see p.214). A CTG tracing during labour will give a continuous reading of the baby's heartbeat and movements, and record the contractions within the muscles of the uterus. Any variations from the characteristic 'normal' pattern on the tracing can be detected quickly by someone experienced in reading CTGs. Depending on the circumstances, it is not always necessary to wear the monitor continuously, as the strap tends to become uncomfortable unless you have an epidural. You do not have to be lying down when wearing the monitor, but can be sitting up on a Swiss ball or in bed to allow gravity to help your labour progress. Some hospitals have also invested in water-resistant monitors, which enable women to be monitored while in the spa or birthing pool.

Taking a CTG trace

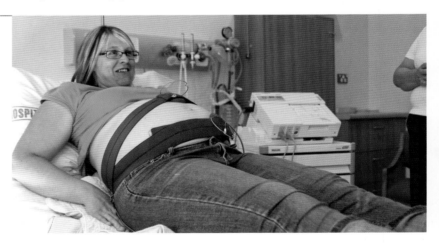

- Using a foetal scalp electrode. If the CTG tracing indicates that the baby may be stressed, and the waters have broken, it's possible to place a small electrode on the baby's head to measure the foetal heart rate more accurately.

- Foetal blood sampling (FBS). A blood sample can also be taken from the baby's scalp to check the acidity (pH) or to do a lactate analysis of his blood. The pH test is a sensitive guide to the baby's well-being, but expertise is required to perform and interpret it, and the measuring equipment needs to be checked every day. The technique, which involves making a tiny cut on the baby's scalp, is not done often, and is warranted only in a very few high-risk situations. Foetal lactate testing is being tried in some hospitals in New Zealand. It requires a smaller blood sample from the baby's scalp than the pH test, and gives a reading within 60 seconds at the bedside.[9]

If, after using one or more of these checks, there is good evidence that the baby is stressed in some way, active intervention in the natural course of labour may be advisable.

Factors that can put extra strain on the baby during labour

- long labour – woman exhausted and dehydrated
- baby in wrong position, e.g. posterior position, breech presentation or transverse lie (these last two positions need to be identified as soon as possible, because of the very different management required; see pp.191 and 278)
- baby (or babies) too small – premature and/or with intra-uterine growth restriction (IUGR; see p.142), or twins
- blood supply to baby poor, because either cord twisted, or around baby's neck; placenta not working properly due to high blood pressure, or 'too old' (overdue baby); or placenta in wrong place, or partly separated from uterus
- contractions very strong, without time for relaxation in between, e.g. when labour is induced too strongly
- unnecessary artificial rupture of membranes

Transition (the end of the first stage)

Transition occurs right at the end of the first stage, when the cervix is nearly fully dilated (10cm) and cannot be felt at all during a VE. Only then can the baby start moving down the birth canal and the second stage begin.

If you start to get a very strong desire to push, associated with really large contractions, then you may be in the transition stage of labour. If you or your support person recognise that any of the signs listed in the box (right) are happening, tell your midwife and ask her if you can push. She may need to do a quick VE at this point to check that you are indeed fully dilated.

It's really important *not* to push until *all* the cervix is out of the way. The last part of the cervix to disappear is known as the anterior lip – pushing on this will only make it swollen and slower to move out of the way. It can be very frustrating if you feel you want to push, but are told to wait – labour seems to be slowing down just when you thought you were nearly there. But if you can hold off pushing, the cervix will usually dilate fully and allow the second stage to begin.

If the waters haven't broken by this stage, they probably will do so now, usually with quite a rush. Because labour nearly always progresses faster once the waters break, your LMC may suggest doing this artificially to help you get through transition and into the second stage.

Second stage of labour

A normal second stage can last from a few minutes to one or two hours. It tends to be much longer in first labours than in subsequent ones.

Contractions often feel quite different once the baby starts to move down the birth canal, because the force exerted by each contraction is now directly pushing the baby rather than stretching open the cervix. With this change in contractions, you may feel very different too. Suddenly the end is in sight, and often there comes an incredibly strong desire to push the baby out.

Some indications of transition

- big, strong, and even more frequent contractions
- multiple contractions with two to three peaks to each one
- sweating and shivering
- vomiting
- strong desire to push down and/or pass a bowel motion
- feeling out of control, shouting, swearing, crying, wanting to have the baby taken out of you

Now you may find yourself calling on new reserves of energy you didn't know you had. With each contraction, you can really help push that baby down towards the vaginal opening by following what your body is telling you. You can push as hard as you possibly can. This is really hard work, requiring all your mental and physical energy. Second-stage contractions tend to be longer than first-stage ones, but they are also less frequent. This is normal, and gives you a bit more time to gather your strength for the next push.

Forces exerted by the uterine muscles during labour

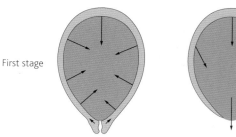

First stage

Second stage

Positions are important too, and you will work out what is best for you only at the time. Lying flat on your back is a particularly hard position in which to push; squatting, semi-squatting, and being on hands and knees are easier positions. A special birthing stool can be used to help maintain an upright position and make pushing easier. Your midwife may also suggest sitting on the toilet to get the full feel of pushing, and then moving back to the pool/bath, bed or mattress where you plan to give birth to your baby.

In some second and subsequent labours, the second stage progresses so rapidly that the perineum doesn't have time to stretch properly. Lying down may slow things sufficiently to allow this to happen. Lying on your side, particularly the left side, can also be a very good position for pushing, ensuring that your baby is getting sufficient oxygen and enabling your LMC to see the perineum and provide support while the head is being born.

If the contractions begin to 'get on top of you', you may find it helpful to use Rescue Remedy, a homeopathic remedy that has no confirmed research basis as yet but has been found helpful by women in labour. Entonox (gas) can also be useful, particularly just at the peak of a contraction. It will help take the worst of the pain out of the contraction, but allows you and the baby to be alert within a few seconds of taking the mask off or removing the mouthpiece.

Once the baby's head has negotiated the pelvic outlet, it's usually possible to see a small portion of it at the vaginal opening during each contraction. With each successive contraction a little bit more of the head should be visible, and the perineum starts to become thin and stretched. It can be tremendously encouraging to see all this in a mirror, and your support person or midwife can hold one for you. If you're having trouble with your pushing technique, a glimpse of your baby's head in the mirror may be all you need to concentrate your efforts.

In most women, the perineum will stretch more and more with each contraction to allow the baby to be born without tearing or splitting, as long as the head or shoulders do not come through the vaginal opening too quickly. Sometimes the baby's head or shoulders are too big or the perineum hasn't stretched enough over several contractions, so that the skin does indeed tear, and in a jagged and uncontrolled way.

Episiotomy

To avoid a large tear, your LMC or specialist obstetrician will sometimes need to make a cut (episiotomy) in the skin and tissue at or near the back of the vaginal opening, using a very sharp pair of sterile scissors, just before the baby's head is born. Local anaesthetic can be used, but often the skin of the perineum is quite numb by this time, and no anaesthetic is required. An episiotomy gives more room if the baby needs to be actively assisted in the second stage. It can be repaired much more easily (see p.273), and heals better than a large, jagged tear, which may affect the deep muscles.

In the past, doctors and midwives sometimes tried to speed up delivery by doing an episiotomy too readily, before the skin was properly stretched. Today, the aim is to avoid unnecessary episiotomies, and there is good evidence that routine use of episiotomies is not justified.[10] However, there will always be some situations where an episiotomy is necessary, such as a very long second stage with a baby in distress, if the shoulders get stuck, or for a breech, forceps or vacuum (ventouse) delivery. You should discuss episiotomies and how best to avoid one if you can with your LMC early on in labour, as well as at an antenatal visit.

Certain birthing positions may make large tears and/or an episiotomy less likely, as they encourage maximal stretching of the perineum. These include being on hands and knees, squatting, and using a birthing stool during the second stage of labour.

Episiotomy

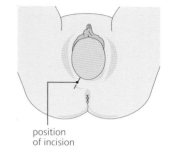

position
of incision

Cord around the baby's neck

If the cord is around the neck, it could strangle the baby if it tightens as the body is born. The LMC will watch carefully, and if the cord tightens too much it will be clamped and cut straight away before the next contraction. If the cord is not cut, it is sometimes (but not always) possible to use a 'somersault manoeuvre' to keep the baby as close to the mother's pubic bone or thigh as possible while the body is being born, ensuring that there is not much tension on the cord. Once the baby is fully born, the cord can be unwrapped from around the neck. This means that the cord doesn't have to be cut until after the birth, allowing the baby to receive the benefit of the extra blood usually left in the placenta.[11]

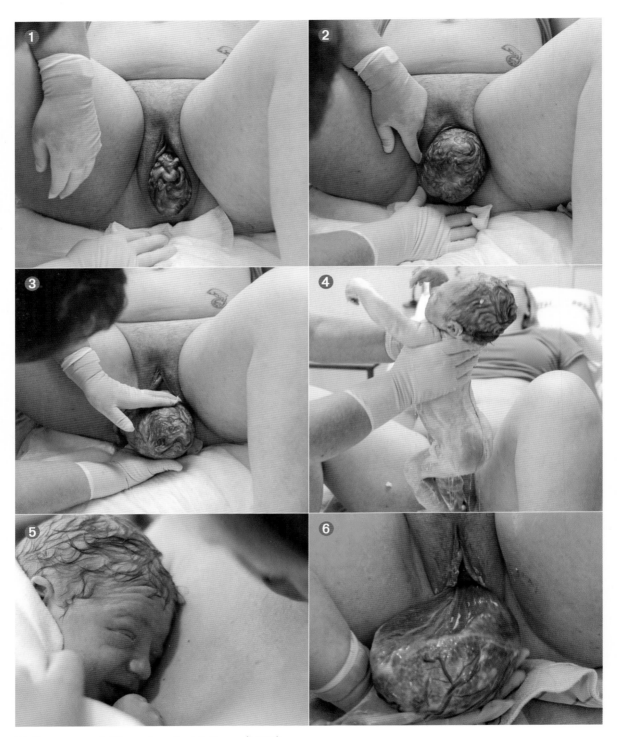

Birth sequence 1: Normal vaginal delivery (NVD)

❶ The baby's head crowns, and **❷** is born. **❸** The midwife gently steadies the baby's head as the shoulders are born. **❹** The baby is born. **❺** Baby has skin-to-skin contact with mother. **❻** The placenta is born.

The birth

The sensations that accompany the stretching of the perineum are intense. Even with an epidural, there will often be some sensation, although it is much diminished. Feelings range from 'white hot pain' to 'almost orgasmic' as the perineal skin stretches. Such feelings are an indication of good stretching – and of the fact that your baby is very nearly born!

At this point, pushing is usually no longer required – your LMC will often tell you *not* to push, and to do 'panting' breathing to help you achieve this. Not pushing when you have a strong urge to do so can be really difficult, but there is less risk of tearing if the baby's head can emerge through the vaginal opening as gently as possible. If you do tear or have an episiotomy, you will not feel it – the skin is so stretched that the nerves do not carry the normal pain messages.

The baby's head is usually born during a contraction. Your LMC will apply just enough pressure to the head to guide it through the vaginal opening, checking the baby's neck as they do so to ensure the cord is not wrapped around it. The moment when the top of the baby's head emerges at the vaginal opening is sometimes called 'crowning'.

The baby's head is usually facing towards the woman's back as he is born, and then rotates to one side. Mucous often streams out of his nose and mouth. This is normal, as the airways prepare to take in air for the first time.

But before the baby can take his first breath, the shoulders must be born, usually with the next contraction. Again, this needs to happen as gently as possible to avoid tears in the perineum. First one shoulder (the uppermost, or anterior) emerges through the vaginal opening and then the other. The rest of the body then follows, sliding out easily. Your baby is born, and the second stage is over.

Your new baby!

Your baby is born and breathes in deeply. For the first time, his lungs fill with air, his skin feels direct touch, and his eyes see light and dark. For the first time, you can see exactly what your baby looks like. You can see whether 'it' is a girl or a boy. You can be amazed and overwhelmed that a real live baby has just emerged from inside you. Suddenly, instead of a large lump in your abdomen, you have a baby to touch, to cuddle and to love. It is a very special moment, and one that you, your partner and/or support person and your baby can share and treasure.

In most cases, babies breathe entirely of their own accord and need no assistance. Some need a little gentle stimulation and to have mucous sucked out of their mouth and nose, but suctioning is done only if there is meconium in the mucous, and the baby is not breathing and is floppy (see p.288). Some babies benefit from a little oxygen. Some take their first breath immediately, while others take several seconds to breathe. They sometimes cry, but quite often they don't.

Birth sequence 2: Using water in labour

❶ Checking the baby's heartbeat while the mother labours in water.

❷ Out of the water, the mother is lying on her side and pushing the baby.

❸ Mother moves onto her back and can see the baby's head in the mirror.

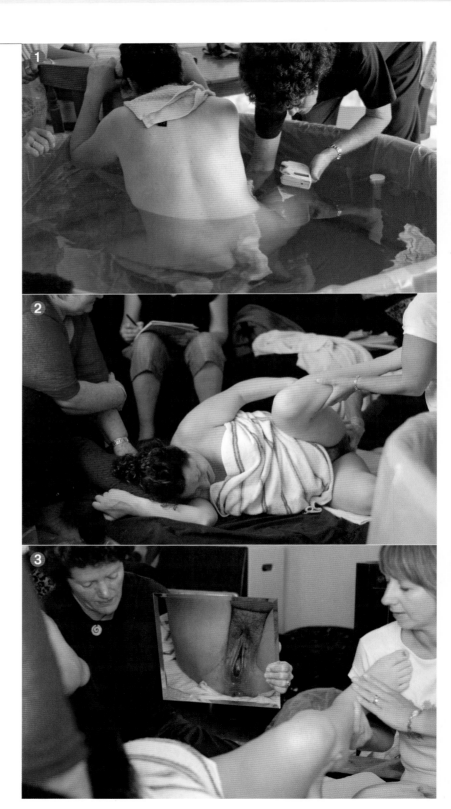

If you want, your baby can go straight onto your tummy or thigh so that you can see and touch him, even before the cord is cut. He does need to be dried, as he will get cold very quickly, but this can be done while he is lying on you, skin to skin. At the same time, your baby's need for active assistance can be assessed by your LMC. If a baby is not breathing at all, and/or is very floppy with no responses, he may need immediate, active resuscitation within the first five minutes after birth.[12]

In recent years the Apgar score has been commonly used to measure how well a baby is at birth. Heart rate, breathing effort, colour, muscle tone and reflex responses all contribute to a score out of ten, measured first at one minute and then at five minutes after birth. By five minutes, babies should be breathing well, have normal colour, a normal heart rate and good muscle tone (i.e. are not 'floppy'). In practice, your LMC will assess these crucial factors quickly, without necessarily recording them formally as an Apgar score.

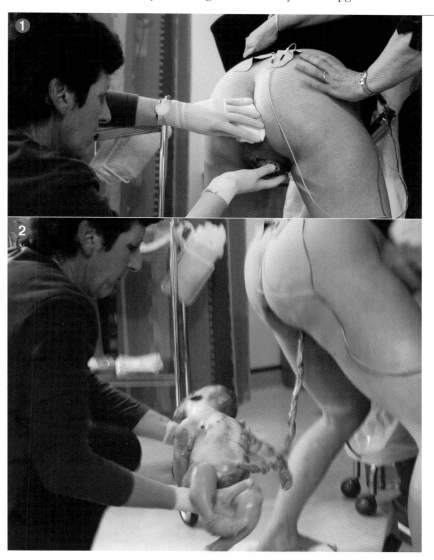

Birth sequence 3: Birthing in the standing position

❶ Baby's head crowning, with mother in standing position.

❷ The baby is born.

Giving birth in water

Some hospitals have baths that can be used for water births. As long as the woman and her baby are healthy and labour is progressing normally, giving birth in water can have considerable benefits.

Giving birth in water significantly lessens the need for other pain relief, particularly in the first stage of labour (see box on p.255). Pushing in the second stage may also be easier, and healthy babies born under water do just as well as any others. The evidence of benefits in the third stage is not clear, so you may need to get out of the water if there is any delay in delivering the placenta.[13]

Whether you are having a water birth at home or in hospital, there are a few important points to bear in mind.

- The water temperature should be increased to no more than 37°C for the actual birth.[14]
- The water should be kept as clean as possible, so have a sieve handy for removing blood clots or stools.
- The baby should be born completely under water, with no air contact until the body is born and the head is then brought gently to the surface within a few seconds to a minute. This prevents the baby taking a breath and inhaling water.
- Once the baby is out of the water, he should lie with his head facing downwards to assist drainage from his mouth and nose.
- If the cord is around the baby's neck it should not be clamped and cut until the baby's body has been born and brought to the surface.
- After the birth, once the baby has been brought to the surface and taken his first breaths, he can be kept warm by immersing his body in the water up to his shoulders. A warm air temperature is also essential to ensure he does not become cold.
- Your LMC will monitor your well-being and that of your baby while you are in the water by checking your temperature, the water temperature and your baby's heart rate.
- If at any time you do not feel comfortable in the pool, you should tell your LMC and get out of the water.

Birth sequence 4: A water birth

As soon as the baby is completely born under the water, he is brought to the surface to take his first breath.

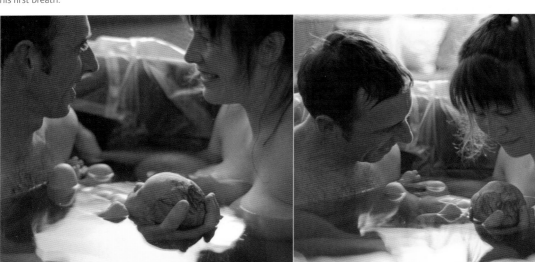

Cutting the cord

Once the baby breathes air, he has no further use for the placenta. However, the cord should not be cut straight away but allowed to pulsate for one to two minutes. Once the cord has stopped pulsating, it can be clamped with forceps in two places and cut between them with a pair of sharp, sterile scissors.

If you want, you, your partner or support person can cut the cord. There is usually no need to hurry, and the baby can receive the benefit of up to 80ml of blood through the cord from the placenta after birth. This also enables the baby to obtain valuable extra iron, which is at a premium in the first year of life.[15] Even for babies born before 35 weeks of pregnancy, where active assistance with breathing is more likely to be needed, it is beneficial if up to 45 seconds are allowed to pass before the cord is clamped.[16]

Once the cord is cut, a small clip is placed onto the cord close to the baby's umbilicus (tummy button), and the excess cord removed.

Then you can place your baby just where you want him. As long as the room is warm, he will be quite all right in direct body contact with you, preferably covered by a warm soft towel or blanket to prevent him cooling down. You may want to put him to the breast immediately, or you may want your partner or support person to hold him.

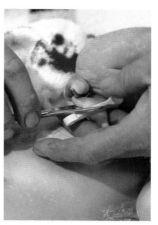

Cutting the cord

For partners and support people

You may very much want to hold and cuddle your new baby too: be guided by your partner's needs, but also by your own. Many women are more than happy to have their baby held close by his father or grandmother or other support person at this time, while they finish the business of labour (the third stage). The baby will need to be kept warm if he's not in direct skin-to-skin contact, so make sure he's well wrapped up.

Third stage of labour

Delivery of the placenta

In the excitement of the baby's arrival, it's easy to forget that labour is not over yet. The placenta must also be completely expelled from the uterus, along with the remnants of the membranes. This often takes only a few minutes, although anything up to 20–30 minutes is quite normal.

Usually the placenta separates from the wall of the uterus as the baby is born, and the uterus must then contract firmly to prevent bleeding from the place where it was attached. A naturally occurring hormone, oxytocin, is produced within the woman's body to help this process.

Expectant (or physiological) management

For some women, the natural production of oxytocin will be all that is needed to cause the uterus to contract and the placenta and membranes to separate. If a woman is not overly tired or dehydrated, she will often have an urge to push, the uterus will usually contract strongly, the placenta will be quickly expelled within a few minutes, and bleeding will be minimal.

Active management

Sometimes, natural oxytocin alone is not enough to expel the placenta efficiently and to contract the uterus. In such cases, a small dose of synthetic oxytocin can greatly aid the natural hormonal process and prevent subsequent haemorrhage. This is usually done by injection into a muscle (or into an IV line, if you have one) about 1 minute after the baby has been born or very shortly afterwards. This injection helps the uterus to contract down very firmly.

With several contractions, the placenta is pushed down into the birth canal and out through the vaginal opening. Often this is hardly noticeable compared with the hard work of pushing out the baby, but sometimes it does need a few pushes to get things going. Your LMC will help you deliver the placenta by very gently pulling on the cord and supporting your uterus just above the pubic bone. This active management of the third stage of labour significantly reduces the risk of post-partum haemorrhage (PPH) and the need for a blood transfusion (see p.282).[17]

After the delivery of the placenta

Once the placenta is expelled, it needs to be inspected to make sure it is complete. Your LMC will do this, but so can you or your partner – it's worth taking a look at this amazing organ, which was literally the life-blood for your baby throughout the pregnancy. If you want to keep the placenta, remind your LMC and others present so that it can be put aside for you or your support person to take home.

The special significance of the whenua (placenta) as a life force has long been recognised by Māori (see box below). Proper burial of the whenua in a culturally significant place, often in a family cemetery or on ancestral land, gives that person a 'place always to come home to'. Many people place the nutrient-rich whenua in a pot and plant a shrub or tree over it, so they can take it with them if they move.

Whenua

Whenua is the common Māori name for the placenta that is primarily responsible for nurturing your baby inside your womb. Apart from this practical role, the whenua has customary significance concerned with wairua (spiritual, psychological and emotional well-being) and whakapapa (ancestry). Today, tikanga (etiquette/protocol) around the time of childbirth and specifically for the whenua are being reclaimed by some Māori women, because such practices were forgotten or nearly lost, partly due to the influence of Western ideas that dominate childbirth ideology in New Zealand.

Tikanga often has common elements across whānau but there may be differences, so each woman needs to explore the unique practices of her own whānau. You may be the first woman in your generation to renew significance to the whenua. If so, it is useful to talk to members of your whānau or other Māori women before or during your pregnancy, so you can carefully consider and plan what you would like to do with the whenua and why.

Hope Tupara

Repairs to the perineum

Your perineum and vaginal opening need to be carefully checked for any cuts or tears. Achieving good bowel, bladder and sexual function after childbirth relies on good healing of the perineum. Superficial tears and bruising will nearly always heal rapidly and naturally just by being kept clean and rested. However, if there are any deeper tears and/or an episiotomy, they will heal much faster and more completely if they are surgically repaired. This is nearly always done by your LMC as soon as the placenta is delivered. Some local anaesthetic is injected into the skin and surrounding tissue, and dissolvable stitches are used to repair the muscles and the skin of the perineum. A cleanly cut episiotomy takes only a few minutes to repair; a very deep or jagged tear may take considerably longer.

Finally, your doctor or midwife will check your abdomen to make sure the uterus is hard and lying below the level of your tummy button. This indicates that it is contracting well, and that there should be only a little further bleeding.

After the birth

Once this is all over, you will need to be cleaned up. Your partner or support person and your midwife can help you into the shower if you wish (although you can do this later once you have had some more time with your baby), or they can sponge you down, change the bedding and give you a sterile sanitary pad to wear. You will need to empty your bladder, too (see p.318).

Now that you're clean and comfortable, and the hard work of labour is over, there is time at last to spend with your new baby. This can be a very special family time; your professional caregivers should be able to give you time alone now with your partner, your support people and your baby. In the hour or two after birth, newborns are very alert, taking in the sights, sounds, touches and smells around them; this is especially the case if they do not have any analgesic drugs used during labour in their systems. They may want to start tasting, too – some are keen to feed straight away or at least within the first hour after birth. Others are content to gaze at you wide-eyed, grasping firmly at your finger or the edge of a blanket.

For partners and support people

The period immediately after birth is a time to be treasured, a reward for all your hard work as well as your partner's. Don't be in a hurry to rush away – take time to start getting to know this new son or daughter, grandchild or friend. Most women find this time a real emotional 'high', especially if labour has been long and difficult; a very few women may want everyone to leave, but most want to share the experience. Later, most women will want and need to sleep, so perhaps that is a good time for you to start telephoning family and friends.

If your baby has been taken into the neonatal unit or intensive care for any reason, your partner will especially need your love and support. You can almost always go together to the nursery and be near your baby, although you may not be able to hold him.

4. Complications and interventions

There are, and always will be, situations in which normal labour and delivery are not possible. Today, modern obstetric care offers many effective ways of salvaging a potentially disastrous situation, but unfortunately not all situations are salvageable.

It is also important to remember that intervention is not always appropriate. Intervention always carries a risk – though usually a small one – and should be undertaken only when the benefits outweigh the risks. Every single birth is different, and sometimes it is very difficult to decide whether the benefits do in fact outweigh the risks. Often the decision must be made quickly. It is your choice whether or not to accept the active management being suggested, but to make that decision you must be quite clear about the consequences. Accepting active management means you have to place considerable trust in your health care professionals – not only your own LMC, but also the team of health professionals that your LMC will now need to work with, often in a larger hospital with obstetric services. This is easier if you and your LMC have already discussed possible complications before you go into labour.

When complications do arise, the skills of a specialist obstetrician are invaluable. They are experts in the safe and effective management of abnormal labour and birth; they can discuss options and give advice, as well as undertake the more complex interventions that might be required. In addition, highly skilled hospital midwives, nurses, anaesthetists and paediatricians are all available in hospital to help with complications that arise during labour and birth.

When home birth is no longer advisable

There are times when a home birth has been planned and labour has started, but unforeseen complications arise.

If this happens, it may be you, your partner/support person, or your LMC who suggests transfer to hospital. There is not always time to discuss this fully. Often decisions must be made very quickly, and you need to have talked about this possibility with your LMC beforehand. It is advisable to have worked out a birth plan that allows for transfer to hospital if complications arise.

In general, any situation where active intervention becomes necessary is better managed in hospital, where emergency back-up is readily available. The most common reasons for transferring to hospital are prolonged labour, very slow progress, baby in distress, or delayed delivery of the placenta and/or bleeding after birth. Although these things are unlikely to happen, you have to be prepared to change the birth plan if they do, so that you and your baby can maintain the best possible health.

Usually your LMC can accompany you directly to hospital and stay with you for the rest of your labour and delivery, although a hospital midwife may attend you as well. However, if they have already been at your side for many hours, it may be wise for them to hand over care at this point, as they may be too tired to care for you safely. Depending on what the problem is, your LMC may want to seek the help of a specialist obstetrician and/or transfer your care to the hospital's specialist obstetric team. Your LMC will discuss this with you at the time, even if you have already talked about it when developing your birth plan. In most cases, you and your baby can return home within a few hours of delivery, where your LMC can once again care for you.

Induction of labour

In most pregnancies, labour starts spontaneously within about ten days of the expected date of delivery, triggered by a complex interplay of hormonal changes in both the woman and her baby. Normally, the spontaneous onset of labour is preferable to an artificial induction, as there is a lower associated rate of complications and interventions.

Occasionally, however, a situation may arise where the health of the woman and/or her baby may be at risk if pregnancy continues. In these cases, labour can be induced artificially. There are several ways of doing this, and the choice will depend on how far advanced the pregnancy is and the reason for the induction. Induction of labour is almost always done in hospital because of the higher risk of complications. In some cases, your LMC will stay and care for you, while in other cases your care may be handed over to the secondary or tertiary care team in the hospital.

Artificial rupture of the membranes (ARM) (see also p.260)

ARM will stimulate labour in many women, and contractions often begin within a few hours. It can be done only if the cervix is sufficiently open to reach the membranes. It involves using a small sharp hook (a bit like a crochet hook) during a VE to make a hole in the membranes. The membranes themselves have no nerves so there is no pain, but the VE is likely to be uncomfortable.

Prostaglandins: pessaries or vaginal gel

Special vaginal pessaries or a vaginal gel containing the hormone prostaglandin can be inserted high into the vagina. Prostaglandin is gradually released around the cervix, and this stimulates contractions. The most common method is to insert one pessary or one applicator of gel and wait several hours until contractions start. Usually, labour can then progress quite normally.

This method is only effective near the end of the pregnancy, when the cervix is 'ripe' (see p.226) and almost ready to go into labour anyway. For women who are having their second or subsequent baby, it is often all the stimulation they need.

Intravenous (IV) line with syntocinon

An IV line is inserted into a vein in the woman's arm and some special salt solution is slowly 'dripped' into her bloodstream. A small amount of syntocinon (synthetic oxytocin) will have been added to the salt solution. This will stimulate the uterus to contract, but must be carefully monitored to make sure the contractions don't become too strong. Usually, a special syntocinon pump is used to control the dose.

This method is sometimes combined with an ARM (see above), and tends to be used mainly when the woman is having her first baby or when labour is induced prematurely. In a first labour it is often more difficult to stimulate contractions, and they can sometimes start and then stop in the early stage if the syntocinon is discontinued.

Some reasons for inducing labour

- pre-eclampsia, or worsening hypertension of pregnancy
- diabetes in pregnancy (see p.140)
- IUGR (see p.142)
- baby definitely overdue (usually at least 10–14 days past the confirmed due date)
- membranes ruptured over 24 hours previously with no signs of labour and baby at risk if not delivered

Depending on the reason for the induction, your usual LMC may manage your care initially, and if all goes well will continue to care for you throughout the induction, labour and birth. They will however consult the hospital team, so that extra assistance can be readily obtained if needed.

Whenever labour is induced, it is important that the baby's health is closely monitored. You may need to wear a CTG monitor continuously, especially if syntocinon is used.

In a very small number of pregnancies, attempts to induce labour may fail: sometimes the cervix is just not ready to open. In such cases, a Caesarean section may be necessary (see p.282).

Augmenting labour

Sometimes, labour starts spontaneously but then slows and stops. If this happens early on and the membranes are still intact, the wisest course may simply be to accept that this was a 'false start' and let things be.

First-stage delay

However, labour can sometimes slow and stop during the first stage once the cervix is well dilated. This is much more likely to occur in a first labour than in a second or subsequent one.

When a first-stage delay occurs, it is important to find out why. The baby may be in a posterior position. In some cases, all that is needed is for the woman to rest on her side to help turn the baby, and have some food and fluid; labour may then restart more strongly and progress normally. Otherwise, an ARM and/or syntocinon drip will usually stimulate labour successfully.

Delays may also occur if the uterine muscles are contracting in an unco-ordinated manner, which makes progress very slow and exhausting. Each situation must be assessed individually, and specialist obstetric advice is likely to be advisable. A syntocinon drip and an epidural may solve the problem, but sometimes a Caesarean section is necessary, in which case the specialist obstetric team will need to take over your care.

If, however, labour is obstructed for some reason (such as a previously undetected sizeable ovarian cyst), then a syntocinon drip will not help and can make the situation worse – the uterus will be contracting but the baby will be making no progress towards being born. Urgent specialist obstetric advice and a Caesarean section are likely to be necessary.

First stage: some reasons for labour slowing and stopping

- abnormal position of baby, e.g. head extended (i.e. not flexed, with chin well tucked in), posterior position, breech baby, transverse lie
- obstruction in the pelvis, e.g. misshapen pelvis, ovarian cyst
- muscles in the wall of the uterus not coordinated properly, so contractions are ineffective, or muscles lack the energy they need to contract effectively
- intense fear and worry
- the presence of someone the woman does not want to have there, e.g. someone she is in conflict with, or someone who is abusing her or has abused her in the past

Second-stage delay

Labour may also slow and stop once the second stage is reached. Again, the cause of the delay needs to be identified so that it can be managed most effectively. In some situations, if the baby is in no distress, it may be quite appropriate to wait a little; contractions may start again spontaneously. In other situations, rupturing the membranes and/or an episiotomy is all that is required. Occasionally, a syntocinon drip and/or a forceps delivery (see p.280) may be necessary.

Second stage: some reasons for labour stopping

- any of the reasons in the box opposite (first-stage delay)
- baby's head too large or in an unusual position
- woman's pelvic outlet too small
- no apparent cause

The 'posterior' baby

A baby in the uterus is said to be in the posterior position when the head is down, but facing the woman's front instead of her back (the more usual 'anterior' position). This is especially common in first pregnancies, possibly because of the woman's firm abdominal muscles.

Many babies lie in the posterior position in late pregnancy, but turn to the anterior position early in labour. A small number remain in the posterior position during labour, which makes several things more likely:

- The baby's head seems to 'ride higher' than usual at the pelvic ring.
- The membranes may rupture spontaneously before labour begins.
- The baby's head doesn't press firmly on the cervix.
- The baby tends to 'go overdue'.
- The cervix dilates more slowly, making for a much longer, less efficient labour.
- Backache often occurs as the baby's back presses on the woman's spine.
- The baby's head doesn't descend through the pelvic ring, or it gets into the pelvis but has trouble getting through the outlet.

Helping yourself with a posterior baby in labour[18]

- Move around as much as you can.
- Position yourself on your hands and knees to take pressure off your back. Sitting or leaning forwards against a chair can also help.
- Get someone to massage your back to help ease the backache.
- If, despite your best efforts, you are beginning to feel overwhelmed by contractions, consider whether some extra pain relief now might keep you more comfortable and help relax you so that labour can progress a bit faster.

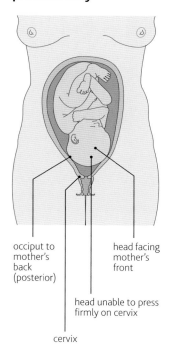

Position of posterior baby

occiput to mother's back (posterior)

head facing mother's front

head unable to press firmly on cervix

cervix

In many cases, especially with a second or subsequent baby, any of these measures may be enough to ensure that labour progresses to a normal delivery. Sometimes the baby's head will rotate spontaneously to the more usual anterior position as it moves down the birth canal, and usually the baby is then born very speedily! Sometimes, when there is plenty of room, the baby emerges unassisted – still in the posterior position, facing his mother's front.

Intervention with a posterior baby

Posterior babies sometimes need help if they are to be born healthy. The contractions have to be stronger to provide the extra power needed to turn the baby around. Active intervention to achieve this can involve one or more of the following (not necessarily in order).

- A drip with a special salt solution can give the extra fluid and energy required for the longer labour.
- An epidural can give excellent pain relief during a long labour and let you relax, allowing labour to progress faster and more strongly.
- A Caesarean section may be necessary if the baby's head still won't fit down through the pelvic ring. This can usually be done under epidural/spinal anaesthetic.
- Once the second stage is reached, forceps or vacuum methods can be used to ease the baby's head through the pelvic outlet, usually by rotating it to a more favourable anterior position. Very occasionally, the baby will emerge still in the posterior position.

Your LMC is likely to consult with a specialist obstetrician if it appears that a forceps or vacuum delivery or a Caesarean may be necessary.

Breech birth

Breech presentation

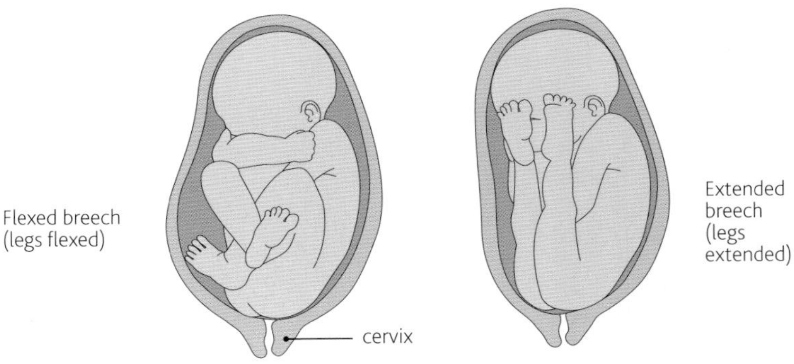

Flexed breech (legs flexed)

Extended breech (legs extended)

cervix

A small number (about 3 per cent) of babies are born bottom or legs first, and head last (see p.191). With good antenatal care, nearly all breech babies should be detected before labour begins. If your LMC finds that your baby is (still) in the breech position when you are 36 or more weeks pregnant, they will consult a specialist obstetrician and discuss with you the options for delivery.

A Caesarean section will usually be suggested, as this is often the safest method of delivery for you and your baby, but vaginal birth can sometimes be appropriate. This will depend on whether this is your first baby, the position of the baby's legs, and a number of other factors. You and your doctor or midwife can then decide on the best method of delivery and/or the options available to help turn the baby.[19] (See p.225.)

Options for delivery of a breech baby

Normal labour and vaginal delivery are perfectly possible for some women with a breech baby, but a number of things are more likely to happen:

- The baby's buttocks or legs 'ride higher' than the head normally would at the pelvic ring, and don't engage properly. An 'extended breech' baby is more likely to engage than a 'flexed' one.
- The membranes may rupture spontaneously.
- Labour may be slow and less efficient.
- The baby's feet, or one foot, and/or the cord may slip through the cervix before it is fully dilated.
- The cord may get squeezed during contractions, which puts extra stress on the baby.
- The baby's head may get stuck coming through the pelvic outlet when the legs and body are already born.
- The breech baby often passes meconium during labour, and may inhale some of it as he struggles to breathe before his head emerges.
- Forceps delivery of the head is usually done to avoid potential damage to the baby's head and neck region.
- A Caesarean section may be advisable to avoid such problems. Premature babies who are breech are nearly always delivered by Caesarean section, as the hips are smaller than the head and the head is in danger of getting stuck after the hips have passed through the cervix. First babies who are breech are also more likely to encounter problems.

Breech delivery

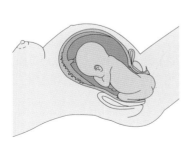

Beginning of second stage, baby's bottom descends through pelvis and is born

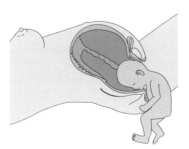

Baby's body is born, but head is still descending through pelvis

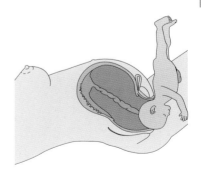

Baby's head is born more easily if body is gently elevated

If there is any doubt, an elective (planned) Caesarean section may be the preferred option. In other situations, you and your LMC, in consultation with a specialist obstetrician, may decide to try for a normal labour and assisted breech birth, but proceed with a Caesarean section if any delays or problems occur (see p.282).

Forceps delivery

Forceps delivery

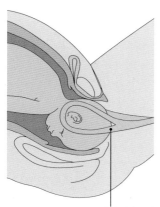

forceps move baby's head to easier birthing position

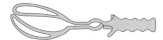

Forceps in locked position

Obstetric forceps can be used to assist a baby during the second stage of labour. They can deliver him quickly if he is in distress, or turn him around to fit through the pelvic outlet. They can also be used to ease a larger baby down through the birth canal, or to deliver a baby when the woman is exhausted and/or cannot push, as sometimes happens with an epidural.

Using obstetric forceps requires considerable skill on the part of the obstetrician. There is almost always time for you to discuss a proposed forceps delivery before it is done. Forceps deliveries are invaluable in some situations, and may be the only solution to some second-stage problems. But they can be used too readily in other situations, where it may be better to wait just a little longer (provided the baby seems in no distress).[20]

Before a forceps delivery, a small tube (urinary catheter) is usually inserted into the bladder to make quite sure it is empty. You will also be given an anaesthetic for the birth canal area, either by setting up an epidural (see p.257) or topping up your existing epidural. Otherwise, you can be given an injection of local anaesthetic directly into the nerves surrounding the cervix. An episiotomy usually needs to be done as well, to allow room for the baby to be delivered with the forceps attached.

The forceps blades, which are like slim metal hands, are then fitted on either side of the baby's head and locked together. They act to widen the birth canal and bring the baby out through the vaginal opening (sometimes rotating him first if he is posterior). The 'locking' of the forceps ensures that the baby's head is not squashed during delivery. Once he is born, the baby may have superficial marks on his head from the forceps. These can look quite ugly at first, but most of them disappear within a day or two of birth.

Very occasionally, a forceps delivery is not successful, especially if the baby's head is higher in the birth canal than was initially estimated. An immediate Caesarean section may then be required, so if any doubt exists, forceps will be used only in an operating theatre already set up for a possible Caesarean.

Vacuum (ventouse) delivery

A 'ventouse' is a rubber or metal suction cup that is attached to the baby's head, allowing the baby to be gently pulled down and through the birth canal. This technique has some advantages over forceps, as it is often easier to use, and can help flex the baby's head if it is hyper-extended or in a posterior position – provided the obstetrician can fit the cup near the fontanelle at the back of the head. The experience of the obstetrician in one or other of these techniques is an important factor in deciding which to use, but the stage of labour and the exact position of the baby's head are also significant. As with a forceps delivery, if a vacuum delivery is unsuccessful, an immediate Caesarean section may be needed. Again, this means a vacuum delivery will usually be done only in an operating theatre already set up for a possible Caesarean.[21]

Babies born by vacuum delivery often have a swelling on their heads where some of their scalp tissue was sucked up into the rubber suction cup. This is known as a 'chignon', and usually resolves itself within a few hours after birth.

Delayed delivery of the placenta

If, despite active management, the placenta is not delivered within 15–30 minutes of the baby's birth, one of several things may have happened:[22]

- The placenta has passed through the cervix but is simply sitting in the birth canal.
- The placenta has separated but is still within the uterus.
- The placenta has broken, so that part of it is being expelled but some remains within the uterus.
- The placenta (or part of it) is still firmly attached to the wall of the uterus.

In all but the first of these situations, the uterus will not be able to contract firmly. Heavy bleeding (post-partum haemorrhage, or PPH; see p.282) can easily occur, either straight away or later on.

Placental problems

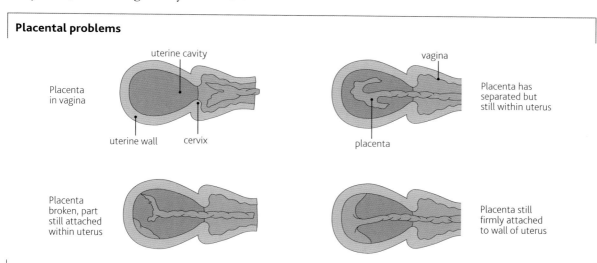

Placenta in vagina — uterine cavity — uterine wall — cervix

Placenta has separated but still within uterus — vagina — placenta

Placenta broken, part still attached within uterus

Placenta still firmly attached to wall of uterus

What can be done?

- Putting your baby to the breast immediately after the birth may help stimulate the placenta to separate and the uterus to contract.
- The first two situations (above) may be resolved simply by controlled cord traction (where your LMC pulls gently on the cord and at the same time presses firmly on your abdomen, just above the pubic bone, to hold the uterus up). If this doesn't work at first, your LMC may decide to wait for 15 minutes or so before trying again; this time, it may well be successful.
- It may be useful to cough, stand up, or sit on the toilet for a while so that gravity can help.

- If, despite all these measures, the placenta is still not delivered completely after an hour or so, it may be necessary to remove it manually from within the uterus. Otherwise, the risk of post-partum haemorrhage is high. Manual removal of the placenta is a specialist obstetrician's skill, and is best done under anaesthetic (general or epidural). It may seem particularly hard to have an anaesthetic straight after your baby is born, but the procedure usually takes only a short while and greatly hastens the effective contraction of the uterus and your subsequent recovery.

Post-partum haemorrhage (PPH)

In some women, the uterus is slow to contract after birth, even though the placenta may have been delivered and syntocinon (synthetic oxytocin) given either as the baby was born or a short time later. If the muscles of the uterus are slow to contract, the blood vessels that supplied the placental area of the uterus will bleed profusely and quick action is required. This problem is relatively common, affecting about one in 20 births. Active management (injection of syntocinon as the baby is born, and easing out the placenta) greatly reduces the risk of subsequent PPH, but does not eliminate it.[24]

> **Some causes of post-partum haemorrhage (PPH)**[23]
>
> - muscles of the uterus don't contract properly (more likely after a very long labour, especially a long second stage, or with a multiple pregnancy)
> - retained placenta
> - complications from IUGR or pre-eclampsia e.g. clotting problems
> - lacerations or big tears in the uterus, cervix or vagina

- If rapid bleeding does occur (over 500ml), more oxytocin can be given into a muscle, although this takes several minutes to take effect.
- The uterus can be rubbed vigorously to get rid of blood clots or any remaining placenta, and to stimulate the muscle to contract. This is very uncomfortable but is sometimes necessary. If the placenta, or a large part of it, is still within the uterus, it must be removed as quickly as possible (see above).
- If not already present, two IV lines need to be quickly inserted, one in each arm, so that copious fluids and/or a blood transfusion can be given. The drug syntocinon (see p.275) can also be given into the drip to help the uterus to contract. Alternative drugs (for example, Syntometrine) can be given too, encouraging a stronger and longer contraction of the uterus. Usually these measures will stem the flow, but very occasionally prompt surgical intervention is required.

Post-partum haemorrhage needs to be taken seriously and treated immediately. Blood loss in excess of 1000ml is potentially life-threatening. In developing countries it is still a major cause of maternal death. However, good, prompt obstetric care will almost always prevent this from happening, or at least rapidly improve and stabilise the situation. All LMCs are trained to deal with PPH, but will want to summon assistance as soon as possible, either from a colleague and/or hospital team members. A specialist obstetrician and an anaesthetist may both be required.

Caesarean section

This is also known as a Caesar, LSCS (lower segment Caesarean section) or C/S. All these terms describe the delivery of a baby through a surgical incision in the woman's abdomen. It is an operation that requires considerable skill on the part of the surgeon (a specialist obstetrician), the assisting midwife or midwives, and the anaesthetist. A paediatrician experienced in neonatal resuscitation will often be present as well.

Within the last 60 years Caesarean section has become a relatively safe and common procedure, but it must be remembered that it is still a major abdominal operation that carries a higher risk than vaginal delivery. It should be done only if the health of the woman or the baby is likely to be seriously compromised by a vaginal delivery; in these circumstances, a Caesarean section can quite literally be a life-saver.

Nevertheless, the number of Caesarean sections being done has risen steadily in the last 20 years in most developed countries, and New Zealand is no exception. This has happened partly as a result of more accurate detection of potential problems before babies are born, partly because women on average are bearing their children at an older age, but also to some extent because of women's choices about childbirth.

Once a woman has had one Caesarean section, she is more likely to have a subsequent baby by Caesarean, regardless of the original reason for doing so.[25] However, vaginal birth after a Caesarean is perfectly possible for many women; and as long as the reason for the Caesarean is not a recurring one, vaginal birth is still preferable. Closer monitoring than usual is required, and advice needs to be sought from a specialist obstetrician well before the due date (preferably before 36 weeks). Good continuity of care during labour is important, as is the ready availability of Caesarean delivery if this becomes necessary. For these reasons, home birth is not usually recommended.[26] Rarely, the scar on the uterus can give way or rupture, requiring urgent delivery by Caesarean section.

A Caesarean section can be 'elective', which means that before you go into labour, it is decided to deliver your baby by Caesarean section on a certain day. Alternatively, it can be done after labour has started.

These days, the operation can usually be done under an epidural anaesthetic, which allows you to be awake to see your baby being born. Your partner or support person can usually be with you. Occasionally, in an emergency or if there is bleeding, you will need to have a general anaesthetic (GA). Your partner or support person may still be able to see your baby being born.

Situations where a Caesarean may be necessary[27]

Woman's health at risk

- position of baby makes vaginal delivery impossible, e.g. transverse lie
- placenta praevia or placental separation
- labour not progressing at all
- woman's anatomy stops baby moving into birth canal, e.g. very narrow or misshapen pelvis
- previous surgery to cervix, uterus or bladder

Baby's health at risk (especially if twins or triplets)

- baby (or babies) in severe distress during pregnancy/labour, e.g. severe pre-eclampsia (toxaemia), long labour
- baby (or babies) in abnormal position, which is creating, or may create, further problems, e.g. breech, posterior position
- baby too big to fit through pelvis
- a loop of cord has come down through the cervix in front of the baby

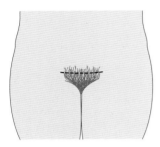

Caesarean incision – most common site

What happens during a Caesarean section?

Preparation

Your midwife will prepare you for the operation by helping you to change into a clean hospital gown, removing your jewellery and watch, checking your personal details on a wristband name tag, asking you to sign a consent form if you have not already done so, and shaving some of the hair around your lower abdomen and pubic area (you may be able to do this yourself). In some hospitals, these preparations are carried out in an area of the operating theatre known as the day of surgery area (DOSA).

Your baby may be monitored using a cardiotocograph (CTG) if there is concern about his well-being. A sonicaid may be used to listen to his heart at intervals until the surgery begins.

You will then be taken in your bed to a room next to the operating theatre, where you will meet the anaesthetist (although if it is an elective Caesarean, you may have already met for an assessment a few days before the operation). Your midwife and partner or support person can nearly always come with you.

You will be given a special medicine and/or injection to help neutralise any food remaining in your stomach. If you haven't already got an IV, the anaesthetist will insert one into a vein in your arm.

You will then be taken into the operating theatre, moved onto the narrow operating bed, and covered with sterile cloths (drapes). If you are having a GA, you will usually be given some oxygen to breathe for a few minutes. Some anaesthetic will then be given to you via the drip and will quickly make you go to sleep. You may feel some pressure on your throat as you drift off.

If you have an epidural/spinal, the anaesthetist will check this and top it up as required, and also measure your blood pressure. A catheter will be inserted into your bladder to make sure it stays empty. If you do not have an epidural or spinal already, one will be inserted in theatre while you are sitting up prior to lying down and being covered with sterile drapes. Once the epidural or spinal is working, a catheter will be inserted into your bladder.

People who may be in theatre during a Caesarean section

- surgeon (a specialist obstetrician or senior registrar)
- assisting doctor (a registrar, house surgeon or your GP obstetrician)
- your own midwife (who may also be assisting the surgeon)
- chief theatre nurse
- assistant nurse
- anaesthetist
- paediatrician (if you are having twins or triplets, there may be a paediatrician for each baby)
- paediatric nurse
- your partner or support person.

All these people have to wear sterile clothes and masks to keep the environment as clean as possible and to minimise the risk of infection. If you are having a general anaesthetic, it is less likely that your partner or support person will be able to be present, because of the extra equipment required for a GA. In some circumstances, however, it may be possible.

First step

The surgeon makes a cut in the abdominal skin, usually horizontally at the pubic hair-line (see diagram opposite). Very rarely a vertical cut is made. The surgeon then cuts through muscle and fat layers until the uterus is reached. The paper-thin wall of the uterus is carefully cut, releasing the amniotic fluid (waters) in a sometimes noisy gush.

The surgeon reaches in and delivers the baby (or babies) through the incision. This requires skill, especially if the baby is large – occasionally, obstetric forceps may be used to deliver the head. Twins or more sometimes require complex manoeuvres for safe delivery.

Mucous and fluid may be sucked out of the baby's nostrils and mouth using a suction tube (this is, however, rarely done these days, and only if there is meconium in the fluid and the baby is not vigorous). If necessary, a little oxygen is given via a small tube. This is often done by the paediatrician on a special warmed table at one side of the room.

If the baby breathes easily and is a normal size, you or your partner may be given him to hold straight away. However, if the baby is very small or has trouble breathing, the paediatrician will actively assist him to breathe. He may need to be transferred to the special-care baby unit. This whole process takes five to ten minutes, or longer if there is more than one baby to deliver.

Second step

The placenta and membranes must be removed completely from within the uterus to allow the uterus to contract. Twins may have had separate placentas, and each must be carefully and completely removed. The anaesthetist will give you syntocinon via your drip to help this process.

The uterus is sewn up with dissolvable sutures (stitches), and a check made for any bleeding. Each layer of tissue is stitched together – sometimes a small plastic tube or drain is left in place to allow any oozing blood to escape. The skin is drawn together and secured with nylon sutures, little metal clips or a dissolvable thread. The uterus is then checked again by applying firm pressure, and any excess blood will pass out through the cervix and vagina.

This phase takes about half an hour.

Afterwards

If you have had a general anaesthetic, you will usually become drowsily conscious at this point and can be transferred back to your own bed. You will probably still have your drip, catheter, drain and epidural/spinal cannula in place to provide you with ongoing pain relief. If your baby is well, you will often be able to have him with you from now on.

You and your partner or support person can now spend time with each other and your new baby. This is a time to be treasured, especially if you have had a general anaesthetic, and can help to compensate for missing out on a normal birth experience.

If your baby is in the special-care baby unit, you can usually be taken straight there in your bed to see him. Sometimes, with twins, one baby will be well and can be with you immediately, while the other needs more special care – you will want to see both babies as soon as you possibly can.

'Hamish was there when they were delivered. He had a look as they were pulling Briar out, and she was all blue and kind of stretched. And he just said, "Ooh-oh", and the anaesthetist suggested he should sit down quickly. So Hamish was still on the floor when Tanner came out, but he saw them straight after they were born and brought them over for me to have a quick look.'

Birth sequence 5: Caesarean

1. The obstetrician surgeon cleans the skin and
2. makes the incision.
3. The uterus is opened, and
4. the baby is delivered, coming out bottom first.
5. The baby's legs and body are delivered, and
6. the head is born last.
7. The cord is clamped and cut.
8. The baby is handed to the midwife (front left, back to camera).
9. The baby is taken to the resuscitation area, watched by the father, before
10. joining the parents.

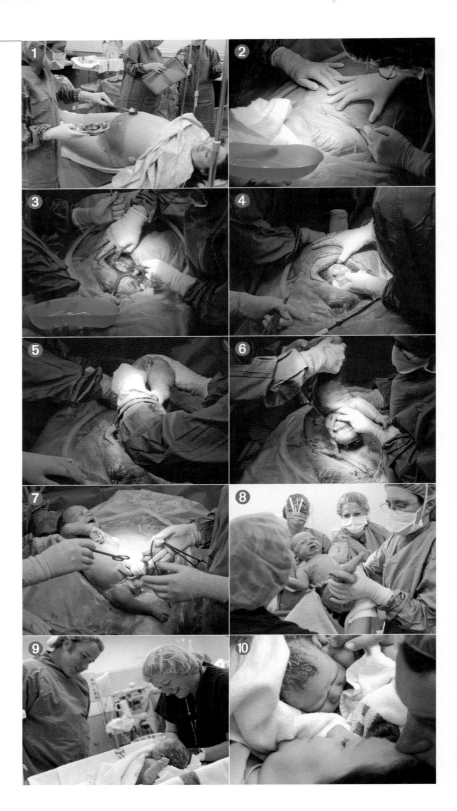

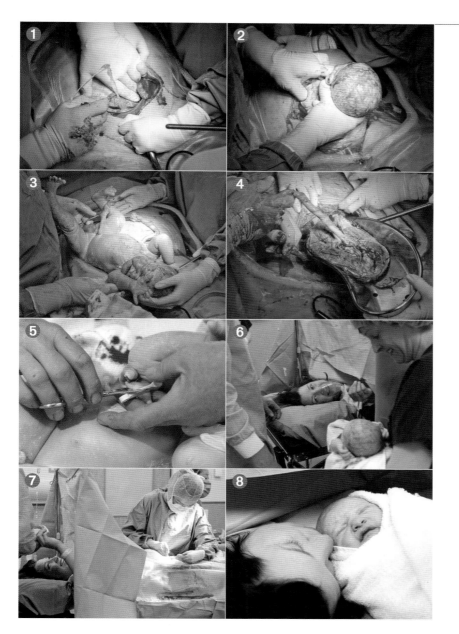

**Birth sequence 6:
Caesarean**

❶ As the obstetrician surgeon makes the incision, the amniotic fluid gushes out.
❷ The baby's head is born, and
❸ the baby fully delivered.
❹ The placenta is delivered.
❺ The cord is clamped and cut.
❻ The mother gets a look at baby as
❼ the surgeon sews up the mother.
❽ Mother and baby share a moment.

Actively assisting a baby to breathe (neonatal resuscitation)

Sometimes a baby does not breathe, or does not breathe normally, once he is born. If this happens, it is necessary to act quickly and skilfully, otherwise the baby may die or suffer brain damage due to lack of oxygen.[28] Specialised equipment is needed to resuscitate a baby, and all delivery suites and midwives attending home births have enough equipment to take immediate action, should this prove necessary.

Basic resuscitation

After drying your baby and placing him on a warm, firm surface, your LMC and/or paediatrician will give him some oxygen with a bag and mask to open the lungs. If this doesn't help, they will check that there is nothing blocking the baby's airway. If there is, it will be cleared and they will try again. All the while, they will be checking his colour, breathing, muscle tone and heart rate. Often these basic measures will be sufficient and your baby will start breathing well on his own. His colour will improve, and his heart rate will rapidly become normal. But if needed, your LMC and/or paediatrician will take other steps, such as chest compressions to help the heart pump blood around the body – especially to the brain.

Advanced resuscitation

If these basic measures do not quickly establish spontaneous breathing, more action may be needed. Using a good light and with the baby in the warmest place possible (in hospital this will be a specially warmed tray at a high table height), an instrument is placed in the baby's throat so that a small, stiff plastic tube can be inserted into the windpipe (trachea). Any obstructive material is sucked out directly, and then a mixture of air and oxygen is given straight to the baby's lungs so that oxygen can start circulating immediately in his blood. This procedure is known as intubation.

If your baby has to be resuscitated in this way, you will not be able to have him with you immediately. But you can be close at hand and be kept informed of his progress. Babies who need resuscitation require expert care in the hours immediately following their birth, and this will mean a prompt transfer to the nearest special-care baby unit, even if you have had your baby at home. If your baby has been born near his due date (i.e. after 37 weeks of pregnancy), your labour was straightforward, and no problems were detected during your pregnancy, his chances of making an excellent recovery from this initial setback are very good with expert care. But even so, this is an intensely worrying time. You will want to go with your baby if at all possible, and be as close to him as you can. Sometimes, extra tests and investigations will be needed to see if there is some underlying problem that contributed to his initial lack of breathing.

Sometimes, in spite of all these measures, babies do not survive. The reasons may be unknown, or there may be some abnormality of the heart or lungs that prevents them from breathing normally. If your baby is very small, either because of prematurity or severe growth restriction, he may just be too undeveloped to survive outside the uterus.

When a baby is born with a severe abnormality

About 1 per cent of babies are born with a significant congenital abnormality, and very occasionally this will not have been suspected during pregnancy. Although more and more abnormalities, especially significant heart problems, can be detected with prenatal diagnostic tests (such as blood serum tests, and the different types of ultrasound scan; see pp.105 and 150), a few may be missed by even the most sophisticated tests. In addition, some women and their families choose not to have such tests, and may have had trouble-free pregnancies. In such situations, even though everyone is aware that the baby could have a problem, it is still an overwhelming shock if this is indeed the case. An abnormality may be immediately obvious after birth (for example, cleft palate) or it may not become apparent until some hours or days later (for example, congenital heart disease).

Either way, coming to terms with this situation is very hard. The birth, far from being a joyous experience, becomes tinged with tragedy, and it may be that the people around you don't know how to help.

Women who have had an abnormal baby nearly always say that it helps to be able to hold the baby or be with him as soon as possible. Imagining what an abnormal baby looks like is often worse than the reality.

Many women have intense feelings of grief as they mourn the 'loss' of a normal baby, and this can take many months to come to terms with. It seems that at least part of this grieving process needs to be worked through before you are ready to love and care for a 'different' baby. Parents who are adjusting to this situation need as much support, love and care as they can get. They need time to be alone, but also time to talk and to cry, and they need support to do these things at their own pace. They need people around them to be as open, honest and accepting as possible about what has happened.

Families and friends can be wonderful, but professional people can be helpful too. Information becomes very important. The more factual information you can find about your baby's condition, the more you will be able to understand and accept the reality of the situation. One particularly helpful group may be Parent to Parent (Matua ki te Matua) New Zealand. (See Appendix: Disability.) This parents' group works to empower 'parents, caregivers and whānau of children and family members with disabilities, health impairments or special needs through the support and provision of information'.[29]

Reflections on the birth experience

Every birth is different, and no one can predict how a pregnancy will end until it is all over. Every pregnant woman wonders just what 'it' will be like, especially the first time around. Some feel sure that birth is a 'mind over matter' situation, and that mental control is all important. Others see physical fitness and suppleness as the key to a straightforward labour and delivery. Still others wish, more than anything, for it to be 'pain-free', and want maximum intervention to achieve this. And then there are those who simply 'take it as it comes'.

If the reality turns out to be very different from what you had hoped, you may have very mixed feelings about the birth. Some women feel they have 'failed' because they accepted pain relief; others feel cheated of a normal birth experience because they ended up having a Caesarean. On the other hand, some women who had long and complicated labours with their first child are amazed and delighted when the second birth is absolutely free of all problems and an ecstatic experience. These birth stories (and those at the end of other chapters) illustrate just how very different the experience can be.

Rhiannon's story: A first birth in hospital

I was ten days overdue, which were the longest ten days of my life! I enjoyed being pregnant for the most part, but by this stage I had really had enough. My body felt huge and unmanageable, all our preparations were done and I was getting about ten phone calls a day from people wondering if the baby had arrived yet.

My midwife was also pregnant and although she was due a few weeks after me, we scheduled an induction for when I was nine days overdue. Although I wasn't keen on being induced, I did want to have her as my midwife for the birth. Anyway, I thought I'd probably go into labour by myself before then since I was trying everything to bring it on – from hot curries to acupuncture and long walks. Two days before the induction date, my midwife phoned to say she had had her baby that afternoon so I would have to have a different midwife! I arranged to meet her on the Friday morning that the induction had been scheduled for. She checked us out and the baby didn't seem in a rush to be going anywhere – she still hadn't dropped and my cervix wasn't even flat. We rescheduled the induction for Monday, so I went home and told my husband that he might as well go out with his friends that night; it would probably be a while before he'd get the chance again!

I still really wanted to go into labour naturally, although I now thought there was little chance of it happening. I planned a relaxing last few days before becoming a parent. As a last attempt to get things started, I went for a long walk on Friday afternoon. Later that evening – about 10.30 p.m. – we were just going off to bed when I felt the first twinge. I wasn't completely sure that things had started and didn't want to worry Elliott unnecessarily, so I didn't mention it. Due to his evening's entertainment, he was soon snoring, but as it happened, I wasn't going to get any sleep that night!

For the first few hours, the contractions were quite noticeable but didn't hurt. They were about 20 minutes apart but I was much too excited to sleep. By 2 a.m. they had got too painful to lie still through, so I woke Elliott up and told him that we were definitely about to have a baby! We got up and dressed and got everything ready to go to the hospital, although it didn't seem to be time to leave. By 3 a.m. the contractions were very painful and just over three minutes apart. We decided to phone my midwife to let her know, and she said that the longer we stayed at home the better the chances for a natural birth; we should phone her again when I was having three 'really good' contractions in under ten minutes. I spent the next two hours yelling 'OWW-WWW!' during each contraction while Elliott held my hand. At 5 a.m. the contractions were closer together and I couldn't speak during them. So we phoned my midwife who repeated that the longer we stayed at home, the better our chance of the natural birth we wanted. She asked if I had tried a hot bath as pain relief, so I hopped in the bath and Elliott went back to bed.

The bath was wonderful; although the contractions were still strong and close together, they were much less painful. This lasted for about 45 minutes, but by 6 a.m. the pain was back and I decided I just had to go to the hospital. I woke Elliott up again and told him to let the midwife know we were on our way to the hospital 'RIGHT NOW!!', and that I thought I might have to have an epidural after all. At this stage, I thought I might only be a few centimetres dilated and would be told at the hospital that I had come in too early. But if that was the case, then labour was going to be too painful and I would need some relief.

When we got to the hospital, they were expecting us. My midwife quickly established that I was in fact 7cm dilated. She congratulated me on my good work at home and asked if I would like an epidural or to try gas. I felt really encouraged by the progress I'd made and tried the gas. It worked wonderfully and I hopped into another big hot bath; the combination of the two virtually eliminated the pain. Elliott and I spent the next hour and a half chatting until the contractions started feeling 'pushy' and a bit painful again. My midwife reappeared just at the time they started to change, and I got out of the bath and went back to my room. I was now 9cm dilated and my midwife said it would be about another three hours; I decided that I could do it without pain relief.

Although the last centimetre of dilation was probably the most painful part of the labour, the pushing was quite a different feeling. It was much harder work than I had thought it would be, requiring all my strength. I was very, very tired by this stage. Elliott and my midwife really got me through it with their encouragement and excitement at seeing the baby's head. Towards the end of the pushing, when I was feeling quite worn out, I changed position so that I was on my knees on the bed with my arms resting on the raised bed head. This was great since I could now feel exactly how far I still had to push.

Before I knew it, our beautiful daughter was born. I was lucky enough to escape any tearing and had very little grazing. This luck continued with breastfeeding, where I didn't experience any problems either!

Moana's story: A first birth in hospital

We had tried for what seemed like ages to get pregnant. When we found out, we were really excited, but I also suddenly felt this overwhelming sense of responsibility for our baby. I found myself quite nervous in the first trimester, hoping that everything would progress normally. I remember reading the list of foods you are meant to avoid and thinking 'Oh no, I've eaten everything on that list.' I felt really tired and nauseous in those first weeks, and so there was no hope of keeping the pregnancy secret.

Despite all my worrying, the pregnancy progressed well and seemed to pass quite quickly after those first 12 weeks. Near the end of the pregnancy, I stopped growing much and there was a little bit of worry about my baby being small for dates. This meant we did some extra scans at the end of the pregnancy, which I found quite nerve-racking as I was worried each time that they would find the baby wasn't growing or that the placenta wasn't working properly. My husband told me to think of the scans as another chance to see our baby, and I found it helped to take friends and family with me, so I could focus on their excitement at seeing our baby.

I was quite closely monitored over the last few weeks of the pregnancy. At this stage I was really glad that I had ended up choosing an obstetrician as my LMC, as I knew that if anything complicated happened I already had a good relationship with the specialist. As it got closer to my due date and baby wasn't growing, there was talk of the possibility of induction. Although my first concern was doing what was best for the baby, I wasn't really too keen on an induction as it felt to me like I was losing control over the birth process to an extent. I was a little nervous too, as I had only heard 'bad' induction stories and didn't know what to expect.

At this point, I remember looking at the birth plan that I had worked out with my husband, birth partner and midwife, which was not based on an induction scenario. The things that were most important to me about the birth were having the people there that I wanted, and having baby's whenua to take home with us – I felt better about things when I realised this was still possible with an induction.

In the week before I was due, I had a couple more scans. Two days before my due date, I remember going in for a scan and I noticed the measurements for baby were smaller than at the last scan. The radiographer also had trouble finding amniotic fluid, so I left there pretty convinced that my obstetrician was going to suggest an induction.

I was determined to try to get things going myself if possible. Up until then I had only had what felt like period cramps, and a VE the day before had showed no dilation or effacement. We decided to go have a spicy lunch (just in case it worked) while we waited to hear back from the midwife. She called me after lunch, and it was decided we would go into hospital the next morning at 8 a.m. for an induction.

I remember it being a really weird feeling knowing when you are going to have the baby – I mean, you go the whole pregnancy knowing that at some stage you are going to give birth, but it felt strange to be given a day and a time. The upside of this was that I was able to let people know and to have all the people I wanted at the hospital there with me.

In the morning driving in to the hospital, I remember that I was mostly just excited about meeting our baby. We got there early, and got settled in our room and hooked up to the monitors. When the obstetrician came in to do the examination before the induction, I was really happy to be told that I was already 2cm dilated and things were already on the way. He broke my waters and pretty soon after that I started to notice contractions. I was on a drip but I was still able to move around quite a lot, and rock through the contractions, which helped. Things seemed to move quite fast and I remember after about three hours I started wanting to push. There was about an hour where the contractions were really intense, and I remember getting my birth partner (a close friend) to ask my family except my husband to leave – I really felt I needed to concentrate. I used the gas a bit during this time, and it helped to give me something to focus on during the contractions.

Once it was time to push, I found the pain was easier to take as you could feel things progressing. I was glad that I had two support people with me, as there were lots of little things they did to help during this stage. After about an hour of pushing, my son was born. The midwife tucked him under my singlet on my chest and it was an amazing feeling. Our friend cut the cord, which meant a lot to me. I really wanted it to be done by one of us but didn't think I could do it myself, so I was really honoured that she did that for us. For me, it also ties her to our son for ever.

Although the birth hadn't gone exactly how I'd planned, I felt really good about it as I had been able to do the things that were important to me and to still have some control. I got to wear the shirt I wanted to wear, to have the music playing during labour that I wanted, to have my family and close friends there, to have my friend cut the cord, and to take bubba's whenua home with us.

As we weren't able to take our son's whenua to where we wanted to bury it straight away, we planted it in a pot until we got the chance to travel to where my husband is from. So it was buried there with some soil from our home, which I like as it ties him to both places.

I know we did some things differently from how we planned and from what other people might expect, but I feel glad that I got to do the things that were important to me in my way – to have my whānau there and my wishes about the cord and whenua respected and not questioned by those involved in my care.

Gabrielle's story: Four home births

I have had four home births, all planned and all a little different. My first girl was born when I was 21, had just graduated and was in a brand-new relationship. I was inspired by my sister to have a home birth and, since I was close to the hospital, decided it was a safe option for me. The idea of being able to stay in my own familiar space, to climb into my own bed as a new family and not to have to comply with hospital rules cemented my reasons.

I was two weeks overdue when my waters burst in the middle of the opening of the art gallery that we lived above. A towel between my legs, I gingerly made my way through 100 guests to my room and waited for someone to notice my absence. The contractions were strong and close together right from the start, and I became tired and despondent rather quickly. This was not what I had envisaged from my antenatal classes. The second stage seemed to take for ever. However, with support from my partner, family, midwife and GP, I made it through with just homeopathy. Eight hours later, I gave birth to my daughter, 8.2lb. I was very sore and bruised and needed stitches for a tear, which meant I wasn't running around doing all the things I'd thought I'd be able to do for quite a while. Riding horses was a wee way off and the thought of intercourse made my eyes water, but eventually both activities were resumed in due course.

My next pregnancy came along about 15 months later. Like the first, it was uncomplicated and something that I enjoyed. Two weeks late once again, my labour started in a more relaxed way, with slow contractions throughout the day. It was late summer and we were living at my family homestead. I felt at home and relaxed; at 7 p.m. another 8.2lb girl arrived. This time, however, she was far from OK. I glimpsed that she was a bluey-purple colour and gasping for breath. No cry came and my midwife, all alone, had to work out what might be wrong. I can remember feeling that I needed her too, as I was shaky and delivering the placenta. After quick thinking from my mother, a neighbouring GP came to our assistance, taking over the baby's care.

An ambulance arrived and we travelled the 45 minutes to the hospital. There, she was found to have her chest full of bowel, her lungs squashed to the far right-hand corner and a hole in her diaphragm. A diaphragmatic hernia was diagnosed. A team was flown from our nearest big centre to collect her, and at 3 a.m. I found myself hobbling (stitched up again) barefoot to a plane in my dressing gown (always prepare your own hospital bag in advance!) This was not at all what I had planned. I was desperate to hold her, panicking that she would suffer emotional repercussions from missing that early bonding. However, as she was in a drug-induced coma, that time was perhaps 'time out of time'. When she woke up two weeks later, we were able to bond with her; she was an emotionally well-adjusted child and fond of cuddles.

Turning up at a big hospital in the middle of the night, without my partner, trying to run after her incubator as it was swiftly wheeled to intensive care, with no one there to meet me and being separated from my precious sick wee baby was a blur of exhausted numbness. One thing that connected me with my absent family were the messages left with various staff from my brother in the city; they were pulled out of pockets and read on the plane, and were there waiting for me at the hospital ward.

After a shaky first few days, where she was given a 50/50 chance of survival, Kate had successful surgery and made a good recovery. All I could do to contribute to her care was to express milk, touch her arm and talk to her over this noisy, beeping environment. We returned home three weeks later, complete with a big bag of expressed milk that the dog wouldn't even drink! Kate immediately preferred it straight from the breast, and finally I was back in my own bed, surrounded by my family with the whirlwind experience behind us. I never doubted my choice of a home birth. My other option would have been a small birthing unit, which was further from the hospital anyway, and the same ambulance trip would have been required. Kate's birth has been reviewed as a case study many times, and the midwives in the region soon adopted a back-up system to ensure they were not alone in such situations.

Eleven years later, now in a new relationship and settled in our own home, my husband and I were expecting baby number three (number one for him). He supported my wish to have it at home. I knew my earlier experience was unlikely to happen again and trusted in my ability to have a safe home birth. One week early, my contractions began slowly and continued through the day. It was school holidays and my 11-year-old wrote down all the times of the contractions. My midwife kept in touch, waiting until things got stronger. At 9.30 p.m., she arrived and things sped up. Throughout this pregnancy, I had used the 'Pink Kit – essential preparations for your birthing body' [a useful pack provided by some midwives] as my antenatal preparation. I was able to visualise the baby moving down, and to breathe and position myself to make the baby's passage into this world open and easy. A back-up midwife arrived at 10.40 and Jay was born at 11.17 p.m., next to our bed. Once the placenta appeared at 11.45, we bundled up into bed with a suckling baby. My girls had popped in as soon as he was born, then returned regularly to see what was happening and to have a cuddle with their new brother. They hadn't wanted to see any 'yucky' stuff and hung out with Granny in their room, one with her pillow over her head in case I made 'weird' noises during labour.

I remember saying to my midwife a few hours after the birth, 'Well that was easy.' Sure, it hurt; but with each step, I could feel the progression and I felt in control of what was happening – and no stitches this time! My midwife settled us and kept a check on our well-being before leaving at 2 a.m., taking any mucky linen with her to be laundered at the community hospital. She returned the next day with fresh linen and checked on our progress. Jay was a little blue and we went to the GP to have his heart checked out. All seemed fine and his colour improved over the next day. He was so content and we all fell in love with him more than we ever imagined.

At four weeks, he was losing weight and we visited a paediatrician for a check-up. Jay was given the thumbs-up and once I realised that he needed feeding beyond his easily satisfied nature, he put on adequate weight. At 14 months, Jay was again referred to the paediatrician due to delayed gross motor development. A blood test revealed an extra 21st chromosome. Jay had Down syndrome! He had some of the characteristics but they were subtle, and in many ways he was keeping up with his peers. After the initial shock and grief, we realised that he wasn't suddenly different or sick; he had always had this extra chromosome and it contributed to some of his wonderful personality. Also it was only one extra out of 24 pairs of chromosomes; we shouldn't discount the contribution of the other 23 pairs that we had given him.

I am glad to have had the diagnosis late as it allowed everyone to treat him as a normal and valued member of our family. Having a diagnosis like this does dramatically change your expectations of what the future may hold for your child. But with any child, we can never be sure what the future holds for them; all we can hope for is that they will enjoy their life and be happy doing whatever they choose.

The fourth pregnancy was much harder than the previous ones due to separated abdominal muscles and dysfunction of the symphysis pubis joint, which gave me pelvic and leg pain. A referral to physio helped a great deal; I was given Tubigrip [a firm circular knitted 'bandage', big enough to go around the tummy for support] and an abdominal belt, as well as instructions on good posture and post-natal care. I felt much less active for a good four months, unable to walk far. I made the most of Jay's afternoon sleeps, using them to rest as well and get in my quota of reading material to last me until I have time to myself again (in my retirement!) A painful bout of protruding haemorrhoids at 35 weeks, followed by a violent tummy bug at 38 weeks, made me feel like I wished the baby would be cut out there and then. But by 40 weeks I was feeling the best I had been for quite a while and I felt confident that I could again have a successful birth at home.

Five days after my due date, contractions began much like my previous labour, quietly building up through the afternoon. By 7 p.m. they were close together and stronger, and my midwife was on her way. I waited for my son to go to sleep, my midwife to get everything laid out and have some tea, and then in a matter of minutes my waters broke with an audible 'pop' (which we later discovered coincided with the eruption of Mt Ruapehu!) Contractions became very strong and I stood, leaning on my husband. My support person massaged my legs to ease the pain during contractions and help me to remain as relaxed as I could. My 13-year-old daughter came and went from the room, getting more hot water and flannels and watching what was happening. I got the urge to push and made use of each contraction, focusing my energy on moving the baby's head through my pelvis. The pressure on my tailbone and rectum was intense, but I remembered that was a good sign that the head was moving down; having a bowel motion was par for the course and also a good sign. My midwife recommended moving into a side-lying position with my top leg supported, and the baby's head emerged a few minutes later. The shoulders were a little stuck, though, and my lack of tummy muscle meant that my pushes didn't have much strength. Once I stood up again, gravity assisted and the shoulders eased out. A big baby girl (9lb 12oz) was handed up to me as I leant back on my husband on the edge of the bed, 45 minutes after my waters had broken.

The baby needed a bit of coaxing with some oxygen to take her first big breaths, and then she let everyone know she had arrived with a lengthy burst of crying. She didn't want to drink initially, but had a strong suck so we waited to see how she went overnight before worrying. I showered and snuggled up in my bed, exhausted. She slept in between us and woke in the night to feed, the strong after-pains in my tummy a good indication that she had latched on well. We hadn't thought about it initially, but then had a look at her and decided she didn't seem to have any Down syndrome features. However, it didn't feel very important in the whole scheme of things. She was doing all that she should be and appeared healthy. What more can anyone wish for than that?

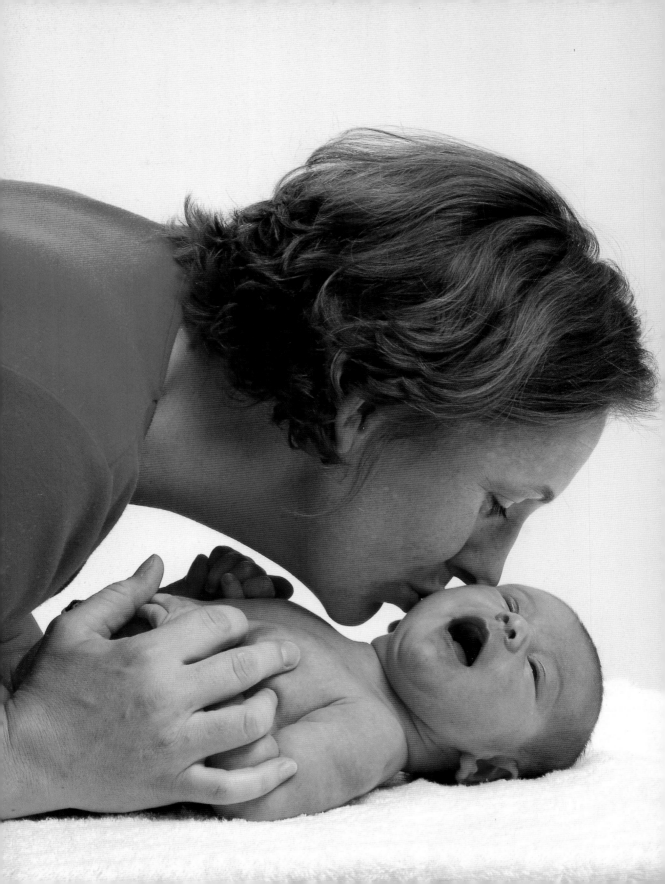

CHAPTER 7

The week after birth

1. The first few hours

As soon as your baby has been born and she is breathing well, you can lie her skin to skin on your tummy even before the placenta is delivered. Your LMC or hospital midwife will dry her off and cover her with a warm, dry towel. You can then just rest with her there while your placenta is born, your perineum gets checked for any tears and stitches are inserted if necessary (see p.273). Then you will have time to sit up and really focus on your baby while your midwife tidies up, writes up the notes on your baby's birth, and organises some well-deserved food and drink for you.

Feelings

'The absolute instant Jane was born, I just knew I loved her to bits – she was bright-eyed and beautiful; but she was my second – it wasn't like that with Timothy, not at all.'

At last the two of you are alone with your partner and/or support people. How do you feel? Relieved? Overwhelmed? Exhausted? Happy? Full of tears that turn into laughter? Proud? Nervous? Shy?

And how does your baby look? How does she feel, sound and smell? Does she seem unbelievably tiny, light and fragile? Or has she a 'been here before' look?

Do you wonder how *you* could have produced such a beautiful baby? How does your partner or support person feel about her?

Take time to look your new baby over. Count her fingers and toes, examine her little legs. Turn her over and look at her squiggly backbone and her little bottom. Feel her hair and look into her eyes. Don't let her get cold – she'll need a wrap or two even if the room is really warm; and cover her head, as that is where she loses the most heat.

Checking on your baby

Your LMC will want to do a thorough head-to-toe check of your baby after the birth to make sure that all is well, and will explain things as they go. They may prefer to examine her in her cot, on the resuscitation table under a radiant heater, on your bed or while she is on your tummy. If you have a preference, just ask. Remember, this is *your* baby!

This check takes only a few minutes, and your baby will not be unduly upset by it. Then you should have her with you so she can continue getting to know you, your smell, your sound and your touch, and the many invisible things that make your body unique.

Vitamin K (Konakion; see also p.138)

A single dose of vitamin K is given to babies shortly after birth, either orally or by injection into the thigh muscle. Even though you will have discussed this previously, you should be asked again about your baby having vitamin K, taking into account the circumstances of the labour and birth.

Vitamin K is essential to the blood-clotting process in humans, and is naturally low in newborn babies. Some babies are prone to haemorrhages around the brain after birth, and there is good evidence that this can be largely prevented by giving a small amount of vitamin K shortly after delivery. Since Vitamin K has been routinely administered, the incidence of brain haemorrhage in newborns has fallen.[1]

Until recently, vitamin K was thought to have little adverse effect, but questions have been raised about a possible link between childhood cancers and vitamin K given by injection. Because of this, oral doses of vitamin K have been tried in some centres. The oral dose has to be given three times to be effective (one dose in the first 24 hours after birth, the next at seven days and the third at six weeks), and has also been shown to be slightly less effective than the injection at preventing brain haemorrhage. As the possible link with child cancer has not been subsequently proven, many obstetric experts are now recommending the single dose of injectable vitamin K once again.

There is little doubt that babies at high risk of haemorrhage (i.e. premature or small babies) benefit from preventative vitamin K, but further work needs to be done about lower-risk babies. Until there is more evidence, most experts recommend continuing to give vitamin K routinely, either by injection or orally, since brain haemorrhage can be devastating, causing serious brain damage or death.[2] You will be asked to give your consent prior to your baby having vitamin K, and it is helpful if you have already considered this (see p.138) – but ask for more information at this point if you are still unsure.

A routine examination of a newborn baby includes:
- checking skin colour, breathing rate and breathing noises
- listening to the chest to check the lungs and the heart
- checking the abdomen for the position of the liver, intestines and stomach
- examining the genital area, the anus and the cord
- checking limbs for appearance, reflexes and muscle tone (floppiness)
- examining the hips
- checking ears, eyes, nose, lips, mouth and palate
- checking fontanelles and skull
- measuring head size, and sometimes length
- noting specific or unusual features in any of the above areas
- weighing your baby

Checking on you

After the birth, your LMC or hospital midwife will most likely check your blood pressure, pulse and temperature. She will also check that your uterus remains firm by feeling your abdomen from time to time, perhaps every half-hour or so, and that there is only minimal bleeding. You will also be encouraged to go to the toilet to pass urine, as you may not be aware that you have a full bladder. A full bladder can relax the uterus, which may cause bleeding to start up again. It can also aggravate the 'after-pains' that some women experience more intensely after the birth of a second or subsequent baby. It is common to pass a lot of urine immediately after birth.

The first feed

If you keep your baby close, skin to skin, she will usually be ready to suckle at the breast within an hour or so of birth. During this first hour she will usually push on your breast, lick her lips and your nipple, and make sucking sounds. You may find that she will move from an upright position between your breasts to lie with her mouth and nose at the level of the nipple and areola, getting herself into position to latch on and suckle! She may well do this without any encouragement or help from you or your midwife, so just follow her lead. (Some babies who have been affected by medications or other interventions in labour may not react quite like this, so just help her to adapt by keeping her close to you; see p.302.)

Most babies will need some nourishment within three to four hours of birth. Whether you plan to breastfeed or formula-feed, your baby will benefit from the colostrum produced within the breast before the milk 'comes in'. Colostrum is a thick, yellowy liquid that can sometimes be expressed from the nipple in late pregnancy or just after birth. It contains antibodies – complex protein substances that help protect your baby against infection in the first weeks of life.

The easiest way for your baby to get this colostrum is by sucking directly at the breast. If this isn't possible (for example, if she is premature), you can express the colostrum, or use the colostrum you may have expressed before the birth (see box on p.232).

Helping to get the baby latched on

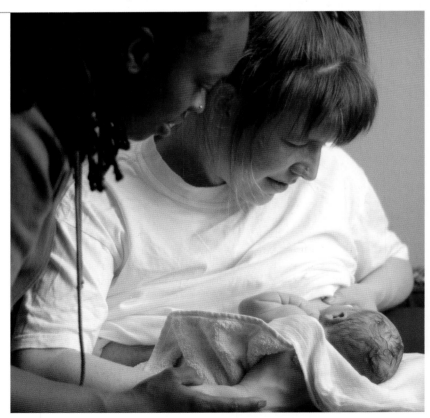

Leaving the birthing area

If you're in hospital, you will be free to leave the birthing area within two to four hours, depending on your condition and that of your baby. You'll be able either to go to a post-natal ward, or to go home.

If you're going to a post-natal ward, you and your baby can usually go together in a wheelchair if you are too exhausted or too sore to walk, and can both be settled into your room. Just when this happens will depend on the time of day, how busy the birthing area is, and what sort of room is available. Your LMC will discuss with you when and how often they will visit you in hospital (visits will be at least daily), and will usually also notify the staff of the arrangements.

You may, however, have chosen to go home at this stage. If everything has gone according to plan and your baby is well, this is quite a good time to make the transfer, provided you have good adult support at home and good childcare for your other children. You do need to feel confident that you can manage with your new baby, and sometimes early discharge is a more appropriate choice for a woman who already has experience as a mother. If the birth has not been as straightforward as you'd hoped, or if you or your baby are unwell, you may have to change your mind and accept a slightly longer stay in hospital.

If you do go home, your LMC is responsible for ensuring that you are visited at home within 24 hours of being discharged from hospital. Either your LMC or a post-natal midwife should call at least daily for the first few days to check on both you and your baby, and to help with feeding and baby care. They will then visit most days until your baby is about two weeks old, depending on need. Your midwife will normally make 5–10 home visits (or more if needed) during the post-natal period (see p.337). However, as they cannot be there all the time, make sure you have someone you can call on at short notice for help and advice in the first few days. It might be a relative or friend who has had a baby, but it must be someone you respect and trust.

Family and friends (for partners and support people)

Sooner or later, you and your partner will want to tell everyone about the baby's arrival. This task usually falls to you, at least in the first instance.

Most hospitals have phones available for short local calls, and you may want to use these to share the news with your closest family. It's probably best to keep the full list until you get home and can talk at length. Most mobile phones can now be used in hospitals, but it's important to check first that your mobile won't interfere with any important medical equipment that may be nearby.

If either of you wants to restrict visiting, either in hospital or at home, make it clear to everyone just when they can visit. Rest and unhurried time with a new baby are important prerequisites for a successful start to mothering. Some women get exhausted with having too many visitors too soon.

Some people put a birth notice in the local newspaper, although new parents are increasingly using email and/or a website to tell everyone the news. Some people wait a few days to avoid being inundated with visitors

'He was pretty wakeful, but even when he was sleeping I always had visitors. I felt I had to talk to them. It was tricky.'

immediately; others prefer to get the information out as soon as possible and to receive all their visitors in hospital, where there is no pressure to produce cups of tea.

How you handle this will depend on your circumstances, but it's worth talking about it before the birth and sorting out some priorities.

Bonding – the mother-baby unit

'You know, quite often, privately to myself I would wonder if she was really mine in those first few weeks. Then one day she smiled at me – just for me; I smiled right back; I was hooked, and still am – ten years on!'

All of the hormonal and emotional changes surrounding birth culminate in one thing – a very special feeling that develops between you and your baby. It's a two-way process – not only do you become 'tuned in' to the sight, smell and sound of your baby, but she becomes 'tuned in' to you.

This process is sometimes called 'bonding', and contrary to popular opinion, it is not always automatic. Looking back, many women say that it took time to 'fall in love' with their babies, especially their first. It didn't happen overnight, but was a gradual process as they spent time feeding, cuddling, changing and 'showing off' their babies. Somehow, this 'falling in love' seems to be compensation for the broken nights, the dirty nappies, and the more restricted lifestyle. If it doesn't happen, parenting can seem a thankless and dreary job.

So it makes sense to help the bonding process, not only between the baby and her mother, but also between the baby and her father and older siblings.

Factors affecting bonding[3]

Things that promote good bonding

- skin-to-skin contact immediately after birth or as soon as possible
- spending uninterrupted time together soon after birth
- being able to feed your baby soon after birth
- being able to have your baby with you as much as possible, especially in the first few days
- being free from pain
- having enough rest in the first few days
- being in surroundings where you feel comfortable

Things that may interfere with bonding

- being separated from your baby soon after birth
- having a very premature baby who is not able to suckle and needs special care
- not having a chance to recover from labour and birth before resuming other responsibilities
- going home, or being at home, without enough good adult support
- having too many visitors
- being in an overcrowded, overheated hospital
- being in pain

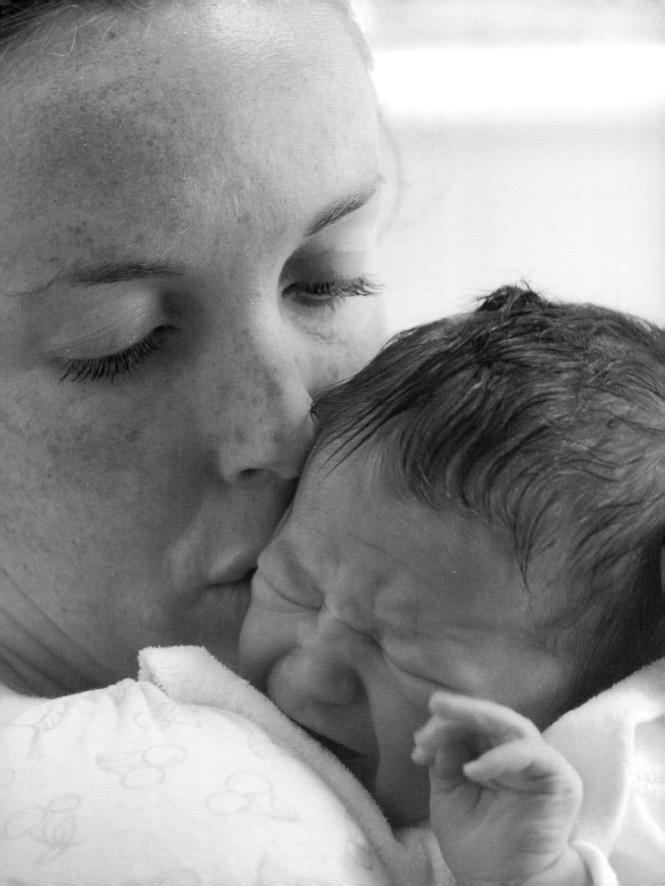

2. What's happening?

Your body – changes after birth

Changes in the circulation and body fluid

The extra fluid your body accumulated during pregnancy will now be lost, most of it within 24 hours of birth and the rest within the next few days. For some women, this may take longer – up to a week – regardless of whether they had a straightforward vaginal delivery or a Caesarean section. The kidney function alters so that a lot of watery urine is produced. This process is known as diuresis, and may start during labour. It is not unusual to pass up to 3 litres of urine within a few hours of birth.

Changes in body temperature

The heat-exchange system that kept your baby at the right temperature is no longer needed. Suddenly the body temperature drops, which is why many women feel very shivery and cold shortly after birth. Within a few hours they adjust, only to have their internal thermostat upset again once their milk 'comes in'. The body temperature often rises slightly until the supply and demand of breastfeeding is established.

Changes in the vagina and perineum

The vagina rapidly shrinks back to a more normal size after birth. It is very elastic and has a rich blood supply, which means it recovers quickly and any superficial tears heal within three to four days. The perineum also returns to its normal size and small tears heal very quickly.

Episiotomies, and deeper tears in the muscles around the vaginal opening, take longer to heal. If they have been well repaired and the edges neatly matched, and if there is no infection, healing can proceed quickly; even within the first week the tissue will knit together well. Problems arise when large tears are not repaired, or are not repaired completely. Then healing is much slower, and there are raw areas that can easily become infected.

There may be bruising around the vaginal opening, especially if the second stage was lengthy or there was a forceps delivery. This can make the whole area very swollen and sore for a few days. Initially, though, the vaginal area may be numb as a result of swelling. Again, because of the good blood supply to the area, most of the bruising will subside within a week.

Changes in the uterus

Immediately after the birth of the placenta, the muscles of the uterus contract firmly and must stay contracted to prevent further bleeding.

Breastfeeding also stimulates uterine contractions in the first few days – these 'after-pains' can be quite uncomfortable, rather like a period cramp. Some women say these after-pains are worse than the contractions of labour.

The place where the placenta was attached is a soft, raw area that takes several days to heal over. Within two to three days it becomes covered in a thick, cloudy, mucous-like layer, which provides temporary protection and is then gradually shed through the vagina over the next 10–20 days. This discharge, known as the lochia, makes the initial red bleeding immediately after birth (normally no heavier than a period) turn to a pinky colour within four to five days. The lochia can take up to six weeks to stop completely, although for most women it stops one to two weeks after birth.

Because of this process, there is potential for infection in the first few days after birth. If harmful bacteria get into the uterus immediately after birth, they can easily spread to the bloodstream and cause puerperal sepsis (fever). In the days before antibiotics, this was a common cause of maternal death in overcrowded hospitals. But with good attention to clean conditions for the birth and after-care, post-partum infection is much less common than it used to be.

Avoiding infection after childbirth

- Use clean, sterile equipment during labour and birth.
- Keep toilet and bathing facilities very clean in the days immediately following birth. This means using disinfectant every time the bathroom is used and thoroughly cleaning the area once a day.
- Dispose of used sanitary pads promptly, and ensure that your sheets, towels, nightwear and underwear are washed promptly and thoroughly.
- Wash your hands well after going to the toilet or changing the baby's nappies.
- Avoid using tampons until a month or so after birth.
- Avoid intercourse for 10–14 days following birth.
- Inform your LMC promptly if you develop a temperature that persists for more than 24 hours or if you feel unwell with flu-like symptoms. Prompt use of the correct antibiotic will usually avert a more serious problem.
- Especially in hospitals, there must be high standards of hygiene to prevent any infection that does occur from spreading from person to person.

Changes in the breasts

For the first two days after birth the breasts seem much as they were during pregnancy, although they now contain a small amount of colostrum, which is very valuable for the newborn baby.

On the second or third day after birth, milk production begins in earnest and the breasts can become swollen and uncomfortable. As this often coincides with the 'third-day blues' (see p.326), it can be a difficult time, especially for first-time mothers. Regular suckling within the first day or two, as demanded by your baby, will have helped stimulate this production. But now you need your baby to feed more often, to make your breasts feel more comfortable.

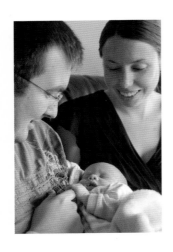

Your baby – changes after birth

Your newborn baby must accomplish many things as she adjusts to life outside the womb. Some of these happen immediately, whereas others take several days or weeks.

Breathing

Your baby must now get oxygen into her bloodstream by breathing air into her lungs. Her heart must beat so that the oxygenated blood will circulate to every cell in her body. All this requires a dramatic change in her circulation, which she usually accomplishes quite easily and naturally. She is likely to run into problems only if she has been abnormally stressed and short of oxygen during labour, or has an anatomical problem with her heart, lungs or diaphragm.

When a baby breathes vigorously after birth, she looks pink (as opposed to blue, or white), is alert and has strong, active limbs, although it may take an hour or two for her toes and fingers to lose their dusky colour and look completely pink. Her breathing is sometimes quite noisy, with snorts and sucking sounds.

Changes in the blood

In all newborn babies, some of the red blood cells are broken down and destroyed. These are special blood cells that were needed before the baby was born and are now no longer required. When the blood cells are broken down, a substance called bilirubin is produced, which the liver normally clears from the bloodstream.

However, in some babies, especially those who are premature, the liver function is still immature and is slower at clearing the bilirubin. When there is a lot of bilirubin in the blood, the skin becomes a yellow or golden colour – a condition known as jaundice.

Healthy full-term babies can also become jaundiced if they don't have enough colostrum or food to provide their liver with albumin (a protein) to clear the bilirubin.

Occasionally, a lot more blood cells than normal are broken down and the bilirubin level in the blood becomes very high. This condition requires active management to avoid the risk of brain damage (see p.333).

Temperature control

Newborn babies have a large surface area in relation to their size. This means that when naked, and especially when wet, they lose heat quickly. Newborn babies must be dried well and covered with a warm, dry towel or blanket. A newborn baby's head will lose a lot of heat, so it needs to be covered as well. Even when wrapped warmly, babies can have trouble maintaining body heat in the first few days if the air temperature is low. So it helps if the room is kept at a fairly warm, even temperature (around 18–20°C).

On the other hand, babies have a limited ability to lose heat in a hot climate or overheated room, particularly when wrapped up. In these situations, uncover them to make use of their large surface area and to let the air circulate freely.

Feeding (see also p.308)

The baby has a very strong instinct to turn towards the breast (the 'rooting reflex') and to suck (the 'sucking reflex'). The ability to suck does not develop until near the end of the pregnancy, and will be impaired if the baby is not fully mature or is having trouble breathing. If labour has been long and difficult, the baby may be exhausted and want to sleep a lot, but she will usually suck quite well with some encouragement.

With the first feed, milk passes for the first time into the baby's mouth, down her oesophagus and into her stomach and intestines. There she digests food for the first time, and fluid is absorbed into her bloodstream. Colostrum and breast milk contain special proteins that help to line the newborn gut. This lining protects the gut against disease and prepares it for a lifetime of digesting food.

Normal healthy babies usually manage the first feed with very little trouble. Some babies are a little mucousy and snuffly, which may make them rather reluctant to feed, although they can usually be persuaded to do so. Babies may swallow some fluid during birth, and this may make them gag a little and vomit up small amounts of mucous in the first few days after birth. But grunting, choking and/or copious vomiting are not normal, and should be checked out promptly.

Passing a bowel motion

Within 24–48 hours of birth, most babies will have passed meconium – the dark, sticky substance present within newborn intestines. Be aware that small baby wipes are no match for sticky meconium; a wet flannel or cloth is often necessary, and you may need to bring a couple from home. A little Vaseline on your baby's bottom may be helpful in easing removal of the sticky meconium. Gradually, the meconium will be replaced by stools that are more brown in colour ('transition' stools), followed by very loose yellow motions that look slightly curdled. This is perfectly normal, and indicates that the baby's digestive system is all in working order. The loose yellow stools usually occur once the milk has 'come in'.

Passing urine

Newborn babies produce a lot of very watery urine, as their kidneys are still immature. This means they can very quickly become dehydrated. Lots of wet nappies are the norm for the first few months. Most babies have 5–50ml of urine in their bladder at birth, and should pass this within the first 48 hours. Right from the beginning, babies should not 'dribble' urine constantly; they should pass urine and then stop completely for a short while.

Why babies lose weight after birth

Nearly all babies lose 100–300g within 48 hours of birth. This is mainly loss of fluid, and occurs because their fluid intake is small in the first couple of days before the mother's milk 'comes in'. Most babies have regained their birth weight within a week, and this temporary weight loss is managed easily by healthy babies.

3. Feeding your baby

Breastfeeding (see also pp.158 and 342)

Getting started

After birth, the mother's breasts do not instantly fill with milk; it usually takes two to three days to start normal milk production. Before this, the breast tissue contains small amounts of colostrum, which is particularly beneficial for newborn babies.

It helps if you can get your baby properly 'latched on' to the breast in the first day or so, while the colostrum is present and before full milk production begins. You will then be well prepared when the breasts fill up with milk and become much bigger on the second or third day.

'Latching' your baby on the breast

For effective and comfortable breastfeeding, your baby needs to suck on breast tissue – not chew on the end of the nipple. This means that the nipple should be right at the back of the baby's mouth, and her lips almost at the outer edge of the areola (the dark part around the nipple). This position seems odd to us as adults, because we're used to taking our food into the front of our mouths. But the baby is quite comfortable with the nipple in the back of her mouth: it allows her to 'milk' the breast, so that the milk ducts are emptied and more milk can flow down from the breast tissue to refill them.

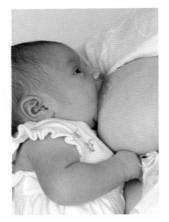

Baby correctly latched on

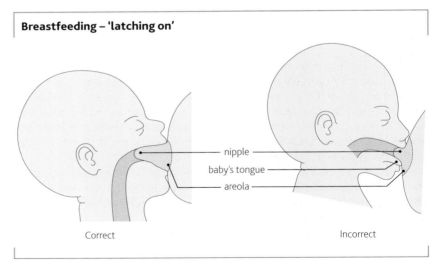

Breastfeeding – 'latching on'

nipple
baby's tongue
areola

Correct   Incorrect

It all sounds fine in theory, but how do you get your baby to do it in practice?

- Get yourself in a comfortable, relaxed position so that you can hold your baby with one arm and have the other hand free.
- Until you get used to it, it's often easier to have your baby firmly wrapped so that her head can't flop about and her hands don't get in the way.

- Get the whole breast area free of loose clothing or blankets, and then place your baby so that her cheek is next to the breast, and her tummy is next to your tummy. This will usually be sufficient to get her to turn her head, with her mouth wide open, towards the breast. This instinctive reaction is known as the 'rooting reflex'.

- Wait until her mouth is *wide* open – not just the lips but the gums as well. Now, hold your breast with thumb and forefinger on either side of the areola and bring her mouth over the nipple and areola. She should not suck the nipple gradually into her mouth with her lips partly closed, and nor should you lean down to get the breast into her mouth. If she is properly 'latched on', she will nearly always start to suck – perhaps tentatively at first, but then more strongly.

- If more than a little of the areola is showing around the baby's mouth, carefully release the suction by slipping a finger gently into the corner of her mouth and pressing on your breast until she lets go. Now, wait until her mouth is wide open and try to ensure that the whole nipple and areola (or most of it) are right inside her mouth.

- If the nipple feels as though it's being bitten, release the suction and try again. When the baby gets it right, you might feel a bit of discomfort for the first minute or so after she starts suckling; but from then on, the suckling should not hurt or pinch.

Don't be discouraged if this seems difficult – it takes practice to get it right. Accept your LMC or post-natal midwife's help, and ask them to check that your baby is latched on properly until you are quite sure. If it feels painful, take the baby off and try again, even if your midwife says it looks right.

Babies vary a lot in how much they want to feed in the first few hours. If she doesn't seem at all interested, try again a little later. If she does want to suck, don't forget to change her from one side to the other after a while, as this avoids putting undue pressure on one nipple. Once your baby is well 'latched on', let her feed. Repeatedly taking her off and putting her back on can make sore nipples worse. Be gentle with your nipples and treat them as you would your lips – keeping them moist (but not wet and soggy) will help prevent the tissue from cracking. Sometimes a few drops of breast milk wiped over the nipples is helpful to keep them moist; creams are not usually needed at this stage, and may cause unnecessary irritation (see p.344).[4]

The sucking action on the breast will stimulate the uterus to contract as the hormone oxytocin is released, and you may feel period-like 'after-pains'. Paracetamol (Panadol) tablets and a hot-water bottle or wheat bag will provide some relief if the pains are very intense.

Taking your baby off the breast

If your baby falls asleep while feeding, you can release the suction by slipping your finger gently into the corner of her mouth. She will sleep equally well in your arms or in her cot, whichever you prefer. Some babies swallow air while feeding, so she may need to be held in an upright position, and perhaps given a gentle back-rub, so she can burp before being put down.

Alternatively, she may let go of the nipple herself and be happy to spend some time looking around, only to nuzzle in again a few minutes later.

'At the hospital, the midwives change shift every eight hours, so you can talk to different ones about feeding – each one will suggest something else. They all have different knowledge. I listened to all of them and then I worked out my own method after talking it through with my own midwife.'

Breastfeeding (for partners and support people)

It can be really useful if you too can learn how to get the baby firmly fixed to her mother's breast. Ask the midwife to show you how to do this. A 2 a.m. feed may then be much quicker, quieter and more satisfying for the baby – and you'll all get a better sleep.

'Breastfeeding was a huge problem initially. After the birth, my breasts were so huge and hard – like rocks! For the first couple of days feeding was excruciating. I had to squeeze or express the colostrum out because breastfeeding was too painful. My midwives told me breastfeeding was the best treatment for engorgement – so not what I wanted to hear! But I was determined that Alena would be breastfed, so with painkillers, expressing, and support from my whānau and midwives it got easier. It took a few months, but I'm glad I didn't give up, because breastfeeding became a wonderful bonding experience later on.'

When she has had enough, she will probably be equally content with you or your partner or support person, or lying in her cot. Some babies like their hands free, while others are more settled when they are firmly wrapped. Always put her down to sleep on her back (see pp.381–382).

How breastfeeding works[5]

Breastfeeding is a complex process, involving many different physical and psychological factors. If you are breastfeeding, it helps to understand how it works so that you can learn to make your own day-to-day judgements about feeding.

Successful breastfeeding involves two distinct processes, which are under the control of two different hormones. Prolactin is responsible for the production of milk within the alveoli of the breast tissue, while oxytocin is responsible for releasing the milk from the alveoli into the collecting ducts for delivery at the nipple (see diagram opposite).

The action of a baby sucking at the breast stimulates the production of oxytocin. This allows the milk to be 'let down' from the alveoli into the collecting ducts, and from there into the nipple and the baby's mouth. Oxytocin also stimulates the uterus to contract, as it needs to do after birth.

As the baby continues to suck, she gradually empties the collecting ducts and the alveoli of the milk they have produced; but even though your breasts may feel empty after a feed, the cells of the alveoli are continually producing milk. As the breast empties, the milk changes in character from a watery consistency (foremilk) to a much thicker, more nutritious milk (hindmilk) with a higher fat content. This richer hindmilk, with its higher calorie content, is necessary for healthy growth and development, especially brain growth.

Once the breast tissue is relatively empty, the hormone prolactin acts to stimulate production again. Over the next two to three hours, the alveoli will gradually fill up as more milk is produced, ready for the next feed.

The more frequently the breast is emptied (or partially emptied), the more the breast tissue is stimulated to produce milk. The milk won't be released, or leak out, until oxytocin production is stimulated.

The stimulation and production of prolactin are relatively stable. Milk production will continue even in women who are ill or malnourished, and the quality of the milk will still be good.

Oxytocin production, on the other hand, can be much more variable. Some women find that their milk 'lets down' very easily, even when they are not actually feeding their baby. For other women the milk let-down is more difficult, and can stop if things aren't exactly right. If the milk is not let down, the breast will not be emptied, the baby will remain hungry – even though she has sucked and sucked – and the prolactin will not be stimulated to produce more milk.

The whole system works on supply and demand. The more milk the baby takes from the breast, the more milk the breast produces. If milk is not removed from the breast, the pressure of the full collecting ducts and alveoli will slow and eventually stop further production.

In some women the system works perfectly, right from the start. In others, it takes some time for the breasts to adjust to the amount of milk actually required. And in some women, it takes a lot of patience to develop a good let-down of milk with every feed.

Lactating breast

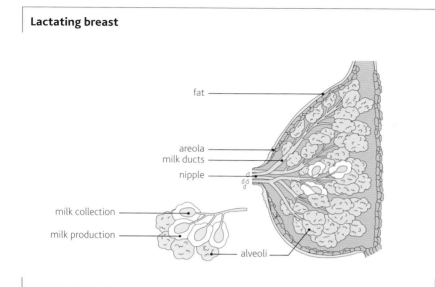

fat
areola
milk ducts
nipple
milk collection
milk production
alveoli

As the milk starts to flow

Somewhere between 48 and 72 hours after the birth, milk production will accelerate and your breasts will quickly become much larger and fuller than before – sometimes dramatically so. It is common for babies to become hungrier at this time as well, and their increased demands mean more frequent feeds. It often takes a few days for the supply and demand system to settle down into a pattern where the amount of milk produced is about equal to the amount the baby drinks.

These few days can be very trying for a new mother, as her breasts may be uncomfortable and so full that her baby has trouble latching on. But the more frequently your baby is fed, the less full and uncomfortable your breasts will feel. It is worth being patient and persevering, as feeding will gradually become much easier.

The let-down reflex

The let-down reflex allows milk to be released from the breast ducts into the baby's mouth. It is governed by the mother's hormones, although it does become an automatic or reflex response to the sound of her baby crying (or even to thinking about her baby) once feeding is established.

The release of milk from the breast can occur even before the baby starts to suck, as the mother anticipates the act of feeding. But it usually occurs once the baby has taken her first few sucks of the foremilk that has collected in the ducts just behind the nipple. Once the let-down occurs, milk flows from all the breast ducts to the nipple and into the baby's mouth.

If the let-down reflex does not occur when your baby starts to feed, she will get only a small amount of watery foremilk, despite sucking vigorously, and she will remain hungry. Some babies will pull off the breast at this point; and unless coaxed back on, they will be unsettled and want to feed again soon afterwards.

The let-down reflex

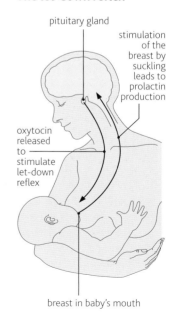

pituitary gland

stimulation of the breast by suckling leads to prolactin production

oxytocin released to stimulate let-down reflex

breast in baby's mouth

Although the let-down reflex is usually a natural, almost automatic response, it is sometimes affected by external factors. It helps to be aware of these (see box below).

Oxytocin production and let-down

Things that may stimulate oxytocin production and promote let-down

- hearing your baby cry
- hearing someone else's baby cry
- thinking about feeding your baby
- baby overdue for a feed
- feeding your baby – the other breast may leak

Things that may interfere with oxytocin production and impair let-down

- your nipple hurts as the baby is put to the breast (often because she is not 'latched on' properly)
- you're scared your nipple might hurt
- you're trying to breastfeed in an uncomfortable position, or in a place that is too public
- you're worried, upset or in pain

The milk 'letting down'

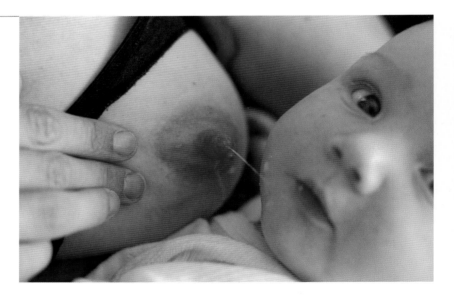

How to tell that let-down has occurred

To start with, you may not be aware of any particular sensation in the breast as let-down occurs. But gradually, as you get more confident about feeding, you may become aware of a relaxing feeling once your baby is fixed on the breast. This may initially seem like relief that you've got your baby properly attached, but as you get used to it, you will recognise a particular sensation – tingling and relaxing at the same time.

For some women, the reflex becomes a definite sensation once lactation is fully established. Others are only vaguely or occasionally aware of it. But if your breasts leak milk freely, either before or during a feed, it is a sure sign that the let-down reflex is working well.

Getting the reflex firmly established can take time. Some women have no problems; others find they need to concentrate on getting the details right, and need lots of support and encouragement in the first few days or weeks of feeding. Any stress or tension can affect the let-down reflex, so make sure you're as relaxed as possible when preparing to feed your baby.

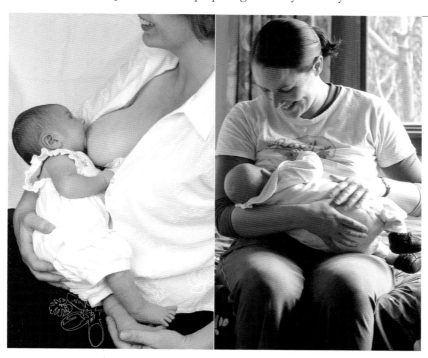

Different positions for breastfeeding

If your baby is hungry and unsettled after a feed, or for hours at a time, there may have been something impairing your let-down reflex at the last feed or feeds (see box opposite). Here are some suggestions for remedying the situation:

- Sit down and relax before feeding.
- Take a warm, relaxing bath or shower.
- Massage your shoulders or try acupressure on a point on your shoulder (known as Jianjing, or GB21).[6]
- Feed in a comfortable position, in a quiet, private place.
- Take some pain relief beforehand if you're in pain, or if you anticipate pain when the baby sucks (e.g. you have a cracked nipple).

If the problem persists, ask for help before it gets any worse – from a support person, your LMC or hospital midwife, a lactation consultant (ask if one is available at the hospital), a practice nurse, a Plunket nurse or a community support group such as La Leche League. (See Appendix: Breastfeeding.)

Breastfeeding twins

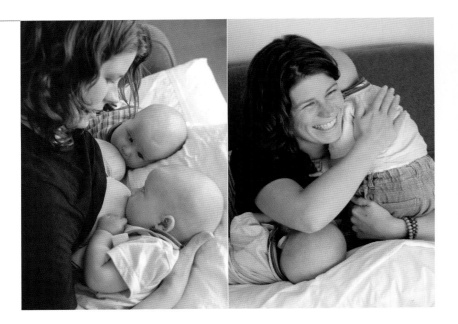

Tips for successful breastfeeding

If you want to promote milk production and continue breastfeeding

- Feed your baby often, in a relaxed environment, always making sure she is properly latched on to the breast. Become aware of the let-down feeling.
- Encourage her to feed before the breasts become very full and hard. Latching a baby onto a very full breast can be tricky.
- If you can't get your baby fixed to a very full, firm breast, try expressing a little milk by hand to ease the pressure. Leave the other breast to drip while you feed on the first side. This will help to relieve the pressure, too.
- At this early stage, don't go more than about four hours, especially at night, without feeding. Wake your baby if necessary, and encourage her to feed from both breasts.

If you have painful, engorged breasts and want to continue breastfeeding

- Feed your baby regularly, especially at night, but try to space the feeds at least two to three hours apart.
- Wear a firm bra (in a larger size than normal), or a breast-binder, pinned firmly to support the breasts but not so tight that it is uncomfortable.
- Get in the shower, and allow the breasts to drip milk to relieve the pressure.
- Place fresh cabbage leaves over the breasts, inside your bra. Many women find the leaves are remarkably effective for reducing engorgement and inflammation of the breasts.[7]
- If your breasts are still really sore, it may be worth expressing some of the milk until they feel more comfortable, but don't take more than a few millilitres (20–30ml) at this stage. You should not do this more than once or twice, as it will only take longer for the supply and demand problem to sort itself out – remember that the more often you empty the breast, the more milk it will produce.

Stopping milk production

Some women are unable to breastfeed, and may need help and support to suppress their milk production. Sometimes mental or physical ill health or certain medications or drugs make breastfeeding impossible. It is also currently recommended that women who are HIV-positive should not breastfeed because of the risk of transmitting HIV to their baby. However, this advice may change as more becomes known about HIV transmission, and treatments continue to improve.[8]

If a baby has died, either in late pregnancy, during labour or shortly after delivery, the mother's milk will still 'come in' unabated, and this can be very distressing until milk production ceases.

If you want, or need, to stop milk production completely

- If possible, put your baby to the breast once or twice shortly after birth, so that she can get the benefit of some of the colostrum.
- Don't feed the baby at the breast again after that.
- Wear a very firm breast-binder for a few days. You will need help to get it fastened firmly enough.
- Take regular pain relief if you need to. Paracetamol (Panadol) tablets (two every four hours) are suitable.
- Medication is available to curtail milk production, but often it is not necessary. While the drugs are effective, they may cause nausea, indigestion or dizziness, and therefore are not commonly used.

Bottle-feeding

Occasionally, there will be good reason to bottle-feed your new baby with formula (see above, and pp.158 and 347–348). If so, it's easy for someone else to bottle-feed your baby initially. However, even if you don't feel up to it, it's worth making the effort to give your baby her bottle yourself as often as you can in these early days – it really helps you to get to know each other and gives you valuable practice while help is at hand. Feeling good about your baby will help you feel good about yourself – an important part of the process of adjusting to being a mother.

Milk mixtures

There are several different artificial milk formulas available in New Zealand especially for feeding babies. All are made into sterilised dried powders, which (if correctly made up) provide newborn babies with a complete, balanced diet. Most of these formulas are made from cow's milk, although some are made from soybean milk or goat's milk.

Straight cow's milk, even if diluted, is not recommended for newborn babies; it is hard to digest and can cause severe stomach upsets and allergies. Straight goat's milk does not have the correct nutrients for a newborn baby, and is not recommended, although goat's-milk formulas can be used safely.

Once milk formulas have been made up, they can very easily become contaminated with bacteria and cause a baby to become ill. This can be avoided if you are meticulous about preparing the milk in sterilised bottles, and discarding any excess milk after each feed.

Feeding with a bottle

- Test the milk temperature by shaking a few drops onto your wrist: if it feels either hot or cold, adjust the temperature until it feels about the same as your skin.
- When feeding, hold your baby in your arms so that she is in a reclining position. Make sure the screw attaching the teat to the bottle is slightly loose, to allow air to enter the bottle. If there is a valve in the teat, it should be uppermost to work properly.
- Place the teat gently in the baby's mouth, well towards the back, and angle the bottle so that the baby can suck firmly.

Bottle in a good position for feeding

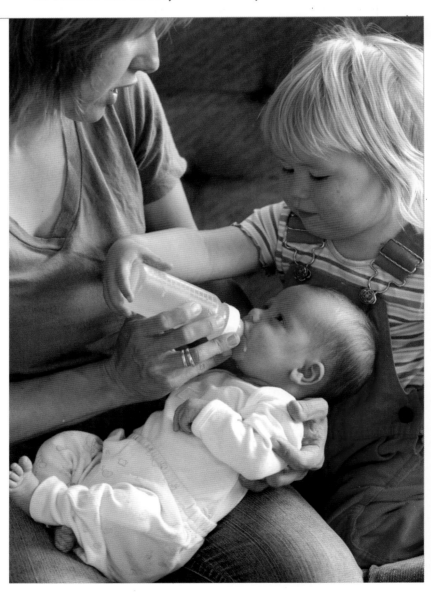

- As the baby sucks, you should see and hear air entering the bottle and forming small bubbles. If not, try loosening the screw top slightly to let more air in.
- You may need to stop several times during a feed with a small baby. Often she needs to bring up wind before she can continue feeding.
- If there is any milk remaining in the bottle after your baby has finished feeding, discard it and clean the bottle as soon as possible.

Sterilising bottles

Boiling

Bottles, teats, caps and any other equipment that comes into contact with the milk can be sterilised by boiling them for ten minutes: they must be submerged in the boiling water. They need to be lifted out with sterile tongs, or the water drained off them, and should be used again as soon as possible.

Sterilising solutions

You can buy a chemical sterilising unit in which bottles, teats, etc. are soaked in a special disinfectant solution before use. This method is easier to manage as it avoids having to boil everything, but the instructions for making and changing the solution must be followed exactly.

Preparing milk mixtures

All milk formulas must be made up with water that has been boiled for ten minutes, and using sterile equipment. The water should be measured into the bottle first before the powder is added to ensure that the mixture is of the correct consistency – neither too weak nor too concentrated. A weak mixture will mean that the baby is not getting all the nourishment she needs, while a mixture that is too concentrated may make her constipated.

Once the mixture is made up, it can be kept for 24 hours, as long as it is refrigerated until required. When travelling longer distances you should store any prepared milk in a chilly bin with an icepack – even better, put only cooled boiled water in the bottle, and take the tin of formula along as well. When a feed is due, you can then add the correct amount of powder to the water, shake it up to ensure it is well mixed, heat the milk if necessary and feed it to your baby. This will ensure that bacteria do not grow in the made-up formula, especially if you are travelling in summer.

Most parents who bottle-feed their baby find it is easier if they have enough bottles and teats (eight is usually sufficient) to prepare a whole day's supply at one time, while their baby is asleep. Then, when the baby wakes for a feed, you can simply retrieve a prepared bottle from the fridge and heat it until the milk is at blood-temperature. A microwave is ideal for this, but an electric jug works well too. If you use a microwave, give the bottle a good shake afterwards before testing the milk on your wrist to ensure that the temperature is even throughout. Another option is to heat the bottle in a saucepan of boiling water – the milk will usually be the right temperature if you place the bottle of cold milk from the fridge in a saucepan of cold water from the tap, and then heat until the water just comes to the boil. Make sure you check the temperature of the heated milk on a sensitive part of your arm to ensure that the baby does not get burned.

4. One day at a time (days 1–4)

First day

Feelings

Now that the flurry of activity surrounding the birth is over, you can begin to collect your thoughts and reflect on the past 24 hours or so. You may have mixed feelings about whether you would prefer company or not. You will probably feel tired even if you have had the opportunity to sleep; many new mothers feel too excited to get much sleep after their baby's birth.

Even if your labour has been quick and straightforward, you will almost certainly need rest on this first day. Let everyone else do the worrying and the caring, and just take things very easy. Your sole aim in this first week should be to get to know your baby and learn how to work as a unit, so that you're sufficiently attuned to each other to face the world – together.

Rest versus visitors

Rest is very important, and all your caregivers and visitors should realise this. You need to make the most of this short time before your milk comes in, when your baby is likely to be relatively undemanding.

This doesn't mean that you have to be in bed all day, though you should be lying down for a good part of it. But don't let the need for rest make you feel isolated. Try to get a good mix of time alone sleeping, and time to be with your closest family. Older children also deserve time on this first day – time to see and touch their new sibling, and time to be reassured that you are still their mother, too.

Passing urine

This is obviously important, but you may hesitate if your bottom is sore. The pressure of a full bladder is very uncomfortable though; it's better to go earlier rather than later. If you're having real trouble, it may help to run a bath and go in there.

Care of your bottom

If you keep the whole area free from infection, any stitches or small tears will heal remarkably quickly. Each time you pass urine or move your bowels, wash the area gently with warm water. A bidet or detachable shower-head is ideal for this, but a plastic drink bottle used to squirt clean, warm water onto the tender areas will work just as well. Then gently pat the area dry with a disposable towel and put on a new sanitary pad. It's also quite safe and very relaxing to have one or two baths a day, as long as the bath and the water are clean. Salt can be added if you wish, as it's a good disinfectant: use about a cupful in a shallow bath.

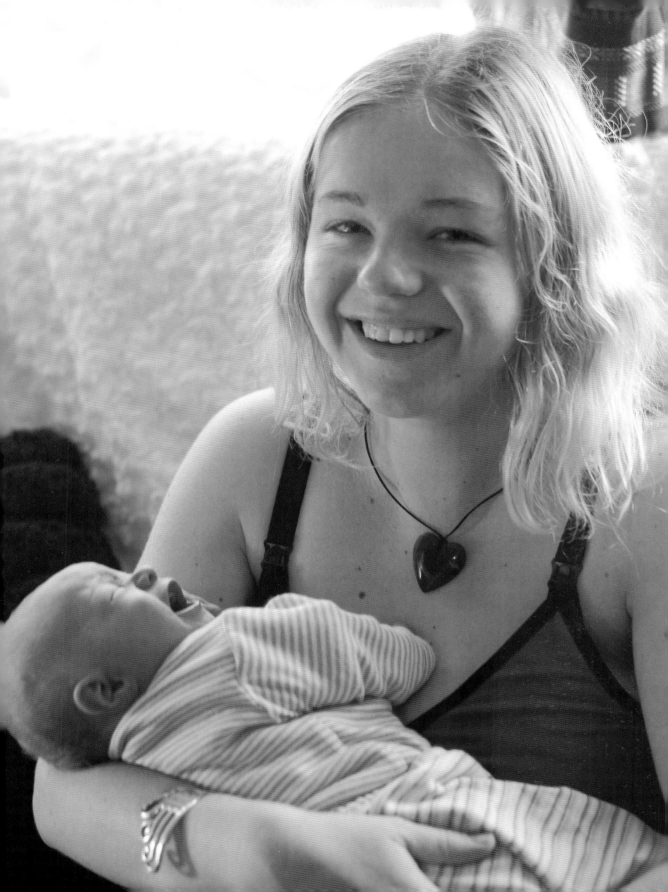

The first day breastfeeding your baby (see also p.314)

The most important thing on this first day is getting your baby properly latched onto the breast. Sore nipples, especially during feeding, are a fairly sure sign that the baby is not on properly.

Once your baby has latched on well, she should get enough fluid to satisfy her and be fairly settled for several hours at a time. Normal, healthy full-term babies seem to demonstrate one of two patterns of behaviour in the day or two after birth: some will have a good feed after they are born, and then sleep for six to eight hours; others will want to feed often in the first 24 hours and then have a long sleep.[9] It is difficult to predict which pattern your baby will follow, but it's useful to be aware that wake-sleep patterns vary. With a baby who has been born full term and has had no major problems during the labour and birth, there is no need to disturb their natural pattern. However, premature or jaundiced babies need more frequent fluid intake, and may need active encouragement to feed.

If your baby wants to feed often in the first 24 hours, follow her lead, ensuring she is properly fixed to the breast. If you intend to continue breast-feeding, introducing any other type of feed at this stage may upset the supply and demand system on which breastfeeding is based. Keep in mind that newborn babies have small stomachs with a capacity in the range of 15–30ml (about 3–6 teaspoons).[10] This means that they do not need large volumes of milk in the early days but will be satisfied with small, frequent feeds. (The amount of colostrum in your breasts will also be small, but quite adequate to meet your baby's needs.)

Ask for help, support or advice if your baby is unsettled or you are unsure if her behaviour is normal or not. If you're at home, ask your LMC or post-natal midwife, as often as necessary. Your partner or support person may need to help if your midwife is not there. If you're in hospital, ask an experienced midwife to help you. It's really useful if you can be helped by the same person for two or three feeds in a row. Be aware that post-natal wards can be very busy places and are sometimes understaffed; you may have to be assertive to get the help you need. Don't be afraid to ask if there is a lactation consultant available at the hospital if you are still having trouble getting your baby latched on and feeding comfortably.

Nappy-changing

See Chapter 8, p.358.

Food for you

If you're in hospital on this first day, and especially if you've had your baby in the afternoon, a meal may not have been ordered for you. You are likely to be hungry, so have some pre-packaged snacks in your bag, and/or get your support person to get some food for you.

Second day

Feelings

It's quite normal to feel very up and down emotionally in the first few days, and many second-day mothers find they are unusually sensitive to small things that go wrong. The elation immediately after the birth can soon be replaced by feelings of vulnerability and inadequacy, especially if your baby is a bit unsettled. It's easy to be in tears over seemingly small things; having someone else's competent arms to hold the baby for half an hour can help a lot. Rest, eating and drinking well, and trusting your own instincts as a new mother will help you get through this emotional rollercoaster. Allow your support people to help you as much as they can; don't try to be a super-mum, and don't expect to manage the household as you did before the birth or as a career woman manages her work life. On the other hand, if you don't experience such ups and downs, don't think you are abnormal!

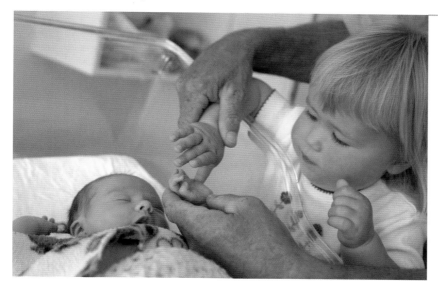

Meeting baby for the first time

Eating and drinking

Producing milk is an energy-intensive process, so you will need to eat more high-energy food than usual. Many of the hormonal changes that occur at the time of birth stimulate the appetite, and most new mothers have no trouble eating.

For those women who suffered from nausea and vomiting in pregnancy, food now tastes especially good! Make the most of this, and eat plenty; but don't forget to eat well, too. All the guidelines discussed in Chapters 1 and 4 still apply.

If you're in hospital, you may need to ask for double helpings – the standard hospital meal is designed for those who are ill, not for healthy new mothers. Most hospitals provide a daily menu that you are expected to complete the previous night. Make sure you tick as many of the items on the menu as you may need, even if you don't eat all of them at that meal. A kitchenette is also provided for new mothers to help themselves to extra bread, butter, spreads, tea, Milo and coffee while they are in hospital.

Drink plenty of fluid, too; breastfeeding women need at least 10–12 glasses of fluid a day. About eight glasses of fluid a day is the normal requirement for body and bowel function, so a breastfeeding woman needs more than this. A useful rule of thumb is to have a drink every time you breastfeed. Water is best, but trim milk, fruit juice and tea in moderation are all fine.

Myths abound about what breastfeeding women should and shouldn't eat, but some women do find that coffee, alcohol and large quantities of certain fruits and vegetables may make their babies unsettled. If certain foods upset your digestive system or increase your wind, they may also do the same for your baby. But even if a few foods seem to upset you or your baby, don't let that stop you eating plenty of other fresh fruit and vegetables, and keeping high-fat and high-sugar foods to a minimum.[11]

Moving your bowels

This may seem impossible if you have stitches and a sore, bruised bottom. But getting constipated will make going even more uncomfortable and may aggravate haemorrhoids (piles) that have occurred during pregnancy or birth (see p.195). So eat plenty of fresh fruit and vegetables and wholegrain bread, and drink plenty of water: these will all help to make the motions softer. Kiwifruit are especially good, and you could also try the pulped kiwifruit drinks that are available in most supermarkets.[12]

Make the effort to go to the toilet if you feel like going – don't 'hold off' until later. It will be uncomfortable, but as long as you don't strain hard, you are unlikely to damage any stitches or healing tissue.

Sitting well on the toilet is important. Your knees should be slightly higher than your hips (a small footstool can be used if necessary). Keep your back straight and your shoulders slightly forward, with your head held high. Let the tummy muscles relax forward. The ideal bowel motion is soft and does not require any pushing or straining. But if you do need to push, keep your tummy relaxed and gently blow through a cupped hand: feel how your waist widens. You will be amazed at what a difference this toilet position will make. Don't be afraid to support your perineum (the area in front of the anus) with a clean pad, and do take pain relief if you need to, rather than have the pain stop you from passing a bowel motion. This toilet position is also a good way of emptying your bladder; in fact, try to make it a habit always to sit on the toilet this way.

It's quite common to develop piles in late pregnancy or during labour itself, but they will generally settle down with time if you don't get constipated and don't strain. Various creams and lotions can help if the piles are sore (for example, witch hazel). Resting with a warm, moist wash-cloth on the area is also soothing.

Managing after-pains

These cramp-like tummy pains felt while breastfeeding are not usually a problem with first babies, but can be quite intense with second and subsequent babies. They are a good sign that the uterus is contracting properly and the baby is feeding well, and will subside within a few days. It may be useful to take two paracetamol (Panadol) tablets before a feed, especially if the anticipation of pain prevents you from letting down your milk. The paracetamol will not affect the baby. Acupressure on a point on the inside of your lower leg, about four fingers above your ankle bone (the point known as Spleen 6), can also help relieve after-pains.[13] Keeping your bladder empty will help too.

Cord care

Within a few days of birth, the umbilical cord will shrivel and become dry, then drop off from the baby's tummy button. Infection can occur if any part of the cord remains moist, so the quicker it shrivels and dries, the better.

Generally, if the cord is simply dried and left alone, it falls off quickly (usually within five to seven days after birth) and with few complications. It may bleed a little, become moist, and smell a little during this process. Keeping the cord free of the nappy will help prevent it becoming moist and smelly.

Occasionally, the area does become infected. The skin around the baby's tummy button looks very red and/or swollen, or there may be several small red spots. If this seems to be happening, seek medical advice promptly. Antibiotics may be required to prevent a far more serious infection.

After the cord has come off, a shiny red lump or two may appear at the place where it was attached. This is most commonly granulation tissue, which sometimes forms during the healing process, and is not to be confused with the more generalised redness of infection. If there is only a small amount it can be left alone, but if the lumps seem to be getting bigger, your midwife may suggest treatment with an applicator stick containing silver nitrate. She will apply it initially, then leave you some applicator sticks to continue treatment as required. Very occasionally, continued redness and moisture can indicate a more serious problem with the abdominal wall. Your midwife or Plunket nurse may refer you to a paediatrician for review and an ultrasound to confirm the cause.

Bathing your baby

See Chapter 8, pp.365–367.

Exercise (see also pp.126–133)

With shorter hospital stays, women are getting up and moving around a lot more quickly than they did in the past. You'll generally feel better for it, and it will help keep your muscles and circulation in working order; but make sure you also get the rest your body needs. Some women feel more inclined to be active if they get up and get dressed into some comfortable clothes – and most women enjoy the novelty of being smaller around the middle.

Most hospitals offer daily physiotherapy for women who have just given birth – do try to get to at least one session if you can. It's much easier to have expert personal instruction in these exercises than trying to follow written directions. If you're at home, you have to be really motivated to get started, or perhaps your partner or support person could act as coach.

After childbirth, your body deserves some special attention. It has worked hard for you during pregnancy, labour and birth; now the big muscle groups need some recovery and rejuvenation. Three main groups need particular care: the abdominal muscles, the pelvic floor muscles, and the back muscles, which affect your posture.

Abdominal muscles (see also pp.128–129)

It will help if you can support your tummy muscles in the early days after delivery. Wearing some kind of external support – such as bike pants, sports pants or more supportive trousers – can help the muscles to recover better, especially if you have a separation (diastasis) of the long abdominal muscles as described on p.129. You may still have the stretchy tubular support that was given to you during your pregnancy; if it's now too loose, ask for a new one.

Have another look at the section on the pelvic floor and abdominal muscles in Chapter 4 (pp.126–129). Think about how these two muscle groups work together, and start the following exercises early, ideally between 24 and 48 hours after birth.

Tummy tucks (see also p.128)

Start doing these lying on your side. Place your hand over your lower tummy. As you breathe out, very gently and slowly pull your tummy away from your hand. Hold this position as you continue to breathe normally. Do this tummy tuck every time you lift your baby or walk along your hallway. Start practising when you are out walking with your buggy or pram, going upstairs, and when lifting anything.

Pelvic floor exercises (see also pp.126–127)

If you didn't get around to learning these when you were pregnant, start now. It's never too late! If you want to avoid problems with leaking urine, especially when you laugh, cough or sneeze, your pelvic floor muscles need attention after giving birth. You will also help prevent long-term problems with prolapse, leaking urine and/or holding in a tampon. Good pelvic floor muscles also improve sexual enjoyment, so do the exercises on p.127 as diligently as you possibly can.

- Rest your pelvic floor for 24 hours after birth, then begin. Whether or not you have stitches, start gently, but do start; exercising the pelvic floor helps reduce swelling and aids healing.[14]

- It's best to lie on your side so you're not working against gravity.

- Try to do the exercises three times a day. The thing you will probably find most difficult is maintaining a steady hold. Start with two or three at each session; as you improve, keep adding another until you can do 8–12 strong pelvic floor contractions three times a day.

- Make this your aim for the first 8–12 weeks after your baby is born. You get the best results if you work hard early on, and it's surprising how easy it is to maintain this level of strength with just a few sessions a week.

- If you do have any 'stress incontinence' (a small urine leak when you cough or sneeze), remember to tighten your pelvic floor whenever you feel a cough or sneeze coming, so that this becomes as automatic as covering your mouth and nose. This deliberate action is sometimes called 'the knack' (see p.127). If stress incontinence is an ongoing problem beyond 8–12 weeks after birth, seek help from a women's health physiotherapist or continence adviser.

Promoting good posture

Stand tall and sit well at all times. Make sure you have a surface at suitable working height for changing your baby: are you able to stand tall to protect your back? If not, it may be better to get down on the floor instead. Do everything you can to avoid straining your back in these early days and weeks; you need to be fit to care for your baby for many months to come.

Resting on your front

Relax with a pillow under your tummy while lying on your front, using an extra pillow under your neck if your breasts are sore. Resting like this helps to relieve a sore bottom and encourages your uterus to return to its normal position within the pelvis.

Getting up from lying down

First, do a gentle tummy tuck, with your knees bent, then use your top arm to push across your body as you drop your knees to the side. Use your hands to push up to the sitting position as you lower your feet to the floor (see photos on p.129).

Foot and ankle exercises

These are helpful especially if you have any residual swelling of the feet and ankles. When sitting or lying, keep your legs still but move your feet firmly up and down several times. It's easier to sustain the movements if you move one foot back while the other moves forward. To work the muscle thoroughly, move your feet up and down strongly, and keep going for several minutes. Elevating your legs (to a horizontal or above-horizontal position) can also help when doing these exercises; when resting, put your legs up on a sofa, stool or bed, and then get your feet going vigorously back and forth.

Exercise feet and ankles

Move feet up and down vigorously.

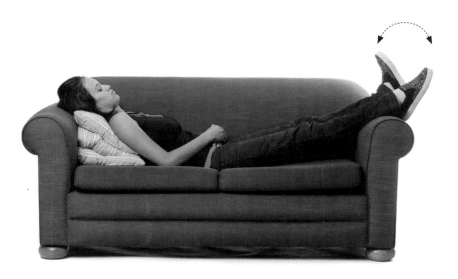

Finally – what *not* to do

- Avoid sitting with crossed legs or feet.
- Avoid lifting with a bent back.
- Avoid doing sit-ups or curl-ups for the first three months or so after giving birth. Before you try these, you need to have reasonable recovery of your pelvic floor and deep abdominal muscles. If done too early, they just stress the already weakened pelvic floor and discourage the abdominal muscles from coming together. Remember, too, that a curl-up works only the superficial abdominal muscles that help movement; the large 'deep corset' muscle (see p.128) is the one that plays the most important role in stabilising and protecting the spine and pelvis along with the pelvic floor. This is why there is such a strong emphasis on tummy tucks and pelvic floor exercises after birth.

Third and fourth days

Feelings – 'third-day blues'

Many women feel rather down emotionally three or four days after giving birth. This feeling often coincides with having painful, engorged breasts and a baby who may be more unsettled than she was before. This emotional fragility is entirely normal, and is no indication at all that things are 'only going to get worse from now on'. Third-day blues are not to be confused with post-natal depression (see p.377).

This first week after birth is not a good time for making major decisions about anything. Choosing names for the baby and birth announcements are two common causes of distress, but you can avoid both by a bit of planning before the birth, or by delaying the whole issue for a good week or so.

Some suggestions for minimising 'the blues'

- Get more rest. Broken nights have to be compensated for by extra sleep during the day. Try to sleep, or at least rest in bed, for a minimum of two hours during the day. Get used to sleeping when the baby sleeps.
- Limit visitors. Give priority to the people you really want to see, rather than those you feel you ought to see. Seek help from your partner or support person if you find this difficult.
- Have a whole day where you simply concentrate on learning to enjoy feeding. Have someone else do the nappy-changing, the bathing and the calming of an unsettled baby.
- Spend time with your older children, but in short bursts. They need plenty of activities and outings at this time – but let someone else organise these for a few days.
- Get up and get dressed into some comfortable but attractive clothes. Do something you enjoy (reading, watching TV, being outside in the garden) to take your mind off babies and sore breasts for an hour or two.

When the milk comes in (see also p.311)

For most women, somewhere around 48–72 hours after the birth the breasts fill with milk as the hormones responsible for milk production become fully 'switched on'.

Nearly all women will notice a significant increase in breast size, and for some the breasts become very uncomfortable. This normal physiological process will happen regardless of whether you plan to breastfeed or bottle-feed. Fortunately, the discomfort usually lasts only a day or two, and will settle as you continue to feed your baby on demand – even if this means you demanding that your baby feeds when your breasts are really full and uncomfortable

Going home from hospital

The timing of this will vary tremendously. At present, most first-time mothers go home on the second or third day if they have had a normal vaginal birth, although some will have gone home a few hours after the birth. Your LMC will discuss with you your readiness to go home and the follow-up support you will get there. The timing of your discharge from hospital will depend on your condition and that of your baby, but it is ultimately up to you to decide. Don't be pressured into going home if you don't feel ready.

Whenever you decide to go home, there are a number of things you need to consider first.

- *Feeding.* Do you feel quite able to cope with breastfeeding on your own? If you're bottle-feeding, are you comfortable about making up the milk mixture and keeping everything sterile? Either way, you should contact your LMC or post-natal midwife if you run into problems or need more advice. Other people who can support and advise you include your mother, a friend, a Plunket nurse, the La Leche League or a lactation consultant. (See Appendix: Breastfeeding.)
- *Baby care.* Do you feel confident about nappy-changing, bathing, dressing and generally caring for your baby? If it's winter, do you have some way of heating at least one room in the house so that it's maintained at a warm and comfortable temperature?
- *Other children.* Do you have someone to help you with your older children for the first few days, and to take them off your hands for at least part of the day?
- *Domestic workload.* Do you have someone at home – your partner or another support person – who can take charge of the cooking, washing and general housework, at least for the first week?
- *Transport.* How are you going to get home? Have you got a car seat for the baby? It's best to get someone to collect you and give you a hand with the baby, the car seat, your bag and so on. A car or taxi is easiest.
- *Your baby.* Has she had all her checks and any immediately required vaccinations (see pp.328 and 396)? If not, who will do these for you? Have you received a *Well Child/Tamariki Ora* health book from your LMC? (This free handbook, produced by the Ministry of Health for the parents of all newborn babies, allows you to record your baby's progress and gives helpful information about growth and development, common problems and first aid.) Is it filled in? Do you know your options for selecting a

Well Child care provider (e.g. Plunket or Tamariki Ora) in your area? Your LMC will usually notify your chosen Well Child care provider about two weeks after the birth, so ask your LMC if they have not already discussed this with you.

Well Child checks

All new babies are routinely examined shortly after birth, usually by your LMC. They will usually do another routine examination at about five to seven days after the birth to check for any previously undetected problems.

In some hospitals, a member of the paediatric staff will check all newborns, and a member of the orthopaedic staff will do a hip examination. In other hospitals, or at home, your LMC will do all the necessary checks.

There are a number of conditions that are very important to detect early, and these are routinely checked for.

Congenital dislocation of the hip (CDH)

When a baby is born, the long thigh bone (femur) is held into the shallow cup in the hip bone (ischium) mainly by ligaments and tendons. As the baby grows, the cup becomes deeper and the head of the femur comes to sit firmly within it, giving the hip joint the stability required for walking.

Sometimes, however, the head of the femur is not held in place firmly enough and the hip joint develops in an unstable way, making normal walking impossible. This situation is known as congenital dislocation of the hip (CDH). It can often be detected within a few days of birth by a special examination of the hips. This check should be done at least once within the first week, and several times during the first few months.

A Well Child nurse or midwife will do a hip check

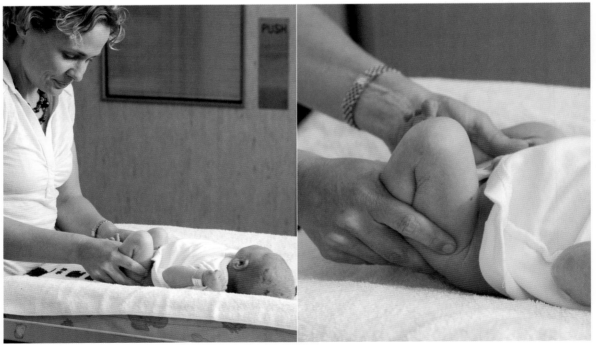

If CDH is suspected, future problems can be entirely prevented by making sure that the baby's hips are constantly held in a frog-like position until the joint is stable. This can be achieved in one of the following ways:

- using double nappies folded in a special way
- placing a foam pad over the nappies
- putting the baby in a special rubber splint.

The method recommended will vary according to the severity of the problem, so assessment by an orthopaedic surgeon and/or paediatrician is usually required to determine the level of treatment and follow-up that will be needed.

Congenital heart disease (CHD)

Occasionally, a baby's heart develops slightly imperfectly during early pregnancy. Usually, this is not a problem until after birth, when she uses her lungs for the first time. Congenital heart disease (CHD) may be picked up during pregnancy, either during the routine anatomy scan at about 20 weeks, or at another diagnostic scan (see p.150). The most common congenital heart conditions involve abnormal holes between different chambers in the heart, although a variety of other problems can also occur.

Often these conditions can be suspected after birth by a doctor or midwife listening carefully to the heart with a stethoscope, although other tests are needed to confirm them. Many of these defects disappear on their own as the baby grows, but others need to be repaired by a cardiothoracic surgeon, using very sophisticated skills and equipment. In a few rare cases, the defects are so major that complete or even partial repair is not possible, and the baby may die after birth.

Inborn metabolic disorders, such as phenylketonuria (PKU) and hypothyroidism

These rare biochemical disorders are caused by a lack of particular enzymes or hormones in the body. If left untreated, these conditions will result in severe mental retardation. However, if they are detected and treated, brain damage can be avoided. For this reason, routine testing is offered to every newborn baby in New Zealand. Originally the test (sometimes known as the Guthrie test) was limited to a small number of rare disorders, but the range of conditions tested for has expanded greatly since the introduction of a new testing technique (tandem mass spectrometry) in 2004.[15]

The test is best carried out three to five days after birth. A small blood sample is collected from a heel-prick and put onto a special card, which can then be analysed for over 20 different inborn errors and some other genetic disorders. The test may be inaccurate if done too early, if the baby has not had a sufficient milk feed since birth, or if she is premature. If you are at home at this stage, your midwife will need to do the test. At present, because of the large volume of tests and the very small number of uncertain or abnormal results, the sample may take several weeks to process. Parents are notified only if a possible problem is found. If you wish, you can request that the card be returned to you after it has been tested; write a short letter, and ask for it to be enclosed with the card when it is sent off to the national testing centre. Otherwise it will be kept on file in case further testing becomes advisable for your child in years to come.

The Universal Newborn Hearing Programme[16]

From 2007, the Universal Newborn Hearing Programme is being introduced in New Zealand. It offers all newborn babies an early screening test to check their hearing. In New Zealand, between 160 and 180 children a year are found to have a significant hearing problem. Hearing loss is difficult to detect until children show delays in their language development, at which time their hearing can be tested. But if the problem is discovered much earlier, it's possible to overcome the child's communication difficulties so that normal development is not affected.

The programme has already been introduced in some parts of the country, and will be available in all areas by 2009. The testing can be done in hospital when your baby is only a day or two old, or at an outpatient clinic before she is three months old. After that, different tests are required.

There are two types of screening test, one or both of which may be used. You will be given the results straight away.

- *Otoacoustic emissions (OAE).* A small, soft-tipped earpiece is placed in your baby's outer ear. This makes a clicking sound, and a computer shows how your baby's ears respond.

- *Automated auditory brainstem response (AABR).* The same soft sounds are played through an earpiece or ear cups. The response from your baby's hearing nerve is picked up through special sensors placed on her head.

The screening test is best done when your baby is settled or sleeping. If you are attending a clinic, you might find it helpful to delay your baby's feeding or sleeping until you get there, and allow plenty of time to settle her when you arrive. Once your baby is settled, the test should take about 20 minutes.

For most babies, the test result will be quite normal, but a small number may require retesting. If a problem is detected, a lot can be done to overcome it, especially if the problem is picked up as early as possible.

Circumcision

Nowadays, this operation (the removal of the foreskin of the penis) is not often done on newborn baby boys. If you have strong religious or cultural reasons for wanting it done in the first few days, you will need to discuss it with your LMC well before the birth. Your LMC may be able to arrange for you to see a surgeon who will do the operation; this may involve travelling to a main centre.

Routine circumcision has fallen into disfavour in recent years, for a number of reasons. The foreskin is there for a good reason: it protects the end of the penis from nappy rash and infections in infancy, and enhances sexual enjoyment for adults. Also, in newborns, the operation has to be done without any anaesthetic – it is not possible to use local anaesthetic, and a general anaesthetic carries a significant risk at this age.

Sometimes, later circumcision is required for cultural or medical reasons (for example, if the foreskin is too tight or becomes infected). If so, current thinking suggests that it can be done at two to three years of age, when a general anaesthetic can be given much more safely. The foreskin has also completed its development by this time, and can easily be separated from the tip of the penis (the glans). This means that the operation can be done more safely and easily, and the job finished more neatly.

5. When a baby needs special care

The special-care unit

The care of unwell and premature babies requires sophisticated equipment and specialist skills and knowledge. The staff who work in this area are highly trained nurses and doctors who have specialised in neonatology.

Not all special-care baby units (also called neonatal units) can provide the full range of care available, and sometimes very small or very sick babies have to be transferred from one part of the country to another. In New Zealand, fully equipped units in the main centres act as referral units, taking babies from other regions when necessary.

The degree of care required depends a lot on individual circumstances. Very premature babies need to be in special care for several weeks, other babies for only a day or two.

Most babies are cared for in incubators – special perspex boxes in which the temperature and oxygen concentration can be controlled to provide the best possible environment for recovery, growth and development. Incubators have 'portholes' to allow staff to care for your baby, and often you can hold or touch your baby through these portholes, too. As soon as your baby is well enough, you will be able to cuddle her outside the incubator for short periods, and also feed her.

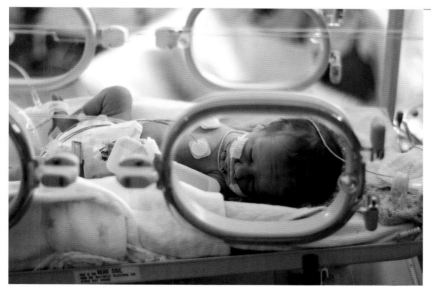

Premature baby in an incubator

Sometimes very small or sick babies have to be artificially helped to breathe with a ventilator. If so, the baby may be placed on a special open tray. Here the temperature can still be controlled, but access to the baby and the complex equipment of the ventilator is easier. In this situation, you may be able to touch your baby only briefly at first, but you can look at her as much as you like. As soon as she is able to come off the ventilator, you can have more contact.

Most staff in neonatal units are well aware that you and your baby need to be together as much as possible. As soon as circumstances permit, they will encourage you to touch, cuddle and feed her. They also understand how much you want a healthy baby to take home, and will do their very best to achieve this for you. But it is important to remember that very small or very sick babies are fighting 'against the odds' for survival, and sometimes the task is impossible. Occasionally, despite the very best modern neonatal care, babies do die in the first few days or weeks. This will sometimes be caused by prematurity or infection, but may also be due to major congenital abnormalities in one or more of the major organs, such as the brain, heart or kidneys (see p.289).

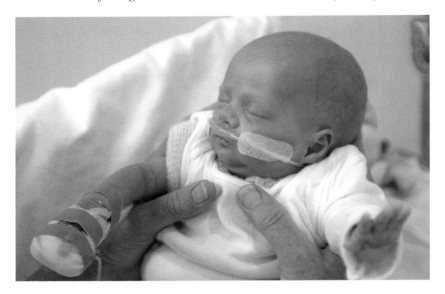

'It's a bit like make-believe parenting when your babies are in the neonate ward. They're not in a crib beside you, and you could just go off and do your own thing if you wanted. I was feeding them and expressing milk as well, which they were fed through naso-gastric tubes.'

What about feeding?

Premature babies are unable to suck at first, as the sucking reflex does not develop until near the end of normal pregnancy. In the special-care baby unit, babies can be given nourishment either through a tiny drip or, if they are big enough, through a little tube put straight down into their stomach through the back of their nose (naso-gastric tube). Only when their sucking reflex has developed can they be fed at the breast or with a bottle.

If you want to breastfeed, you will need to start hand-expressing your milk soon after your baby is born in order to collect the colostrum, which is good for all babies but particularly beneficial for those who are premature or sick. You will need to continue expressing five or six times a day to stimulate the milk production (see p.346). Once your milk comes in, you will be shown how to assemble and use an electric breast pump, which will speed up the process a little. You may find that the milk flows more easily if you have a photo of your baby in front of you. Even if you can't feed her directly, your milk can often be given to her via the naso-gastric tube.

It's hard work expressing milk this often, but most women who have persevered say it was all worth it once they finally held their baby in their arms and put her directly to the breast.

Going home

If your baby has to be in special care for several weeks, you may want to go home before her. This can be a very difficult time for the whole family, especially if you have other children. If you do go home, it's important that you get to the hospital as often as you can to keep in contact with your baby. Don't feel guilty about asking friends and family to look after your other children while you do this.

If you and your baby have been transferred to a hospital in another town, it may be possible for you to stay nearby in the nurses' home, a Ronald McDonald house or a motel. Ask about these options – the nurses in the neonatal unit are a good place to start. Financial assistance is available for families having to travel to other centres for their baby's birth and to cover accommodation costs while their baby is being treated in hospital. Ask your LMC about this assistance.

Getting support

Having a baby who requires special care creates stresses and strain for any parent, especially if the need arises unexpectedly. It is a time when mothers particularly need lots of love and support from their partner, family and friends, and also from health professionals.

It helps a lot if you have plenty of information on exactly what's wrong with your baby; it also helps if the staff are honest and open with you about the situation. If you don't feel you're getting enough information, keep asking. Don't be ashamed if you don't understand what the experts are telling you at first – after all, it's taken them years to learn about neonatal care.

Sometimes, it can be really helpful to talk to a social worker, hospital chaplain or counsellor. Sharing your worries and fears with a caring professional can make this stressful time easier.

Treating jaundice (phototherapy)

Jaundice is a condition that occurs when the bilirubin levels in the blood rise, causing the skin and eyes to become yellow. Mild jaundice is common in newborn babies and soon disappears (see p.306). But if a baby becomes very jaundiced because of high levels of bilirubin, brain damage can occur. Active intervention is needed to lower the bilirubin levels as soon as possible.

One way is to expose the baby to strong light (blue light) in a special phototherapy incubator. To get the best exposure, the baby needs to be naked but with her eyes covered, as they are too sensitive for the amount of light required. Most jaundiced babies need intermittent exposure over 24–48 hours to bring their bilirubin down to a safe level. 'Bili' beds and 'bili' blankets may be used in some hospitals instead of the lights.

In rare cases where the bilirubin level is very high, phototherapy is not sufficient and a special blood transfusion (called an 'exchange transfusion') is necessary. This is likely to occur only if there is Rhesus disease (see p.206).

'The twins were taken off to neonates as soon as they were born, and that made me feel quite detached from them. I'd had a Caesarean and it was a good hour or so by the time I came out of recovery. They took me down to neonates on a hospital bed and I had a little look, but Tanner was in an incubator and we couldn't hold him and Briar was asleep on a camibed. I was taken back up to my room and I sent off texts to everybody, letting them know.

It felt quite surreal – I actually had two babies, but they weren't there with me and I felt like I couldn't really do a great deal for them. And because my uterus was still contracting, it felt like I still had them in my stomach, as if they were kicking. That was really odd.'

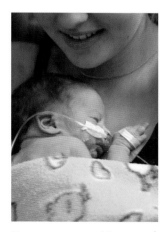

Kangaroo care: skin-to-skin contact

6. After a Caesarean

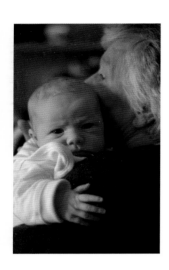

The first few days after a Caesarean section are a bit more complicated than after a vaginal delivery, but knowing what's likely to happen will help to make things easier.

When you first come back from the operating theatre, you are likely to have an intravenous (IV) line still in your arm, a catheter (see opposite) in your bladder, possibly a drain emerging from your wound, and probably an epidural cannula still in place. You may also have a padded dressing over the wound in your lower abdomen, which may be feeling sore. You may have your baby with you in your room, or she may be in the neonatal unit.

The midwives on the post-natal ward are experienced in caring for Caesarean patients and will do their very best to remove all the drips and drains as soon as they feel you can do without them. Most women are ready to go home four to six days after a Caesarean, and some even sooner.

Post-operative pain relief

After any major operation, some pain relief is necessary to keep you comfortable and hasten your recovery. If you're feeling comfortable, you'll be able to get up and move around sooner and feed your baby more easily.

Epidural pain relief

If you had your Caesarean under epidural/spinal anaesthetic (and most Caesareans are now done like this), the cannula can sometimes remain in place for 24–48 hours. This enables pain-relieving drugs, such as pethidine or a long-acting anaesthetic, to be given directly around the spinal cord to keep you comfortable. This is usually very effective. The cannula will be removed as soon as you no longer need it.

Narcotic pain relief

If you had a general anaesthetic, regular injections of pethidine or morphine are recommended for the first day or so. They are usually given into your bottom, and can be given just after, or some time before, a breastfeed so that your baby is not affected.

Oral pain relief

After the first day or so, pain can usually be controlled quite well with tablets – for example, diclofenac (Voltaren), paracetamol (Panadol), soluble aspirin, or paracetamol plus codeine (Panadeine) – taken on a regular basis. Some hospitals provide you with the tablets, and advice on how to use them, and then let you take the tablets when you need them. Minute quantities of these compounds may pass into your breast milk, but the amount is not sufficient to affect your baby. When you go home, you may still need to take these drugs from time to time for a week or two.

Intravenous (IV) lines, drains and catheters

Your IV line (drip) can usually be removed within 12–24 hours of the operation, once there is no longer any risk of haemorrhage and you are able to drink fluid yourself.

Similarly, the catheter in your bladder can be removed once you are producing a good amount of urine and can sit up or get up to go to the toilet (this is usually possible within a few hours of the operation). In the meantime, the catheter keeps the bladder empty and prevents it from pressing on the wound, which can be very uncomfortable.

If you have a drain from the wound, any internal oozing of blood can be collected in a little vacuum-sealed container at the end of the drain. This oozing usually stops within two days and the drain can be removed.

Feeding your baby after a Caesarean

It is perfectly possible, and indeed highly desirable, to start breastfeeding straight after a Caesarean. The only reason for a delay will be if your baby has to spend any length of time in the special-care baby unit. Even then, you can express milk in preparation for breastfeeding (see p.346).

The stress of the operation may cause a slight delay in your milk coming in, especially if your baby was born prematurely. If you have received large volumes of fluid intravenously during labour (which will usually be the case if you had an epidural or spinal anaesthetic), your milk may also be delayed. Putting the baby to the breast or expressing milk frequently will usually stimulate milk production satisfactorily. Occasionally, the delay may be enough to affect your baby's nutritional needs, and other fluid or food may be needed in the interim. Even so, the more you feed your baby at the breast, the more quickly your milk will come in and full breastfeeding can get under way.

If you are bottle-feeding (see p.315), position yourself so that you can still keep in close contact with your baby. The suggestions in the box below for breastfeeding can be used equally well for bottle-feeding.

Breastfeeding after a Caesarean

- You need to be comfortable enough to be able to relax and allow the let-down reflex to work. This means having good post-operative pain relief.

- You will find it easier if you are in a position where the baby is not going to press directly on your wound. A midwife should help you each time for the first day or two unless, or until, you feel confident. Two good positions are: sitting very upright, with your baby on a pillow on your lap or at one side; or lying on one side with your baby lying beside you. You may need someone to hold the baby while you change sides.

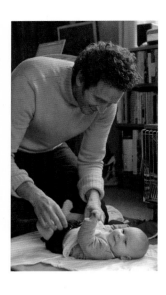

Your Caesarean wound

Any operation where the abdominal area is opened up puts a lot of stress on the body, and a Caesarean is no exception. There are several different layers of tissue that must mend, and it takes time for even the best repair job to heal completely. The skin may look healed after a week or two, but the other muscle and tissue layers heal more slowly and are not strongly 'knit' until about 12 weeks after the operation.

Nevertheless, for most women the skin has healed sufficiently after five or six days for any non-dissolvable skin stitches (sutures) or clips holding the skin together to be removed. The procedure for removing sutures varies a little depending on what has been used, but it usually takes only a few minutes. At this stage, the wound often looks like an ugly, prominent, thick red line on your abdomen, but it will fade, shrink and become much less noticeable with time. There may also be blue and yellow bruising around the wound, and this too will eventually disappear.

Exercises after a Caesarean (see also p.402)

Initially, you will need to get out of bed by rolling slowly to one side, and then continuing to roll off the bed. If you need to cough or move your bowels, try holding a pillow firmly over your tummy.

Don't despair if it seems impossible even to stand up straight for the first two or three days. Try to get yourself slowly into an upright position, holding your tummy with your hands if you want to. Walk just as far as the toilet and shower initially, with assistance if you need it. Then try going a little further afield, keeping your back as straight as you can. It's not easy at first to pull your tummy in when you walk, but by about the third day it's usually possible, and it does get easier each time you try.

All the post-natal exercises described earlier (see pp.323–326) are suitable after a Caesarean section, and you may find you need to use your pelvic floor to help with doing the tummy tuck. See if you can manage the tummy tuck within a few days, as the muscles can easily forget how to work with the wound being in this region. Start gently, doing just what you can manage without causing pain. Even doing a few exercises for five to ten minutes twice a day will make you feel better in yourself and help you to heal faster, as well as starting to firm up slack abdominal muscles.

One of the advantages of having a Caesarean is that your bottom will not be sore, and there will be no stitches in your perineum. So pelvic floor exercises (see p.127) should be easy – and you should still do all the other recommended exercises. Your abdominal muscles and pelvic floor have been under strain during the last few months of pregnancy, so take the opportunity to get them back into shape now.

7. Looking after a new mother

Midwife visits

If you had a home birth, or came home from hospital soon after the birth, your midwife (either your LMC or a post-natal midwife who works with your LMC) will visit you within the first 24 hours, and may well visit daily for the first five to seven days. If all is going well, you can then expect to have a weekly visit until four to six weeks after the baby's birth, with more visits if you need them and/or if problems arise. Most women need, and should expect, five to ten home visits during the post-natal period to assist their own recovery and to have help with feeding and baby care.[17]

Precise visiting times are often hard to give, and your midwife may call at any time during the day. But she can usually give an approximate time if you need to plan your day around this. If you know you're going to be out when your midwife may call, ring her the day before and leave a message.

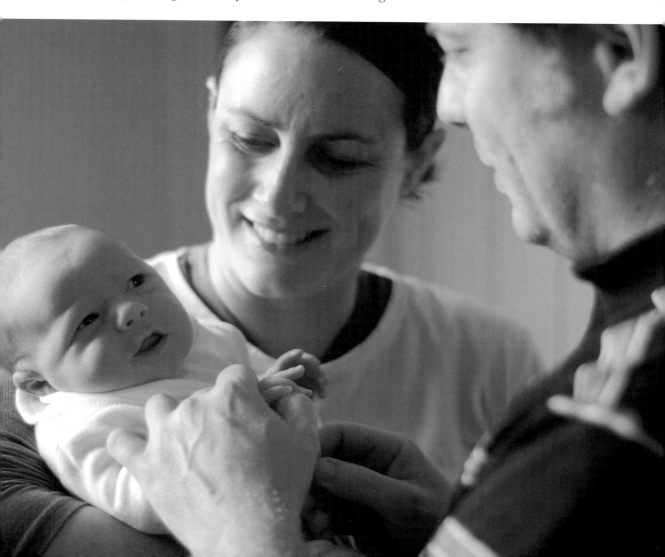

For partners and support people

Before the baby arrives, arrange who is going to be the main support person during this first week after the birth. Many partners take a week or two off work in order to fulfil this role. If this is not possible or appropriate, a trusted family member or friend will be needed.

This person needs to take charge of the household for a week or so, organising the cooking, cleaning, shopping and child-minding, as well as tending to the new mother's needs and helping with the baby.

If you're not used to doing all this, it might be worth making a list of tasks that need to be done, and writing down important things you may forget.

Answering the phone and the door

Be fair but firm with visitors. If it looks as though you might be overwhelmed, arrange for people to come when it suits you rather than them. You may decide to have a 'visiting time' each day and encourage everyone to come then, or it may be easier to ask people to come at different times.

If you want to make sure that precious rest times are not interrupted, try switching the answerphone on and the mobile phone off, and put a 'Family resting – please do not disturb' notice on the front door.

Caring for other children

Small (and not so small) children have a natural desire to be with their mother or usual caregiver. They tend to seek her out, especially when they're tired or hungry or upset. She may find it difficult to rest or feed the baby if the other children are constantly demanding, so it's worth sorting something out to keep everyone more or less happy. Here are some tips to make things easier:

- Try setting time aside at least once or twice a day for some particular activity with the older children. It might be a visit to the park or the shops, or a woodwork session in the garage.
- Make sure the children get some food and drink at reasonably regular intervals – at least every three to four hours. Hungry children tend to be grizzly children.
- Let them spend time with their mother and the baby at frequent intervals during the day, but try to make each visit short. Be quite firm that 'it's time to go out' or 'it's time for lunch', and so on.
- After the first two to three days, try to organise things so that an older child can spend some time each day with her mother reading stories or playing games, without the baby intruding on the scene. Keep an eye on the baby yourself, and be ready to pick her up if she wakes.

One of the advantages of home birth or early discharge is that older children can be active participants in the exciting first few days with a new brother or sister. But it's easy for that advantage to turn to disadvantage if the new mother gets constantly hassled by an exuberant two-year-old and can't concentrate on her new baby or her own special needs.

Terri's story: Four Caesareans

I'm 27. My four children have all been born by Caesarean – two emergency and two elective. Our first, Maynard, was two weeks late. He was posterior, I had high blood pressure, a fever, and we ended up with him in foetal distress, and nothing happening after a long induction. Eventually, an emergency Caesarean was needed.

I remember feeling scared, not knowing what was happening. I was just exhausted too, sobbing and crying. It was awful, really awful. My sister and my mum were there, and they'd both had natural births – I'm one of seven and my sister's got three children. They didn't really understand what was going on, either, and I think maybe they thought I wasn't trying. We found out later that Maynard had his cord around his neck, which was why his head wouldn't come forward.

Vaughn was two weeks late again, he was posterior and the same thing happened – he got stuck, with a really long cord wrapped around his body. The obstetrician said afterwards she'd never seen anything like it – there was no way he was going to come out by himself. So that was another emergency Caesarean.

When I became pregnant with Rachael, things felt different. I had been quite sick with both of the boys – I threw up every day for the first and third trimesters. But this time I wasn't sick at all, just really tired. And that's when we thought, this one's probably a girl.

This time having an elective Caesarean and knowing that she'd be born on a particular date was really weird. As it got close, I felt more as if I was going in for surgery than having a baby. With an emergency Caesarean, it all happens in a rush because the situation isn't good for the baby or the mother – you know you just have to do it. But this was so planned and medical. It was quite bizarre actually.

During the Caesarean itself, I had a spinal anaesthetic so I was awake. And all I could feel was this tugging sensation – which, again, was very strange. There were a lot of people in the operating theatre, but a happy, excited sense in the room.

The recovery from this elective Caesarean was far harder than the two emergency ones, even though people say recovery is much faster when it's all planned. But it wasn't for me. The scar was really sore on the outside and the inside. I got an infection, and experienced some terrible pain. Managing the stairs was really hard, and the baby ended up sleeping downstairs during the day, because I couldn't go upstairs.

It took a good 10 weeks before I could move properly, which was hard with the other children. Even after six months, it was still really tender. I wouldn't go for a run or do sit-ups or anything like that. Looking back, I probably should have stayed in hospital longer than just three or four days. I didn't feel under any pressure to go, but I got to the stage where I just really wanted to come home and see the other kids. It was quite lonely, really.

I got pregnant soon after with our fourth baby – they were born 14 months apart. This last pregnancy was very tiring, emotionally and physically. I had a lot of scar pain throughout, and I did not feel that my body had been able to heal fully from the surgery. I stayed in hospital for four nights, as long as I could cope being away from my family. I kept breastfeeding my daughter throughout the pregnancy, and am now tandem feeding both. They have a lovely relationship already with each other being so close – but it is a busy household with four kids six and under. After Diana was born, I forced myself to take it easy, gratefully accepting all help, and not thinking I could do it all myself. It's funny when you have a Caesarean, other people seem to forget that you've had major abdominal surgery AND have a new baby to look after.

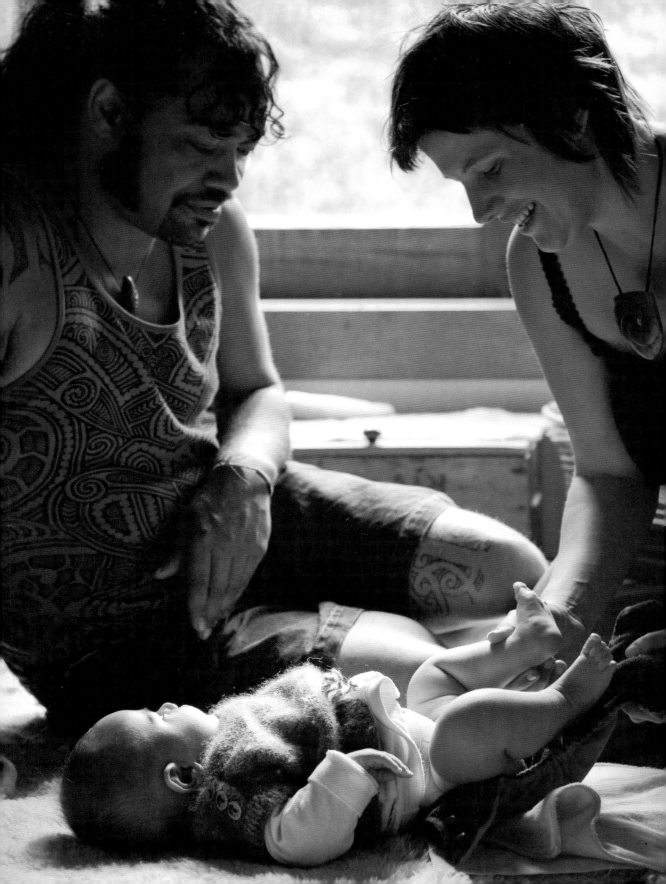

CHAPTER 8

The first three months with a baby

1. Feeding your baby

Most women in New Zealand breastfeed their babies initially, recognising the benefits of breast milk as an ideal infant food. Some continue for many months; others find that, for a variety of reasons, they or their babies wish to stop or reduce breastfeeding after the first few months. This may coincide with introducing solids, using more expressed milk, using a combination of breast milk and formula by bottle, or switching directly to a cup.

Breast milk is the best possible food for a baby until he is at least six months old, after which time solid food can be gradually introduced.[1] But in circumstances where breastfeeding is not possible or desirable, infant formula made up in sterile conditions provides a very good second-best.

For many women, breastfeeding becomes a pleasure and a time to look forward to. Once the art has been learned, breastfeeding becomes easy, convenient and enjoyable. It is an excuse to sit down and relax, and enjoy your baby without interruption – a treat, especially if there are other children to cater for.

It seems that women who actively enjoy breastfeeding (as opposed to merely appreciating its benefits for their babies) continue to breastfeed for longer than women who get little pleasure from it.[2] Many women say that early problems did not put them off breastfeeding, and they came to enjoy it once they got through the first few days. Support and encouragement from health professionals, partners, families and other mothers during the difficult times are very important if new mothers are to persevere with breastfeeding.

Women who decide to formula-feed also need to be supported in their decision. Formula-feeding can be enjoyable too, especially if free from constant pressure to let other people 'give the baby his bottle'.

Breastfeeding in weeks 2–6 (see also p.308)

Balancing supply and demand

After the first week of breastfeeding, the supply and demand system of milk production will gradually settle down and your breasts will become more comfortable. Now, the baby latches on without difficulty, sucks well on the areola to compress the ducts behind the nipples, empties the breast tissue of all (or nearly all) the available milk, and then has enough energy to do the same on the other breast. Milk is continually produced within the breast tissue, ready for the next feed several hours later.

For some women, this natural rhythm will establish itself very quickly, but for others it takes longer. For first-time mothers, lactation takes four to six weeks to become fully established. For mothers who have breastfed before, this happens much more quickly.

During the first month or so, the supply and demand system can quite easily become upset. If your baby becomes unsettled for any reason, he may not feed as well as usual, so that the breast is left partially full and becomes engorged. Or he may be hungrier than usual, emptying the breast completely and then wanting to feed again only a short time later, before the breast has had time to refill. If this hunger persists for a few days, it will act to increase your milk supply. Once this has happened, he will usually become more settled again. Don't become too disturbed if this sudden hunger lasts for 24–48 hours. Babies often have a growth spurt at about three weeks of age, and another at five to six weeks. During these times, avoid giving additional food such as a bottle of formula; if you do so, your breasts may not be stimulated to produce the increased supply your baby needs. You could end up feeling that you do not have enough milk, and give up breastfeeding totally.

Increasing your milk supply during a growth spurt
- Have an afternoon rest with your feet up.
- Have some extra-early nights. Resting will allow the blood supply to the breast area to increase, which will help produce more milk.
- Drink plenty of fluids (at least 10–12 glasses a day).
- Eat well. Don't skimp on meals, and eat larger portions than usual.
- Be prepared to feed your baby more frequently, especially in the early evening.

During these early weeks, your baby may vomit or 'spill' some of his feed. A small amount of spilling is normal, and some babies do this until they are on solid food. Simple things like keeping him more upright after a feed or while changing him (place a small pillow or folded blanket under his head) can often help to reduce spilling. Major repeated spilling is not normal, and needs to be checked out with your midwife, Well Child nurse or GP.

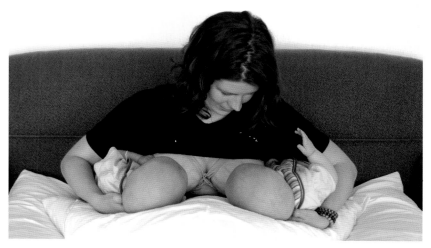

Breastfeeding: using a pillow to keep babies more upright

Despite their best efforts, some women do get sore nipples and other problems while breastfeeding. These are more likely to occur in the first few weeks, but can happen at any time if the supply and demand system is upset. If you encounter any of the problems described below, seek help early from your midwife, Well Child nurse, practice nurse or doctor. In some areas, lactation consultants are available to visit you at home, and many women find the La Leche League's support network invaluable. (See Appendix: Breastfeeding.)

Sore or cracked nipples

The key to preventing sore or cracked nipples is to position and latch the baby onto the breast properly at every feed. Once he is latched on properly, let him feed until he is satisfied – avoid too much latching on and letting go.

It's also helpful to keep your nipples soft and supple, as you would your lips. After each feed, express some breastmilk, rub it on the nipple and allow it to dry. It's probably best to avoid putting any creams onto the nipple, as some may make mastitis more likely.[3] However, if you really do have to use a cream to soothe the nipple, choose one that contains pure anhydrous lanolin and doesn't have to be washed off before your baby can feed. If you are allergic to lanolin, which is contained in a number of products, the allergy is usually related to 'wool alcohols'.[4] Ask your LMC, GP or pharmacist to suggest a product that does not contain wool alcohols and can be used on your nipples if needed.

You can relieve pressure on a sore nipple by:

- feeding your baby in different positions
- offering the least sore breast first
- making sure the baby is properly latched on
- feeding before the breasts become full and sore.

A cracked nipple can become infected, especially with thrush or other bacteria. Get your LMC or Well Child nurse to check both you and your baby if things don't improve.

Nipple shields can occasionally help protect sore nipples and encourage the baby to latch on properly. However, your nipples can still be damaged if the baby does not latch on properly. The shields must be washed and sterilised after use, otherwise they will simply act as a source of infection and make matters worse.

Breast infection (mastitis)

Occasionally, one of the ducts within the breast can become temporarily blocked, causing a build-up of milk. The area around the blockage then becomes hard and sore unless the blockage is relieved. Sometimes it is obvious what's happening, as the duct concerned is near the surface of the breast, but occasionally the problem will not be so easy to detect.

A persistently blocked duct will cause inflammation in the surrounding tissue, known as mastitis. A woman with mastitis will develop a sore, reddened area on the breast and may also feel unwell, as if she is getting the flu. Her back and neck may feel achy, making her want to lie down and rest for most of the day. If left untreated, the blockage can occasionally develop into a breast abscess, where an area of breast tissue becomes filled with pus. This is a very painful condition, which can be almost entirely avoided if action is taken early and any mastitis properly treated.[5]

If you think you might have a breast infection:

- *Contact your LMC, doctor or practice nurse.* Do this as soon as you have any concerns and let them know what is happening.
- *Keep feeding.* Feed your baby as much as you can, especially on the side that is affected. If you can see or feel a lump, massage the area as you feed your baby for the next few days. Sometimes getting into a warm shower

Early signs and symptoms of mastitis

- feeling very tired and 'off colour', shivery or sweaty, with muscle aches and pains
- a hard, tender lump in the breast
- any distinct redness in an area of breast tissue, especially around a lump or sore spot

and massaging the breast while under the flowing water will help relieve the blockage.

- *Rest.* Go to bed straight away. Take the baby with you if necessary. Get someone to look after your other children.
- *Fluids.* Drink plenty of fluid, preferably water. Aim to have 10–12 glasses a day.
- *Paracetamol.* Take two tablets every three hours for up to 24 hours. This helps to relieve pain and also to reduce inflammation and swelling within the breast, which may unblock the duct.
- *Antibiotics.* If you're not feeling better within six to eight hours, and have a temperature of over 38°C, contact your LMC, doctor or practice nurse, as a course of antibiotics will be needed. They may be prescribed for 10–14 days to prevent recurrent bouts of mastitis or the need for much larger doses later on. Several different antibiotics are suitable and are safe for your baby. If you take them correctly and also continue taking paracetamol, you should be feeling much better within 24 hours. If not, contact your LMC or doctor again.

Breastfeeding in weeks 4–6 and beyond

By this time, most babies will be happy and contented with breastfeeding. Your breasts should feel comfortable most of the time, feeling full only when your baby is due or overdue for a feed. The let-down reflex should be working well, with milk being released easily from the breast as your baby starts to suck. Milk production will continue to match the amount your baby is taking.

It is still possible for the supply and demand to get upset, but by now this will probably occur only as a result of a marked change in routine. It is usually possible to express a reasonable volume of milk without going back to engorged breasts or a hungry, dissatisfied baby. It is also increasingly possible to leave the baby to be fed expressed milk by someone else for one or two feeds, without discomfort.

However, problems can still occur from time to time, particularly if you or your baby are unwell. If your baby refuses to feed, or feeds very little, he may be unwell even though he shows no signs of illness. If this continues for more than a few hours, you should seek advice promptly. Your practice nurse, Healthline (0800 611 116) or Plunketline (0800 933 922) can be a ready source of initial advice (see also pp.355–357).

Eating for breastfeeding

Breastfeeding women need even more energy than they did when they were pregnant. Milk production is energy intensive, and even more so for women who are breastfeeding twins or a large, hungry baby.

Because of this high energy requirement, most women do lose weight when exclusively breastfeeding. Even so, many women find they are often hungry. If you respond to this hunger by eating sweets and cakes, you may find you don't lose the weight you expected. But if you continue to eat lots of fresh fruit and vegetables, and just increase your intake of breads and cereals, you will boost your energy levels and still return to your pre-pregnancy weight.

'The only bit of advice I'd give to someone with newborn twins is that even if you're going to breastfeed, try to get them used to having a bottle as well. One of mine won't take a bottle at all and that means I can't go anywhere really. I need my couch and my cushion to be able to feed them properly, and it's quite a rigmarole. Breastfeeding twins is really not conducive to going out in public.'

All the previous recommendations for eating well in pregnancy still apply (see pp.134–138), but you will need larger portions than normal.[6]

Expressing milk

After the first month (or earlier if direct feeding is not possible; for example, with a premature baby), it's perfectly possible to express some breast milk to use later. This can give you a little more flexibility and allow someone else to look after your baby for several hours at a time.

If you express anything more than a few millilitres at a time before about four weeks, you risk upsetting the balance of supply and demand. The result will be either a hungry baby or engorged, sore breasts. Unnecessary or excessive breast stimulation can also increase your milk supply to the point where you experience major leaking or recurrent bouts of mastitis. Your baby may fight at the breast or spill excessively.

If expressing milk by hand, gently squeeze the area behind the areola (the darkened area around the nipple) and then squeeze the milk down into the nipple. You can collect it in a container, making sure that your hands are washed and clean and that the container is sterile. You also need to consciously relax and think about your baby or look at a photo of him to encourage the milk to let down. This method can be slow – you may find it takes 10–15 minutes to collect even 10–20ml (2–4 teaspoons). But for some women, hand-expressing can be fairly efficient and convenient.

A breast pump can speed up the whole process, but you do need a bit of practice. A variety of pumps can now be purchased; some are hand-operated while others run off electricity or batteries. Choose one that suits your needs. For example, if you are planning to return to work and want to express breast-milk for your baby to be fed during the day, a large double electric pump would be preferable. The cost of each type of pump varies, so shop around to find the best price. Don't forget to ask about the warranty.

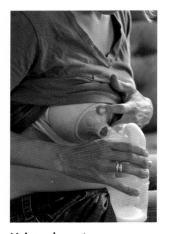

Using a breast pump

Using a breast pump

- Before you begin, read all the instructions carefully. Each type of breast pump is different, so even if you've used one before, check how this particular one works.

- Sterilise and drain all the pieces you're going to use, then let them cool down and dry off.

- Wait until your baby is asleep and it is an hour or so since you last fed him. Milk production varies throughout the day, and you will need to experiment to find out when you can express most easily.

- Follow the instructions for assembling the pump.

- Put the large open end over your breast, placing the nipple in the centre of the hole.

- Hold the pump firmly to the breast with one hand, and either switch on the pump if it is battery/electricity-operated, or squeeze the hand lever if the pump is manual. If using an electric pump, start on the lowest setting and increase it until you feel the pressure on the nipple and see milk droplets appearing. Keep the pressure up and think of your baby or look at a picture of him to help the milk to let down.

- After a few minutes you may feel the milk letting down. The milk should then flow more easily in little streams into the collecting part of the pump.

- You can apply more pressure to encourage the milk to flow, but watch your nipple. If it becomes sore or looks blue, you should release the pressure completely and let the normal pink-brown colour return before trying again. Sometimes it helps to try the other breast for a while, before returning to the first side again.

- Once the collecting container is about half-full, pour the milk into a sterile container.

- Reassemble the breast pump and repeat the whole process with the other breast. At first, don't expect to express more than 20–30ml (maybe even less) from each breast. As you become more proficient, you will be able to express more or transfer it directly to a sterile feeding bottle. In most pumps, the collecting part also serves as a bottle.

You may be surprised at how thin and blue your milk looks compared with cow's milk. This is because breast milk, particularly at the beginning of a feed, has quite a low fat content. Once the milk lets down, it looks creamier.

Storing breast milk

You can keep breast milk in the fridge for 24 hours, or freeze it for up to three months for later use. The expressed milk can be stored in sterile bottles, or in bottle bags. Label the stored milk with the date and time it was expressed, so that you use the oldest milk first. When thawing the milk, heat it to blood-heat (37°C) and then give it to your baby as soon as possible. A microwave is very useful for this, but the container can equally well be heated in a pot of boiling water until the milk is the right temperature, and the milk then transferred to a sterile bottle (see p.317). Be careful when heating milk in a microwave, as it may create 'hot spots' in the milk. Mix the milk well, and test it on a sensitive part of your forearm before feeding it to your baby.

Combination feeding

To allow your baby to continue getting the benefits of breast milk, even when you're not around, it's better to feed him expressed breast milk from a bottle rather than introducing formula in the first three to four months. But if this isn't possible, formula can be used (see p.315).

Once lactation is well established, it is quite possible to give your baby an occasional feed of formula from a bottle without upsetting the breastfeeding process unduly. This may be helpful for women who need to be separated from their breastfed baby at times. If you need to return to work while still breastfeeding, combination feeding (using both breast and formula) can work – as long as you breastfeed whenever you can and as much as possible.

Because a nipple has quite a different shape and feel from a teat, some babies will not change readily from one to the other. A breastfed baby may take a bit of coaxing at first to drink from a bottle, and it may be easier if someone else takes over and you are well out of the way. Otherwise your baby may be confused, sometimes not so much by the unfamiliar teat as by the fact that he can still smell you and your milk.

'We decided to try to leave him for a day with my sister when he was about four months old. I tried him out the week before – and he absolutely refused to take that bottle. In fact, he never took to a bottle at all, but used a cup quite well from six months.'

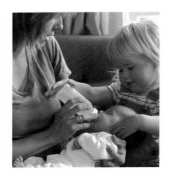

On the other hand, if your baby comes to prefer the teat to your breast, not only will your breasts become sore and engorged again, but your milk supply will eventually decline. When bottle-feeding, hold your baby as you would for breastfeeding, and get him to open his mouth wide and take in the teat as he would your breast. This will lessen the chance of him rejecting either breast or bottle when switching between the two.

Choice of bottle and teats for feeding breast milk

Teats for bottle-feeding vary in size, shape, price, and the material they are made of. Your baby is likely to prefer the softest, most breast-like teat, and you may need to try different types to find which works best. Bottles come in different sizes: the standard is 250ml, but you may find the 125ml size more suitable for feeding the often smaller amounts of expressed milk.

Remember that temperature is critical – milk that's too hot or too cold will usually mean prompt refusal and a disgruntled baby. The milk should be at blood-heat (37°C, or lukewarm to the touch). Always check the temperature yourself (see p.317).

If a baby fails to thrive

Very occasionally, a baby will fail to thrive with either breast milk or formula. All babies should develop and gain weight in the first few weeks, and the growth charts in the *Well Child/Tamariki Ora* health book show the normal range. An important part of any Well Child check is to review growth so that any potential problem is detected as early as possible.

If a baby fails to thrive for any reason, this can have lifelong effects on his brain, and on his general health and well-being. He may be unwell, and need appropriate care. But more commonly, the problem is the feeding process itself. If breastfeeding is not supplying enough milk to the baby, for whatever reason, then formula-feeding (sometimes with a special mixture) may be necessary to help him develop and grow normally. If he is not getting enough nutrition from bottle-feeding using a standard formula, then you may need to change the formula or the type of bottle or teat.

Either way, a thorough check-up by your LMC, Plunket nurse, Well Child nurse or GP can help determine the cause of the problem, and the most appropriate course of action. A referral to a lactation consultant or paediatrician may be necessary.

2. What's happening?

Your body – further changes

Changes in the uterus

By six weeks after the birth, your uterus will have shrunk back to its normal non-pregnant size. The cervix will be small and closed, and the lochia should have stopped. Because the ligaments surrounding the uterus have been stretched, sometimes the uterus may now be tipped backwards within the pelvis ('retroverted'), whereas before it was tipped forward ('anteverted'). This is of little significance, other than occasionally causing a mild low backache with periods, but it is sometimes commented on by a midwife or doctor doing a post-natal check.

The uterus 6 weeks after birth

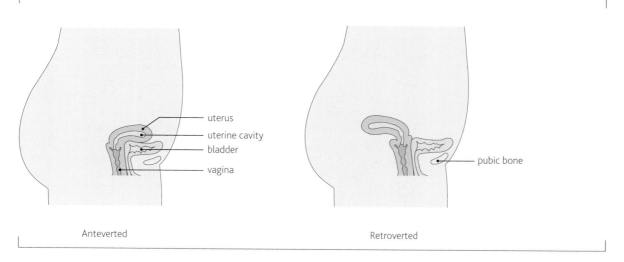

Anteverted   Retroverted

Resuming periods

The main hormone that promotes breastfeeding (prolactin) tends to suppress ovulation and the menstrual period that usually follows, so it is quite common to have no periods at all while you are exclusively breastfeeding.

Once your baby starts sleeping through the night or there are longer gaps between feeds (four or more hours), and/or you start introducing solid food to his diet, your prolactin levels tend to fall. This allows ovulation and periods to resume.

If you are not breastfeeding, your periods will usually start again within six to eight weeks of birth and occasionally sooner, although it would be very unusual to have periods earlier than four weeks.

Your healing bottom

After the first week, any stitches in your perineum will slowly start dissolving. Even if you have had a complicated repair, healing is usually well advanced by this time and, as long as there is no infection, will continue rapidly. Within a month, any bruising will have gone and a healed episiotomy should look like a thin red line. By six weeks, all should be quite comfortable. If the area is still tender, though it seems to be healed, some gentle perineal massage can be a great help (see p.198–199).

Pelvic floor pexercises (see p.127) will also assist with healing and make you more comfortable. Moreover, they will help to reduce any tendency to leak urine in the weeks after birth, and to prevent incontinence in subsequent pregnancies and in later years.

Further changes in the blood

Your blood takes several weeks to return fully to its pre-pregnant state. Some blood is always lost during a normal birth, and in certain circumstances (such as a Caesarean section or a retained placenta) quite a lot of blood is lost. This may mean a loss of valuable iron, so eating iron-rich foods at this time can help replenish your stores more quickly. There is still an increased tendency in the first two to three months for the blood to clot and cause a deep vein thrombosis (DVT; see p.205), so all the precautions mentioned earlier with regard to travel and immobility still apply after birth. If you develop a painful swollen leg, or suddenly have a lot of trouble breathing, seek help immediately to see if a DVT or pulmonary embolus could be the cause. Prompt treatment will generally avoid further complications.

Changes in the abdomen, back and ligaments

The abdominal muscles take 6–12 weeks to firm up again after birth, although you can speed up this process considerably by exercising (see pp.323–326). Any extra fat laid down in pregnancy will also start to disappear over this time, especially if you are breastfeeding and eating a healthy diet. If you put on a lot of extra weight in pregnancy, it will take longer to return to your pre-pregnant size. Stretch marks will gradually lose their red colour and become silvery and much less noticeable. All of these processes will take longer after a Caesarean.

The lower back also had a lot of extra strain during pregnancy, and towards the end of pregnancy the ligaments holding the bones of the pelvis became much softer. After birth, it takes a while to restore everything to its pre-pregnant state (see p.25). All the muscle groups and pelvic ligaments take several months to regain their full strength, so looking after your back is still really important. Minimise lifting as much as possible; and if it can't be avoided, make sure you lift properly (see box on p.202).

Some women find they get a sore upper back from holding their baby while feeding. You can help yourself by positioning yourself comfortably, supporting the baby on a pillow, and bringing him up to you (rather than you leaning over towards him) while feeding. Feeding while lying down can also be relaxing and take the pressure off a sore back. But if, despite trying these suggestions, you still get a sore back after feeding for a while, try standing up and placing one hand between your shoulder blades. Now stretch the shoulders back, bringing your shoulder blades together. Repeat four to six times. Take care with your neck posture too. It's easy to spend lots of time looking down at your baby as he feeds, thus putting strain on your neck muscles. Again, bring your baby up to you rather than leaning over him.

Another quite common problem with a new baby is pain at the wrist. This can be caused by strain on the wrist ligaments from holding the baby, in which case changing positions frequently may help solve the problem. Persistent wrist pain can also be caused by mild fluid retention both during and after pregnancy, and during breastfeeding. Because one of the nerves in the wrist passes through a narrow area (the carpal tunnel), even a small amount of extra fluid can slightly compress the nerve, causing pain and sometimes tingling in the thumb and index finger. This is carpal tunnel syndrome (see p.194). A physiotherapist can help with this problem, and may recommend minimising hand- and wrist-flexion activities, using resting splints at night, and exercises to keep the fingers mobile and to improve the movement of fluids in the area.[7]

Sex after childbirth

The very thought of intercourse may seem an impossibility for the first week or two after giving birth. You may wonder how that bruised and swollen bottom will ever feel good again. But just as your bowel and bladder functions return to normal after childbirth, so does your vagina – and all the more quickly if you start pelvic floor exercises early.

Women (and men too) vary widely in their feelings about resuming sexual activity after birth. The whole situation is made more complex by the new hormonal balance that is necessary for breastfeeding. High prolactin levels (see box on p.310) can result in a rather dry vagina (which may make intercourse uncomfortable), suppression of ovulation, lack of menstrual periods, and less interest in sex. And if you're tired, worried or frustrated with an unsettled baby as well, your interest in sex may be non-existent.

Yet sooner or later, all couples who are new parents need to find ways of keeping their own relationship alive and fulfilling. You need time to talk and enjoy each other's company, as well as time to resume a physical relationship free from your baby's immediate needs. Even if you're not feeling like sex, just talking together about how you feel can be helpful.

Some suggestions for resuming sex after childbirth:

- Find time to spend together when you are least likely to be disturbed, perhaps shortly after you've put the baby down to sleep following a good feed.
- Find time to spend together when you're not exhausted – make the most of mornings or afternoons.
- Take things slowly and gently at first.
- Have some water-based vaginal lubricant on hand (not Vaseline, as it can irritate the tender vaginal lining, and may cause the rubber in condoms to perish).
- Avoid anything that's uncomfortable, and enjoy the things you find pleasurable.

'After my second child, I was quite comfortable about sex within about three weeks – it was great – but it was easy because there were no stitches, no bruises.'

'The doctor asked me at my six-week check about intercourse. I just stared blankly, then said faintly, "Intercourse? Oh, no, not yet ..."'

- You may well be surprised to find that sex is much better than you thought it would be, and that you're both much more relaxed once you've broken the psychological barrier of 'the first time after…'.
- Many couples resume intercourse within four to six weeks of delivery, but there is a wide range of what's normal. Sex after childbirth is not only possible – it can be pleasurable, too. Don't forget about contraception, though (see p.395).

Your baby – growth and development

During the first three months of life outside the womb, your baby grows and develops quite remarkably. He learns to use his eyes to recognise faces, colours and movements. He learns to use his sense of smell to identify his mother. He learns to use his ears to hear voices, music and other sounds. He learns to respond to his environment with smiles and gurgles, as well as crying when he's hungry, uncomfortable or bored.

Growth

On average, babies will have doubled their birth weight by four months of age and tripled it by 12 months. But there is a wide range of normal, and a baby who was on the large side at birth may gain weight much more slowly. Babies who weighed under 2.5kg at birth may get heavier in fits and starts as they overcome some of the problems associated with being small at birth.

The actual amount of weight gained in any one week is less important than the whole pattern of weight gain over several weeks. This is why a graph, such as the one in the back of your *Well Child/Tamariki Ora* health book, is useful.

Example of baby's weight graph

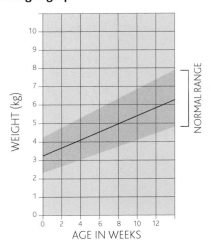

It is also important to remember that, although the graph shows normal weight gain as very even, individual babies may gain weight rather unevenly. Again, it's the overall pattern that is important, not each individual change.

There is cause for concern, however, if a new baby is not gaining any weight or gains very little weight over several weeks. There could be a feeding problem, or something else may be wrong. Your LMC or Well Child nurse should detect this when they weigh the baby each time he is checked. They will either suggest strategies to help your baby gain weight or, if necessary, refer you to a lactation consultant or paediatrician. Once your LMC has discharged you and your baby from their care, you should seek early advice from your Well Child provider or GP, and ask for specialist paediatric advice if you're still concerned.

Measuring length is another guide to progress, although it is often difficult to do accurately in the first few months. Length is not usually measured in the first four to six weeks after birth unless you request it.

Head circumference is measured because there are several conditions that cause the skull to grow too rapidly or too slowly. If abnormal growth is detected early (see box below), treatment can often be started before any permanent damage to the brain occurs.

Three causes of abnormal skull growth

- *Hydrocephalus.* This occurs when there is a build-up of extra fluid because of a blockage in the normal drainage system for the cerebrospinal fluid around the brain. This causes the skull to grow too quickly. The extra fluid also puts increasing pressure on the soft brain tissue, and unless the blockage is promptly relieved with neurosurgery (by inserting a shunt system to drain the fluid), brain development will be severely affected.

- *Cranial stenosis.* This is a condition where the bones of the skull are fused together at birth or shortly afterwards, so that expansion cannot occur and the skull grows too slowly. Again, unless the problem is promptly corrected with surgery (where the bones are separated to allow growth), brain development will be affected.

- *Plagiocephaly (flat head).* This is a positional problem, which (unlike the conditions discussed above) does *not* affect normal brain development. It is largely preventable, and early treatment is relatively simple (see pp.368–370).

Development

Every child follows a natural sequence of development throughout childhood, and the first three months are no exception. Again, there is a range of normal, and each child will progress at his own rate. Your baby may develop at a similar rate to either you or your partner at that age, so check this out first with your parents or your partner's parents if you are concerned. Babies who were born prematurely take longer to reach each stage, particularly early on, as they make up for the time they should have spent in the uterus.

If a child is behind for the odd milestone, this is not usually significant. If he is a lot behind for most of the milestones, there is possibly cause for concern. Ask your Well Child provider about this when you go for your baby's checks. Because developmental assessment is complex, you may also need to seek advice from a specialist paediatrician.

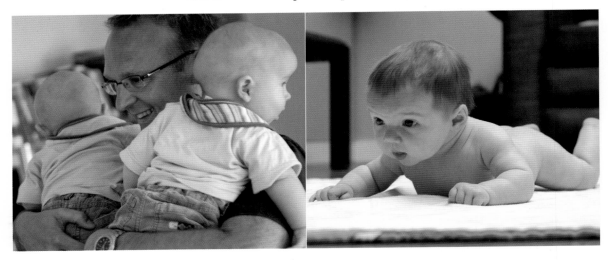

Some major milestones in the first three months

Birth (at full term)
- has rooting reflex (see p.307)
- has grasp reflex (automatically grasps anything placed in his hand)
- is able to suck.

4–6 weeks
- smiles if he sees you smile
- can turn his head from side to side
- follows a bright light with his eyes
- starts to lift his head when lying on his tummy.

3 months
- lifts his head when lying on his tummy
- supports his own head when sitting, although it may still bob a little
- looks towards a sudden noise or voice
- has lost the grasp reflex but has started reaching for an object.

You will notice your baby reach many other milestones each week, and some will reach particular stages much earlier than is suggested here.

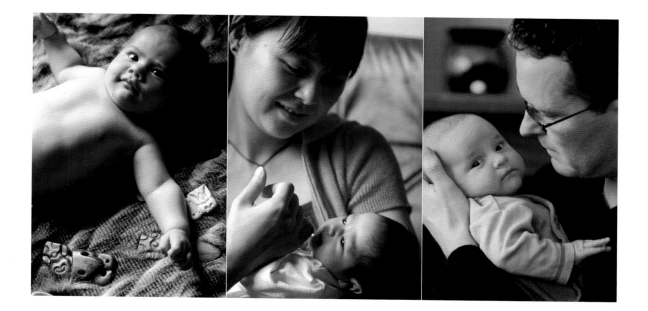

Your baby – ill health

Protecting against infections

Immunoglobulins are complex protein substances in the bloodstream that help the body overcome infection. For at least the first 12 months, babies lack the ability to manufacture these efficiently. The mother's immunoglobulins are transmitted in her breast milk for the first six months after birth, giving breastfed babies good protection against common colds and other infections. But if infection does occur, small babies have only a limited ability to deal with it. If your baby gets sick, he may want to feed more often, especially if he has a sore throat or blocked nose. (A few drops of breast milk can be very effective in clearing a blocked nose, allowing the baby to breathe while feeding.)

Protecting babies against infection

- Keep babies away from crowded, stuffy environments as much as possible.
- A smoky atmosphere makes it more difficult for babies to breathe and to fight infection, so keep your baby well away from cigarette smoke.
- Don't expose your baby unnecessarily to people with coughs and colds.
- Have your baby vaccinated against the more serious illnesses (see p.396).
- Watch carefully for any signs of ill health, and seek advice promptly from your Well Child nurse, GP or practice nurse if you're at all concerned.

Dealing with a sick baby

Babies can become unwell relatively quickly, and the signs of ill health are often more difficult to detect than in older children or adults. One of the things they may do when unwell is to stop feeding, or to feed less, so they can quickly become dehydrated: this compounds the effect of even a mild illness. As you become more experienced as a parent, you will find it easier to sort out which symptoms are more important. Even so, parents of small babies often need to seek urgent health advice. This is to be expected; it is always better to have a baby checked out promptly than to ignore potentially serious symptoms.

To make sure you can get urgent health care when you need it, you should be enrolled with a local primary care general practice (see p.27). Ready access to experienced GPs and practice nurses is invaluable with a small baby, so enrol with a practice that you like and that is close to where you live. During clinic hours, most practice nurses can be contacted by phone for advice. If, after talking to you, they have any concerns about your baby's health, they will organise an urgent appointment – often immediately. Out of hours, Healthline or Plunketline can be ready sources of advice from trained nurses. You may also need to visit an after-hours service; these services vary depending on where you live, so find out about them before you need them (see p.399).

Possible signs of ill health in young babies

If several of the following symptoms appear within a short space of time (even just an hour or two), and seem to be persisting, this is more likely to indicate a serious problem. Seek advice without delay:

- failure to feed properly
- excessive grizzliness or crying
- unusually pale or quiet
- unusually hot and/or red in the face
- unusually cold
- breathing much faster than normal
- difficulty in breathing
- vomiting repeatedly
- frequent watery bowel motions
- persistently dry nappies
- floppiness, or unusual drowsiness

Meningitis

Of all the illnesses that can affect babies and children, meningitis is one of the most serious. Left unchecked, it advances rapidly and causes death, so you should always be aware of what to look out for.

A number of different micro-organisms can cause meningitis. The current vaccination programme provides protection against some, but not all, of these. Although there has been a well-publicised vaccination campaign in recent years (now finished) for one of the common types (meningitis B; see p.397), the MeNZB vaccine used provided only short-term protection to deal with an epidemic, and did not protect against other types. Several of the micro-organisms that may cause meningitis are carried in the throats and noses of otherwise well people. When transmitted to a susceptible person (and babies are particularly susceptible), they spread rapidly to infect the membranes that cover the brain (meninges), and/or the blood (causing meningococcal septicaemia). Fortunately, most types of meningitis can be successfully treated with high doses of antibiotics in hospital, but only if treatment is started in the very early stages (i.e. the first few hours) of the illness.

Because the early signs of meningitis are not very specific, it's best to err on the side of caution and get symptoms checked out promptly. If things don't improve rapidly, even after a check by a doctor or nurse, take your baby back to the clinic or practice and insist on an urgent reassessment. This is not necessarily a criticism of the doctor or nurse you have just seen; reassessment may be required simply because babies' symptoms change so quickly, and meningitis can progress rapidly in just an hour or two.

Early signs of possible meningitis

- failure to feed properly
- continual whimpering, moaning or unusual crying
- unusually pale or quiet
- unusually hot or red in the face
- unusually cold, or hot but with cold hands and feet
- rapid onset of a rash of dark red spots that don't fade when pressed (see 'The glass test' below)
- diarrhoea and/or repeated vomiting
- floppiness, or unusual drowsiness
- a baby who seems stiff, or doesn't like being handled
- other signs of ill health as above

The glass test[8]

The rash of meningitis is not always present. If it is, it can change rapidly from a few dark red pinpricks to more widespread purple-coloured bruising. Get a clear drinking glass and press it against your baby's rash; if it does not fade when pressed, this could be one of the first signs of meningitis. As this is more difficult to see on darker skin, check lighter areas such as the palms of the hands and soles of the feet. If you do notice this type of rash, or any of the other signs listed in the box above, seek immediate medical attention.

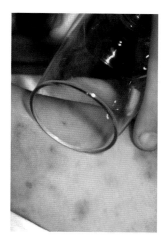

Meningitis: the glass test

www.mediscan.co.uk; 003812

3. Baby care

Nappy-changing (see also pp.172–175)

Changing a baby's nappy is not as easy as it looks, and you'll need a bit of practice to do it efficiently. Modern reusable nappies and disposable (single-use) nappies are slightly easier to manage, but even the newborn sizes don't always fit a small baby very well.

Nappies need changing quite frequently with new babies, especially as they tend to move their bowels with each feed. The combination of urine and faeces is especially irritating to their skin, and is liable to cause rashes. But most babies will be fine in a damp nappy as long as they're warm, and many parents find that changing after each feed, or every three to four hours, is sufficient unless the nappy is dirty or very wet.

Everyone develops their own style with nappy-changing, but here are some suggestions to get you started.

Preparing the nappies

All-in-one reusables and disposables

These are ready for use, but make sure you select the best-fitting size possible. A disposable nappy that is too small may mean that the sticky tabs come into direct contact with the skin and cause a red, raw area. Any reusable or disposable nappy that is too large may not fit around the legs very well, and cause leakage. The better the fit around the leg area, the less likely leaks are to occur, but make sure the border isn't too tight and that plastic and elastic don't irritate your baby's skin. If using a liner, place this flat on the nappy before changing.

Pocket nappies

Lay the nappy flat and open the pocket fully, then place the insert so that it is flat and completely open, extending as far as possible to the edges of the pocket. If using two inserts together (useful at night as babies get older), put them both in at the same time if you can, making sure both are lying completely flat before closing the pocket. If the insert is not flat before you put the nappy on, it can become uncomfortable and is more likely to leak. If using a liner, place this flat on the nappy before changing. Getting several pocket nappies ready in advance makes nappy-changing easier.

Nappy-changing: pocket nappies

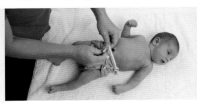
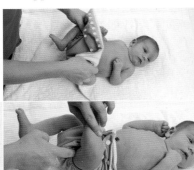
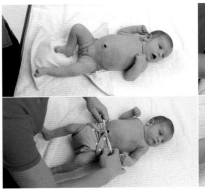

Traditional flat cloth nappies

A cloth nappy needs to fit firmly but comfortably, stay on, and avoid (or at least minimise) leaks. As your baby grows, you may find it's better to fold the nappy in different ways. Here are some of the more common ways of folding flat cloth nappies:

- *Triangle method.* Lay the nappy flat. Fold it in half diagonally. Repeat. If using a liner, place this flat on the nappy before changing. Good for newborns.
- *Origami method.* Lay the nappy flat. Fold it in half, and then fold again to make a square. Pick up a loose corner and spread it out to one side. Now turn the whole arrangement over, and fold the free flaps to make a pad in the middle. Fasten with one or two pins, according to the baby's size. Good for girls, who need most padding at the bottom and back.
- *Flap method.* Lay the nappy flat. Fold it in half lengthwise. Fold in a third on one side, lengthwise. Do the same with the other side. At one end, spread the flaps out. At the other end, fold the nappy up towards the spread-out end. Good for boys, who need most padding at the front.

Suggested routine for nappy-changing

- Collect a clean, pre-prepared nappy, a soft, moistened wash-cloth, some barrier cream and a change cloth.
- Spread the change cloth out on a firm surface at about bench height. (A high bed is fine, but kneel to protect your back if using a low bed or the floor.) Use the safety strap on a changing table or place pillows on the bed so that your baby cannot roll off.
- Lie the baby on his back. Lift his top clothes well out of the way and take off his lower clothes as necessary.
- Remove the wet/dirty nappy carefully, using the clean corners to wipe his bottom as much as you can. Gently lift him by the hips, and thoroughly wipe the whole area with the moistened cloth. Lifting him by the feet is not recommended, as it may worsen any tendency to congenital dislocation of the hip (CDH; see p.328).
- For a boy, check that no faecal matter is left under the scrotum or around the penis. Leave the foreskin well alone (it usually won't retract at this stage, anyway).
- For a girl, check that the lips of the vagina are quite clean, and always wipe gently from front to back to avoid carrying bacteria from the bowel to the vagina and urethral opening. Newborn girls often have a white discharge for just a few days, and a few have a bloodstained discharge. This is because hormones from the mother have temporarily stimulated the genital area.
- Dry the area carefully, and apply a barrier cream if you want to.

Reusable and flat cloth nappies

- Place the clean, pre-prepared nappy (with or without liner) centrally under your baby's bottom, and bring the part nearest you firmly up between the legs. For a boy, check that his penis is pointing towards his feet – otherwise the nappy will remain dry and all his other clothes will be very wet.
- Now bring the two side pieces into the centre, and fasten as firmly as you can. With reusable nappies, there are Velcro tabs, domes, snaps, or hook and loops to fasten securely.
- With flat cloth nappies, safety pins are the most common method of fastening. You can use one or two safety pins, depending on how you've folded the nappy. The pins should be in a more or less horizontal position, with the opening pointing away from the centre of the body – if they do happen to come undone, little harm will result. Always place one hand under the area being pinned to avoid pricking your baby. This also makes it easier to get the nappy on firmly. The pins will go through the nappy more easily if you run the point through your hair first – the oil from your hair acts as a lubricant.
- For small babies, you may not need safety pins if using flat cloth nappies (best folded by the triangle method) with the flaps tucked in, as long as the nappy is firmly secured with pilchers (soft overpants) of some sort – perhaps even an all-in-one reusable nappy – over the top. However, once babies are mobile, it is much more difficult to keep a flat cloth nappy on successfully without pins, unless you have a very secure outer covering.

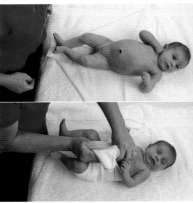
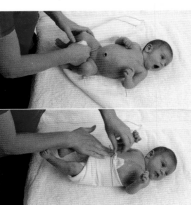
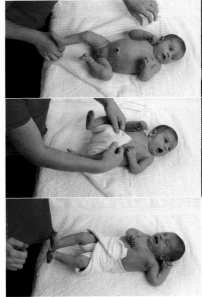

Nappy-changing: flat nappies

Disposable (single-use) nappies

- Unfold the nappy carefully and spread out the ends. Leave the pleats intact in the middle section of the nappy.
- Place the nappy centrally under your baby's bottom, with the plastic side out and tapes away from you.
- Firmly fold the portion nearest you up between the baby's legs (for a boy, check that his penis is pointing downwards). Unfold the sticky tabs carefully, bring them around to the front, and stick them firmly to the nappy, making sure the tapes are horizontal. This keeps the sticky tabs well away from the edge of the nappy and prevents them getting stuck to the baby's skin.

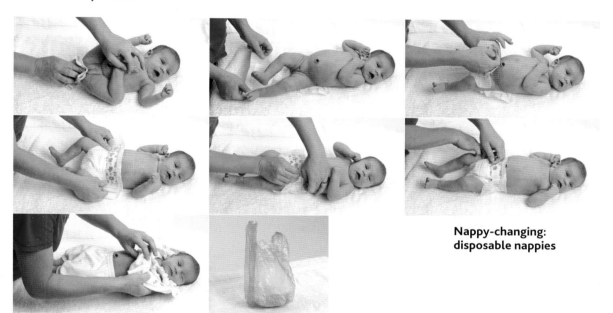

Nappy-changing: disposable nappies

After changing

Put all the baby's other clothes and wraps back on to keep him warm (his outer clothes may need changing too, as leaks are common in the first few weeks). Place him in a safe position in his cot, pram or on the floor. Disposal of the dirty nappy depends on the type being used:

- *All-in-one reusables*. Remove any soiling and rinse as soon as you can. If you're out and about, put it in a leak-proof plastic bag until you get home. Then place it in a nappy bucket of cold water (no bleach or Napisan) until ready to machine-wash (see below).
- *Pocket nappies*. If the nappy is only moderately wet, remove the insert and place it in the nappy bucket, as above. You can often reuse the pocket once or twice before washing. If the nappy is very wet or soiled, remove any soiling and rinse as soon as possible, then soak as for all-in-one reusables.

Getting rid of disposable (single-use) nappies

Getting rid of disposable (single-use) nappies

If you do need to use disposable nappies, make sure you dispose of them as safely and cleanly as possible. Do not flush a disposable down the toilet – this can cause major plumbing blockages.

Remove all soiling into the toilet, including any liner (but check that it's flushable first). Wrap the nappy up, preferably in newspaper and then in a plastic bag; place it in the household rubbish (an outside bin if possible). Disposables can create objectionable roadside waste, so don't be guilty of contributing to this.

- *Traditional flat cloth nappies.* As above, but you can soak them in a bleach or Napisan solution before washing if necessary. If you do a machine-wash on most days, and you rinse dirty nappies before soaking, it's usually sufficient to soak them in plain cold water, without any additives.
- *Liners.* If you've used a liner, either soak it with the nappy and reuse it (many liners will wash at least two or three times), or wrap it well and dispose of it in the rubbish. If it is flushable (check the label), dispose of it in the toilet, but not into a septic tank system.
- *Disposable (single-use) nappies.* See box opposite.

Rinse out or dispose of the wash-cloth, as appropriate. Pack everything away, wash your hands, and then pick up your baby.

Nappy bag (see also p.179)

Regardless of the type of nappy you use, a pre-prepared nappy bag that is easy to pick up and take with you anywhere is well worth having. It can be just as useful around the house as when you are out and about, although most parents also find that a changing table or bench – with room for toiletries, a pile of pre-prepared and/or folded nappies, and a safe storage place for the nappy bucket – makes nappy-changing easier.

What to put in the nappy bag

For your baby

- *Change cloth.* Any piece of soft, easily washable material (such as an old flat nappy) can be used to put your baby on when changing him. Plastic-backed, soft-filled, fold-up cloths sometimes come with designer nappy bags, or can be bought separately.
- *Clean nappies.* Sounds obvious, but it's worth having a selection, depending on what you're using. One disposable (or two if you're taking only disposables), one reusable nappy and two or three inserts are probably the minimum, plus two or three liners if you use them.
- *Wipes.* You will need at least four or five disposable or reusable wipes, preferably damp. Disposable wet wipes come in convenient containers, while damp reusables can be kept in a small plastic bag.
- *Barrier cream.* If you use one when at home, have another small tube or pottle that you keep in the bag.
- *Plastic bag(s) for used nappies.* Again, it sounds obvious, but this is the item most often forgotten. Make sure the bags are leak-proof and large enough to close easily.
- *Spare clothes.* An extra pair of pants, body suit or similar, a sunhat, an extra top and spare socks will cover most eventualities, and save you having a smelly or grumpy baby, or one that's too cold or too hot.

For you (in a separate bag)

Clean breast pads, a spare top and a drink bottle can be invaluable in these first few months. If you are formula-feeding, you will need a pre-prepared bottle of milk if you're out for a short time, or the formula powder and a bottle of cooled boiled water if out for longer. In hot weather, an insulated bottle carrier is recommended.

Washing nappies

Soaking

You need somewhere safe to keep a bucket in which you soak the nappies: a laundry tub is a good place. Once your baby is crawling, the bucket needs to be securely covered and inaccessible, either in a lockable cupboard in the baby's room, or on a bench or in a tub in the laundry. Some people have two buckets – one for wet nappies and one for dirty ones.

As long as nappies are well rinsed to start with, and machine-washing is done most days, soaking in plain cold water is usually sufficient for all types, and is generally best for reusables.

Traditional cloth nappies can be soaked in disinfecting solution such as Napisan, and this is useful if washing has to be delayed for several days. If you use Napisan, it must be made up correctly, according to the instructions. The bucket should not be overloaded, and it must also be really well rinsed out after it's been emptied. Washing-machine manufacturers do not recommend soaking nappies in Napisan in the machine, as this can cause corrosion.

Washing

All modern reusable products, and traditional cloth nappies, are designed to be fully machine-washable, and to dry reasonably quickly after being spun dry. All-in-ones take slightly longer to dry because of their thickness, while the components of the pocket versions (all machine-washable) dry more quickly because the layers are separated. To work efficiently, the stay-dry material that forms the inner layer of reusables needs to be really clean and residue-free, so all reusable nappies must be thoroughly washed and rinsed without using fabric softeners or bleach.

Pocket nappy inserts made from synthetic microfibre wash and dry slightly more quickly than inserts made from natural products such as cotton, hemp and bamboo, but all can be machine-washed.

> *'My one-year-old was a terror. One day he managed to get the lid off the nappy bucket, pulled the nappies out, and then leaned in to touch the water...I turned round to see him head first in the bucket, legs in the air...It was just lucky I was there to pull him out.'*

Washing reusable nappies

- Fold the Velcro tabs back on themselves to avoid collecting lint.
- Soak the nappy and liner in cold water, without bleach.
- After soaking, wash as normal in a washing machine (warm or hot wash), using small amounts of mild soap powder only. Avoid using washing liquids and fabric softener.
- Soak in Napisan once a month or so to get rid of persistent stains.
- Dry in the sun on a clothes-line if possible, or use a tumble-dryer on low heat.

Any soap powder can be used sparingly, although enzyme-based powders for automatic machines will tend to make the nappies rather stiff. Eco-friendly washing powders are a good alternative. (See Appendix: Nappies.) Soap-based powders suitable for hand-washing keep the nappies much softer, but they do need a hot wash and warm rinse to dissolve fully.

Don't be tempted to use lots of washing powder to get nappies clean; it is far better to rinse nappies thoroughly before soaking so that no harmful residue remains. If the nappies have previously been soaked in a disinfectant solution, a cold wash will be sufficient; otherwise, a warm or hot wash is advisable to kill any harmful bacteria. Avoid fabric softeners – they are not good for reusable nappies, and some babies will have a skin reaction to them.

Nappies are best dried outside in the fresh air and sunshine; if bad weather makes this impossible, an indoor line, drying rack or clothes-dryer are good substitutes. Make sure you don't over-dry nappies, as they can become rough and hard.

It takes a little trial and error to find the washing system that works best for you. Your baby's skin will benefit from wearing clean, dry, soft nappies that have been washed with as few chemicals as possible.

Nappy rash

All babies are likely to get a rash in the nappy area at some stage, caused by the irritant effect of urine and especially the combination of urine and faeces. You can usually deal with the problem quite easily, but if the rash seems to be getting worse despite your efforts, seek help promptly.

Hints for minimising nappy rash

- Wash and rinse reusable and cloth nappies very thoroughly – use washing powders sparingly (as described above), avoid bleach and fabric softeners, and rinse well (try using an extra rinse cycle on the washing machine).
- When changing, wash all the urine off the baby's skin with a soft, warm, moist cloth – or try putting your baby's bottom quickly into a small bowl of warm water at each nappy-change (a clean plastic 2-litre ice-cream container is ideal).
- Dry the whole area thoroughly before using any barrier cream. Creams that feel dry on the skin, such as zinc and castor oil, zinc and almond oil, or dimethicone, tend to be better than moister creams. Be guided by your own experience, as some babies react to most of the creams available. It may be best to use no cream at all.
- Greasy petroleum-jelly-based products (such as Vaseline) are fine on normal healthy skin, but don't use them if there is any redness. They can make a rash worse because the skin can't breathe properly. If Vaseline gets onto cloth nappies, it can build up in your washing machine and cause malfunctions.
- If redness develops, try changing the nappy more often, and straight away if it's dirty.
- Leave your baby with a bare bottom for as long as you can at each nappy-change. Fresh air really helps to heal nappy rash. But be careful about sunburn – in the summer, a baby's skin can burn in just a few minutes.
- If redness persists or raw areas develop, ask your midwife, Well Child nurse or GP for advice. You may need some medicated cream to clear the rash up.

Clothes for your baby (see also p.175)

When your baby is very small, it's best to use clothes that make it easy to change his nappies and to dress and undress him. A singlet, then a nightgown, with a nappy and pilcher underneath, is a good combination in warm weather. If the weather is cooler, socks or bootees and a cardigan may need to be added for sleeping, and a shawl when your baby is being fed or held.

Nappy rash – possible causes

- Consider the various chemicals you use for soaking and washing nappies – could they be eliminated, reduced or changed?

- Is a disposable nappy liner causing a rash?

- Are disposable nappies causing a rash around the tummy and legs where the skin is in direct contact with the plastic?

- Has the skin become infected? If so, there will be red spots or crusty areas.

When your baby starts to have longer wakeful periods, it's very useful to have clothes that are warm and minimise gaps. Instead of a nightgown, an all-in-one body suit made from stretch fabric, with buttons or domes down the front and legs, allows for easy nappy-changing; it also keeps all the other clothes in place. In cool weather, an extra singlet, a jersey or cardigan, socks and a hat may all be necessary. In very hot weather, a singlet and nappy may be sufficient, but make sure you also use good sun protection.

It's sometimes difficult to know how many clothes to put on your baby – and overheating is as much a problem as being too cold. Feeling a baby's hands or feet is not always a good guide to his temperature. It's more accurate to feel the forehead or chest, or to watch for sweating or a red face. As a general guide, your baby should wear about the same number of layers as you would if you were sitting quietly in the same environment. If you put on an extra layer or take one off, think about doing the same for your baby.

Bathing your baby

Babies need regular all-over skin care, and a bath is a good way to provide this. A daily bath can also help establish a routine for your baby, and many babies will have their longest, most settled sleep after the exhausting business of a bath followed by a good feed. Traditionally, babies are bathed in the morning, but sometimes it's better to bath them in the evening so that they settle more easily at night.

However, your baby doesn't have to have a daily bath. As long as you gently sponge him all over (especially behind the ears, around the neck and under the arms), it's quite all right to bath him less frequently – perhaps two or three times a week.

Some babies love to get in the bath with a parent and snuggle skin-to-skin, which can be very relaxing. Showering with your baby can also be an enjoyable experience for both of you as long as you ensure the water is neither too hot nor too cold. It's much easier to shower or bath together if you have someone to help you undress the baby beforehand and dress him afterwards.

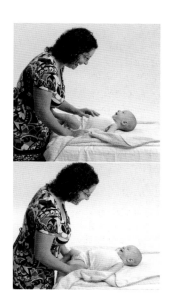

What you need for bathing your baby (see also p.179)

- *Bath* – a plastic baby bath, or any tub, sink or basin that's big enough.
- *Surround* – a firm table or bench under or next to the bath, so that it's easy to undress and dress your baby. If this is not possible, put everything on the floor and kneel down.
- *Towels* – two dry, clean, warm towels – one to fold into a firm pad to cover the surround, and the other to dry the baby with.
- *Wash-cloth* – any small soft cloth will do. A piece of muslin, a disposable nappy liner, or a clean dishcloth will be softer than one made of ordinary towelling.
- *Toiletries* – apart from baby soap or oil to clean the skin, all of the following are optional: baby shampoo (to wash the hair, although baby soap can be used, too); baby talcum powder (for helping to dry the skin folds); baby oil (to rub into any dry skin); and barrier cream (for the nappy area).
- *Clean clothes and nappy* – have a complete set of clean clothes ready, including a dry, pre-prepared nappy.

A suggested bath-time routine

- Make sure the room is warm. Put an extra heater on if necessary.
- Assemble everything you need before you start. Make sure you're not going to be interrupted – leave the phone to ring and turn your mobile off. But if you are interrupted, quickly wrap your baby in his towel and take him with you. Don't leave him alone in or near the bath.
- Fill the bath, sink or basin with 5–10cm of warm water. Check the temperature with your elbow: you don't want it too hot, but nor will your baby appreciate a cold bath. The water should feel slightly warm to your elbow (about 37–38°C).

Bathing the baby

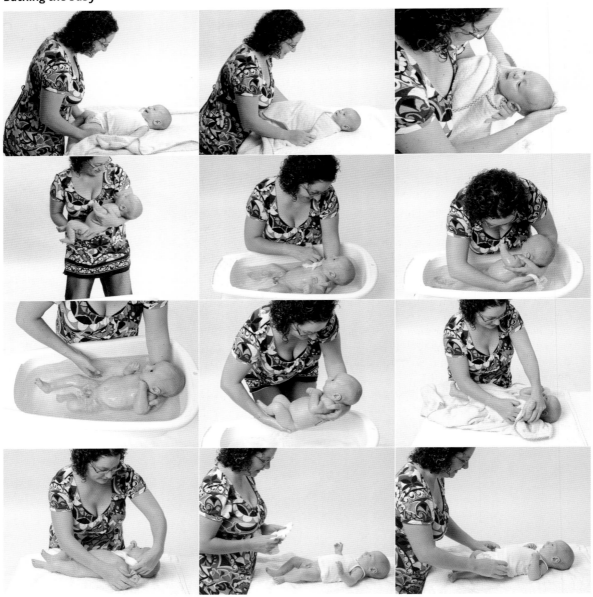

- Using the floor, table top or bench, place your baby on his back and remove his nappy (though you may want to leave his nappy on while you wash his hair – see below). Now undress him carefully, leaving his singlet until last to keep him as warm as possible. Have the wash-cloth warm and wet.

- To wash his hair before putting him in the bath, wrap him firmly in the towel with his head free, and tuck him under one arm, face upwards, supporting his head with that hand. Now, with the wash-cloth in your other hand, gently wash his face, around his ears and under the chin. Dry his face, and then wash his hair with baby soap or shampoo. Don't be scared to rub quite firmly, especially over the top of the scalp. Rinse his hair thoroughly, using the wash-cloth or a small cup, and dry it well. Note that some babies hate this method; they much prefer having their hair washed while they are in the bath, or when they have a bath with you. This is fine if you have someone to help you, but it can be tricky on your own to manage all this with a slippery baby in your arms.

- Put your baby down, unwrap him and take off his nappy (if you didn't do so earlier). Now pick him up with both hands firmly under his arms, and gently lower him into the water. He will probably cry at first. Keep one arm behind his head, holding the arm furthest away from you with your hand. Now gently wash him with the wash-cloth in your other hand (see photo).

- Lean him forward, still grasping his arm firmly with your hand. Quickly wash his back, then rinse him well.

- If he is quite happy, let him kick for a minute or two and enjoy the water; but if he is distressed, lift him straight out and wrap him in a towel. Dry him carefully, patting the large flat areas of the body first, then drying all the creases – especially around his neck, behind his ears, under his arms, around the cord area and in the groin. If you wish, use a little baby powder (on healthy skin only). You can also apply a barrier cream to his bottom. If his skin is dry, baby oil may be useful. A bland vegetable-based oil that is free from petrochemicals, such as almond oil, is good for sensitive skins. (But even the mildest products can be too much for some babies, so if there seems to be any distress or rash shortly after applying a cream or oil, remove the nappy and wash the whole area with warm water before putting on a fresh nappy.)

- Put the baby's singlet on first, for warmth, then a clean nappy, and finally the rest of his clothes. Make sure he's well wrapped, and then sit down in a comfortable seat so that he can have a well-earned feed! You can clear up later.

Bedding

Making up a bassinet or cot (see also p.178)

There are lots of different ways of doing this. Here is one of them:

- Put a firm, well-fitting mattress on a flat base – a cot, bassinet or pram.
- Place a plastic or rubber sheet, a mattress protector or a 'dry cot' blanket across the middle section of the mattress only.
- Place a cotton sheet over the top, and tuck it in firmly around the mattress.
- Cover the head area with a cotton wrap or folded sheet, and tuck it in at both sides.
- In a bassinet, you can place a second sheet right under the whole mattress with two overlapping flaps protruding to tuck in over the baby. In a cot, place the top sheet as if it were an ordinary bed.
- When putting your baby down to sleep, place him on his back, and tuck the sheet firmly around him. Depending on the room temperature, put one to three blankets, fluffy shawls or aircell blankets over him, and tuck them in firmly on both sides. Duvets are good for older babies in cots, but make sure they are the right size and can't inadvertently bunch up over the baby's head.

Bedding care

This varies according to the kind of bedding you're using, but here are some general pointers:

- The sheets need to be changed frequently, especially the sheet under the head area as most babies dribble or spill a little milk.
- All the bedding needs to be aired frequently, especially if you're using a plastic undersheet. Mould can grow on damp plastic within a few days.
- Bedding care is made easier if you have two places for your baby to sleep – a pram or cocoon from a modern buggy makes a good portable sleeping place.
- Even if your baby sleeps with you, it's useful to have somewhere else to put him down during the day. Remember that a baby may not be safe alone in an adult bed. Your own bed will need to be thoroughly aired each day, and changed frequently to keep it free from dust mites (see p.178). However, it's better if your baby has his own bed next to yours.

There have been suggestions that formaldehyde from foam mattresses contributes to SIDS (cot death) in some babies (see p.381), and that this can be prevented by wrapping the mattress completely in polythene. As yet, there is no convincing evidence to back this theory.

Some common problems in young babies

Plagiocephaly (flat head syndrome)[9]

This condition develops as a result of uneven pressure on the soft bones of a baby's head. It does not affect brain development, but in some cases will cause the face and/or head to grow unevenly, changing the baby's physical appearance. Although it is essentially an appearance problem and does not affect overall development, plagiocephaly can still be a cause for concern as children grow older.

Newborn babies often have unusually shaped heads because the bones are soft and flexible. A certain amount of compression in late pregnancy and during the birth process is normal, and most babies' heads naturally return to their normal shape within four to six weeks of birth. But if your baby spends most of his time lying in the same position, a flat spot is likely to develop because of the continual pressure. If this is mild, it will often correct itself gradually as soon as your baby can lift and move his head. But in more severe cases the condition can persist, affecting the face and the position of the ear. Help from a paediatrician and/or specialist physiotherapist may be required to avoid or minimise problems later.

Plagiocephaly is largely preventable by adjusting your baby's sleeping positions, giving him 'tummy time' when awake (see below), and seeking early advice if you notice a flat spot developing. Even though you will always be placing your baby on his back to sleep, try turning his head to alternate sides. If, despite this, he develops a preference for one side, try placing his cot so that there's something interesting on the other side (for example, the window, or a coloured mobile) to encourage him to turn his head in that direction. Change the position of his head by turning him around in the cot, so that one day you place his head at the top end of the cot and the next day at the foot end, making the bed up appropriately. Avoid leaving your baby in the same position on his back when awake, for example in the car seat.

If these simple measures don't appear to be working, or if he seems to have difficulty turning his head in one direction, then talk to your Plunket or Well Child nurse, practice nurse or GP. They will ask what you're doing already, and may suggest a developmental assessment. (See Appendix: Plagiocephaly.)

Tummy time[10]

Babies benefit from spending time playing on their tummies when awake, alert and well supervised. As well as being an enjoyable time with your baby, it helps avoid plagiocephaly (flat head syndrome). It also helps your baby to hold his head up, and builds strength in his upper body and arms in preparation for rolling, crawling and walking.

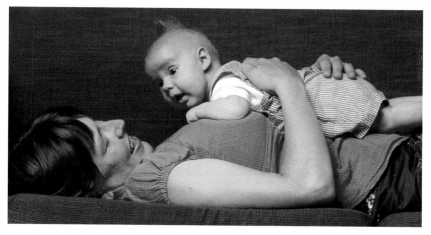

Tummy time helps babies to

- learn to hold their head up
- avoid getting a flat head
- build strength in their upper body and arms
- develop the normal curvature of the spine
- find out about their body by taking weight through their arms
- become interested in exploring their surroundings
- develop balance and coordination for rolling over and crawling

Over the last decade or so, parents have been advised to put their babies to sleep only on their backs to reduce the risk of SIDS (cot death), and this has been very successful (see p.382). The number of babies in New Zealand dying of SIDS has almost halved since the early 1990s, largely because of the change to exclusive back sleeping.[11] There is now no doubt that the back position is the safest and should always be used for sleeping.

But babies also need time on their tummies, preferably when they are awake and reasonably contented. If they are too hungry they will simply be irritable; if too full after a big feed, they may spill and be uncomfortable. Try some tummy time after each nappy-change during the day.

To start with, a minute or two may be enough. Try lying your baby on your chest or on the floor beside you. Smile and talk, playing with him to encourage him to lift his head, gradually increasing the time each day. As your baby gets a little older, place interesting toys or other bright-coloured objects in front of him to encourage reaching and balancing. Some babies will be fascinated by seeing their reflection in a sturdy child-proof mirror.

Cradle cap

This is a common condition in which a build-up of natural hair oil and dead cells forms a crust on the baby's head, and sometimes on their forehead and into their eyebrows. It is a natural occurrence, and becomes a problem only if it gets infected. But it does look unsightly, and the following steps can help to control it:

- Wash your baby's hair (even if he has very little at this stage) every one or two days, and don't be afraid to rub quite firmly. You will not injure your baby's head, even at the fontanelle, by rubbing with your fingers.
- Rinse the soap or shampoo off thoroughly each time.
- If your baby has any hair, brush it daily with a small brush that's not too soft. This will help to distribute the natural oil of the hair.
- If a crust does form, rub it daily with a vegetable oil such as almond oil to soften it, so that the next time you wash or brush the hair, the crust will come away more easily.
- If cradle cap is still a problem, your chemist can provide commercial preparations, including natural organic products containing a mixture of emollient oils. These can be used to soften any crusty areas before they are washed off.[12] But if the right conditions for cradle cap exist, these preparations will only control the problem, not cure it.
- If the skin around the crust becomes red or raw, it may have become infected. In such cases you need to seek professional advice.

Sticky eyes

Small babies often get some thick, mucousy material around one eye. This is usually caused by a blockage of the little tear duct (the lacrimal duct), which goes from the corner of the eye into the nose. In babies, the duct is often very narrow and easily becomes blocked with debris from the eye. A build-up of material then occurs, and hence the 'sticky eye'.

A sticky eye needs to be cleaned frequently – cotton wool and warm water usually works well. Fresh breastmilk, which has anti-infective properties, can also be used. First, clean the eye with warm water, from the inside corner to the outside. Follow this with a few drops of breastmilk placed in the inside corner of the eye.

Sometimes, this mucousy material can indicate bacterial infection or conjunctivitis. The white of the eye will then look red and sore, and both eyes are likely to be affected. A variety of organisms can cause this; it is important to find out which one, so that the condition can be treated appropriately. Seek advice from a health professional.

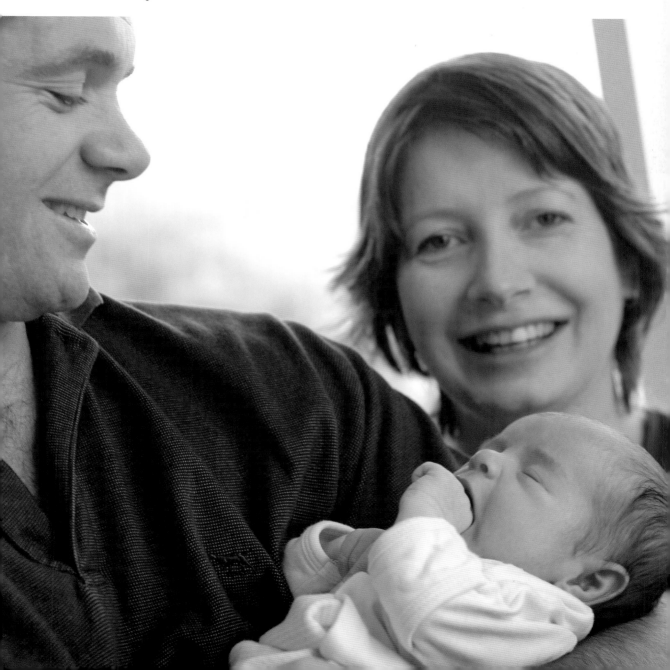

4. Feelings – and feeling in control

Is life beginning to settle down into some sort of pattern? Or are you feeling that you'll never get sorted out with this baby? Are you still on a real 'high' after the birth? Or is being a parent not at all as you imagined?

Gradually, over these first few weeks, you'll come to know just what suits this baby of yours, and what you can and can't manage.

Some small babies are easy to care for. They sleep and feed regularly. They go to sleep after a feed without a fuss. They don't mind being taken out and about. Life seems a breeze.

But other babies are just not like that. Many start to have wakeful periods as early as one to two weeks, and want to be cuddled and amused. This can be very trying at 2 a.m. Some babies are very unsettled after feeds, taking a long time to be satisfied and to go back to sleep. Still others have periods when they are uncomfortable and cry for quite a while, despite being fed, changed, cuddled and rocked.

Nearly all parents with a new baby find it difficult to get enough sleep. Broken nights take their toll, and resting during the day only partially makes up the deficit. This can be especially difficult if your baby is having long unsettled periods at night.

Some people get frustrated if the housework isn't done, and things that used to take only a few minutes now take hours to achieve. But bad days will often be compensated for by good days, and an unsettled period may be followed by a much calmer one.

If you feel 'in control' in these first few weeks, life can seem really good. The house may be a bit messy, but it's easy to cope with that if you're reasonably confident that your baby will feed and sleep without too much trouble.

But if you feel constantly at the beck and call of an unpredictable, grumpy and unsettled baby, the first few weeks can seem awful. Try some of the suggestions below, and don't feel guilty about asking for help – you, and your baby, deserve all the help you can get.

Coping with an unsettled baby

Is your baby hungry?

He may have just been fed, but still want more; this may happen particularly with breastfed babies who tend to 'snack-feed' in the evenings between about 5 and 9 p.m. The aim is to fill him up on the fatty hindmilk so that he will sleep for longer periods at night. Try him at the breast again, or prepare another bottle. Check that you're as relaxed as possible – perhaps the milk didn't let down properly during the first feed. Try going into another room, or getting into a warm, relaxing bath with your baby and feeding him there – often a change of scene will calm you both, especially if other people are around. If you have a clingy toddler, get her to sit up beside you with a book, or with some food and drink of her own.

Has he got wind?

Many babies swallow air as well as milk, especially if they're bottle-fed or if milk flows from the breast very fast. There are two ways of tackling this problem. One is to minimise the amount of air that is being swallowed in the first place, and the other is to help your baby 'burp' to bring up any air he has swallowed.

If you are breastfeeding, try:

- feeding lying down, with the baby either on top of you or beside you to ensure his throat is open in a 'sculling' position (see below).
- expressing a little milk first so that the flow is a bit slower
- feeding before the breasts become really full and engorged
- taking your baby off the breast if he starts to gulp and choke; just let the milk flow into a towel until the flow slows down.

If you are bottle-feeding, try:

- a slower teat (with fewer holes)
- a teat with a valve
- tightening the screw on the bottle a little
- feeding with the bottle in a more upright position.

Either way, pause several times during a feed. Sit your baby in an upright position, put him over your shoulder, or lie him face down across your knee. Now rub his back gently while keeping his body as straight as you can with the other hand. If you have a large milk supply, try to keep your baby generally more upright with his head higher than his tummy – even when changing his clothes or nappy.

Sculling position

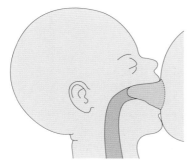

This position reduces the chance of the baby swallowing air while feeding. It ensures good attachment, chin into breast and head back with neck elongated, so milk flows easily down the throat.

Has he got a clean nappy?

Many babies won't settle with a dirty or very wet nappy. Trial and error will tell you whether it's best to change the nappy before or after a feed – some babies seem to need both. Others are best changed half-way through, as they tend to drop off to sleep before they've really had enough milk, and then wake up again ten minutes after they've been put down. Changing these babies half-way through wakes them up and encourages them to feed some more before they drift off to sleep again.

Does he simply want to be awake?

Some babies are keen to start 'exploring' their environment very early. If they're otherwise happy, you can't force them to go to sleep! You can, however, encourage your baby to have his wakeful time during the day rather than at night. A regular evening bath, dim lighting and no talking or playing during night feeds may help. You may find that you need to keep him up for a period during the day, so that he's sleepier at night.

Still unsettled and crying?

Sometimes babies will cry when they want to go to sleep but can't. Some find it hard to settle after a wakeful period.

Some will drift off if they're firmly wrapped and put in their bassinet for a few minutes. Others will not be happy unless they're being carried around; a front pack can be ideal in this situation, as it leaves you with two hands free while he sleeps.

For others, a walk in the pram or a drive in the car will do the trick, or a loud, constant noise such as the vacuum cleaner or washing machine will lull them to sleep. Still others like music or the radio.

Sometimes, perversely, giving your baby to someone else can work wonders. Babies are very sensitive to their mother's (or father's) moods. If you are feeling tense and frustrated, your baby may sense this and, instead of relaxing and going to sleep, will become tense and frustrated as well. So hand him over to his other parent, grandmother or a friend. Go and have a cup of tea, a bath, or some time outside – well out of earshot. A warm, relaxing bath can be an especially good option for both you and your baby when he is unsettled and crying.

If you are by yourself, put him gently in his cot where he is safe and leave him for a few minutes. Simply walking out of earshot for five minutes can really calm you down, so that when you go back, you are feeling a little more relaxed and your baby will be too. Sometimes, even after just three or four minutes, you may find that he's asleep. And if he's not, he may well settle more easily.

Colic

A very unsettled baby who cries a lot for no easily discernable reason is often called 'colicky'. It is widely thought that such babies suffer from spasmodic tummy pain caused by excess wind in the bowel, and this has come to be known as 'baby's colic'.

'That's the point I got to virtually every day for those first crying months, and it was helpful to remember something the Plunket nurse had said to the new mums' group: "They may be hurt if you shake them; they can't die from crying" ... When things got bad I would put the baby down and let him cry while I got my coat and shoes on, then put him in the pram and went out for a walk.'

'Well, I shouldn't really say this, but a box of chocolates beside me, and nice quiet music on the tape, was wonderful for good breastfeeding towards the end of the day.'

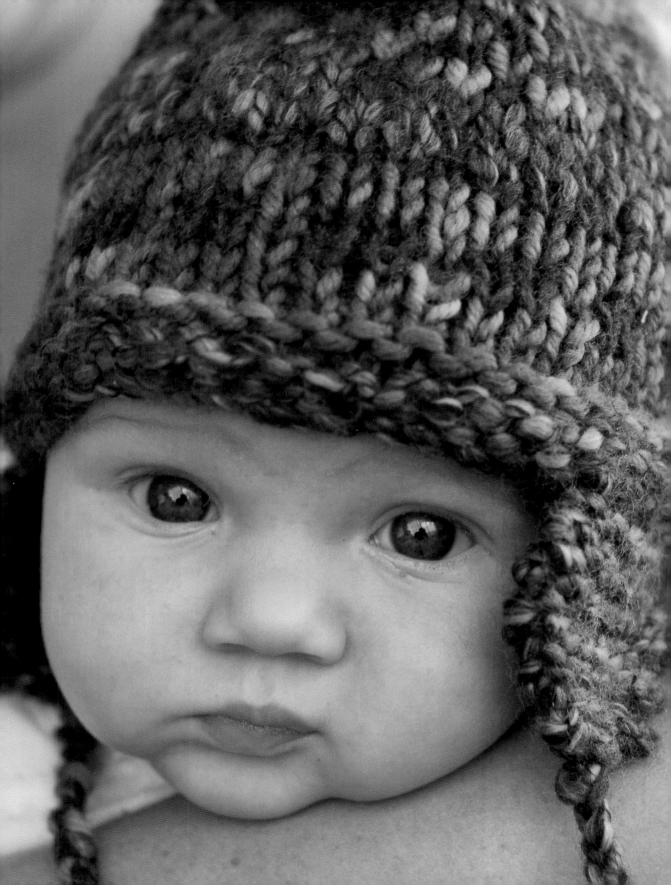

Current thinking, however, suggests that tummy pain and passing wind from the bowel are caused by crying, not the other way around. In the past, many doctors and nurses may have been too ready to label a baby as having colic when, in fact, he may have been unsettled for a variety of reasons. It has also been suggested that babies who cry a lot or are fussy may suffer from allergies or be hypersensitive to substances in their diet (via breastmilk or formula) or even in the air.

Some babies just do cry more than others, especially during their first three months – in spite of being apparently well, and being lovingly fed and cared for. It is especially important that mothers and fathers with unsettled babies receive support and help rather than criticism. Parents in this situation may find it helpful to read a book such as *Crying babies, sleepless nights*.[13]

Asking for help (for all parents and support people)

If you're feeling angry and frustrated, talk with your partner, a trusted friend or family member as soon as you can. This is not always easy, as feeling angry often leads to feeling guilty and inadequate as well.

'When she was very small and the weather was bad, some days I'd feel like I was in prison. Everything was such an effort … I was getting quite low … the Plunket nurse persuaded me to come to a new mothers' support group – what a relief to hear that other mothers felt like me.'

Do you ever feel so angry you want to shake your baby? (For all parents and support people)

All parents and caregivers can feel angry with their children at times – it's a normal reaction to frustrating child behaviour. While we can't stop getting angry and upset at times, we are all responsible for acting safely, no matter how bad we feel. So it's important for every parent and caregiver to have strategies for dealing with anger and frustration. Remember that:

- It is *never* all right to shake or hit a baby. It could seriously injure the baby,[14] and make you feel even worse.
- If you feel yourself starting to pick your baby up roughly and resentfully, quickly put him down in a safe place and WALK AWAY out of earshot.
- Your baby will be fine while you take ten minutes on your own to let your anger subside.
- If you have another responsible adult close by, ask them to care for the baby while you take time out to calm down.
- Think carefully about what has happened, and why it might have happened. Are you exhausted? Are you worried about something else? Are you feeling sad much of the time? Do you feel at risk from someone or something?
- Don't drink alcohol or take drugs to 'forget about it'. They won't help you to work out how you can best deal with the situation.
- If you find yourself on the verge of shaking your baby, even once or twice, it's time to ask for help. Don't wait until it happens again.

You can get help from the Healthline 24-hour phone service (0800 611 116), Plunketline (0800 933 922; available 7 a.m. to midnight), your Well Child or Plunket nurse, or your GP or practice nurse. In some areas (mainly in the cities), there are Plunket-Karitane Family Units open from Monday to Friday, 8.30 a.m. to 4.30 p.m., which provide practical advice and support.

'I'd say that the only difference between "at risk" families and "the rest" is that "the rest" manage to think of one more thing to help the baby. My husband was walking the baby one night, came into the bedroom and passed him over quickly and went out. Later he said that he had been scared because he had found himself starting to shake the baby … '

But often, new parents are surprised at how understanding the people around them can be once the problem is acknowledged. Partners and family members may well be able to work with you to help you get more sleep or have regular time out, and to help with more of the baby care. Accepting their help does not mean you are failing as a parent; rather, if shows you are being a responsible one.

Sometimes, though, partners and/or families are unable to provide support and help. They may be feeling angry and inadequate themselves, or they may have other problems. If that's the case, try one of the individuals or organisations listed in the box on p.376. If you have concerns about your own safety or your baby's, and have nowhere safe to go, Women's Refuge is another valuable source of help. Check out their website or phone them to see what they can offer (see Appendix). Your Internet contact with this service can be hidden if you choose. As a parent, you need to ensure that you and your children are safe from harm. If you are worried about this, it is very important that you seek a safe environment and ask for professional help sooner rather than later.

Especially for stepfathers

If you are a stepfather, or the new live-in partner of a woman with a baby, be aware that you may be particularly vulnerable to feelings of anger. Statistically, stepfathers are more likely than other adults to harm a crying baby. If in any doubt, leave the house before frustration takes over, and seek help. It may be safer to move out, and to visit for frequent short periods.

Getting out of the house

It's very easy to feel house-bound and trapped with a new baby. It seems an enormous effort to get ready to go out, and even more so if you have older children. But getting out of the house can make you feel much better, so try to arrange things so that it's possible even if the weather is not the best.

- Have the baby's car seat, pram or front pack, and a jacket for yourself, ready for use near the front door.
- Put your baby to sleep in the car seat or pram if you want to go out later without disturbing him.
- Have your nappy bag already prepared, with some nappies, cream, wipes and plastic bags for dirty nappies (see p.362).
- Make a definite arrangement to go out in advance. This will spur you on to make the effort.

Post-natal depression and related problems

Society traditionally expects new mothers to be happy, competent and caring, and indeed many women adore being mothers and get much pleasure from their new babies. But for some women, the early months with a new baby are very different. Just as women vary tremendously in their response to the hormonal changes of pregnancy, they also vary in their response to the many hormonal changes that occur after birth.

Some women become clinically depressed after the birth of their baby, and their moods are very severely affected. This seems to happen regardless of how easy or difficult their baby is, whether or not they are back at work, how many children they have, or the level of support they get at home.

'I've come to accept my depression now. After my third pregnancy, I started Prothiaden within a week of giving birth. It seemed crazy – I was feeling fine then – but it completely prevented the nightmare time I'd had with the first one, and thought I'd avoided but didn't with the second one.'

Post-natal depression is caused, at least in part, by complex hormonal changes.[15] These create such significant biochemical imbalances that simply trying to 'pull yourself together' or 'having time out' don't help.

Expert professional treatment from a maternal mental health team (which often includes nurses, doctors, psychologists and social workers) can be of great benefit. The earlier treatment is started, the better the recovery process. Maternal mental health teams are available in the main centres, and most have outreach services for surrounding areas. More information can be found on most district health board websites. (See Appendix: Mental health.)

Post-natal depression has been recognised in part for a long time, but only in more recent years has its importance been acknowledged and effective management been available.

Good support services and anti-depressant drugs, especially in combination with other types of therapy, can be very effective in curing severe post-natal depression. The drugs usually need to be taken for several months, but improvement can be dramatic after the first week or two, if medication is started promptly when symptoms first appear.

Post-natal depression does tend to recur after each successive pregnancy, presumably because the same biochemical imbalances are triggered by the same hormonal changes. Women who have experienced depression before or during pregnancy are more likely to experience post-natal depression. Tell your LMC early in your pregnancy about any previous episodes of depression.

Some symptoms of post-natal depression[16]

If any of the following apply to you or someone close to you, seek help *immediately* from your LMC, GP, or Well Child nurse. They can refer you to one of the maternal mental health teams if necessary. Remember that seeking help is not 'failing as a mother' – it's being a responsible one.

The signs and symptoms of post-natal depression include:

- being unhappy most or all of the time
- being unable to see the funny side of things as you used to
- not looking forward to things as you used to
- not enjoying activities as you used to
- blaming yourself when things go wrong
- feeling anxious or worried for no good reason
- feeling scared or panicky for no good reason
- feeling very anxious that something is wrong with your baby
- having trouble sleeping, even when you get the chance
- feeling sad or miserable quite often or most of the time
- feeling numb and empty
- crying quite a lot
- thinking about harming yourself.

Post-natal depression is not necessarily restricted to the first few weeks with a new baby. It can occur anytime in the first year after the birth,[17] and if left unchecked can affect not only the mother but also her baby. The normal mother–baby bonding process is often interrupted, and this can affect the baby's growth and development, and the mood of the whole household.

It is important to realise that fathers (and partners who are not fathers) can also be at risk of becoming depressed after the birth of a baby. Even though men (or same-sex partners) are not subject to the same pregnancy-related hormonal changes, the stress of broken nights, coping with an unsettled baby and having to care for older children can all take their toll. Just as women with a prior history of depression are more likely to suffer post-natal depression, men who have had previous episodes of depression are also more at risk at this time, and may need extra support.

Post-traumatic stress disorder (PTSD) after birth

Some women who found giving birth very traumatic or difficult may experience an acute stress reaction that is a type of PTSD. This can cause them to have feelings of helplessness, anxiety, fear and horror. Some women have nightmares or flashbacks about the experience, and feel more irritable and less tolerant than usual, and disconnected from other people.[18]

Women who have experienced these feelings often feel very alone and think that no one else will understand. Some have found the Trauma and Birth Stress (TABS) website helpful and supportive. (See Appendix: Post-traumatic stress disorder.) Reading other women's stories and finding that others have had similar experiences can be an important step towards recovery. As with post-natal depression, some women find the expert help available through their LMC, GP or Well Child provider is the best way to get through these difficulties.

Post-natal distress

Only a small minority of women suffer from severe post-natal depression and related problems. But many women and/or their partners find life difficult at times with a new baby, especially if he is unsettled or has trouble feeding, if there are other children to care for, or if there is no other adult support.

In this much more common situation, anti-depressant drugs are usually not appropriate, at least initially. Other kinds of 'new parent support' are better, although it can be hard to find the motivation to organise help for yourself. Partners or friends can be invaluable here, arranging for older children to go out for a few hours, doing some cooking or a bit of house-cleaning, or just taking the baby out for a walk. Often partners or friends recognise that you're feeling 'down' before you do, so if they offer you a break, do try to take it.

Post-natal distress can easily occur when new mothers are at home all day for the first time in an area where they don't know many other people with young children. The switch from full-time paid employment to full-time motherhood is a dramatic one, and it can be difficult to adjust.

Post-natal distress can also occur when women return to paid work within a few weeks of birth, and find themselves juggling the demands of a job, a new baby (and possibly older children) and running a home – often on top of broken nights.

Post-natal depression and post-natal distress are not mutually exclusive; in fact, some people would see them as severe and mild forms of the same problem. Sometimes both professional help *and* extra support at home are necessary for a while.

'I realise now that people did offer to help, but I always put them off: "No, I'm fine thanks", "No there's nothing I need doing"... I didn't realise I was my own worst enemy.'

'A friend did a really nice thing the other day. She rang in the morning and said, "Have the kettle on and the baby fed by ten o'clock – I'll be over to give you two hours out." It was lovely – Tom and I went to see his new kindergarten, and he loved our time together without the baby.'

In New Zealand, many women experience some degree of post-natal distress. But only a small number ask for help, or even tell anyone (including their partners) about their feelings of sadness and frustration. Asking for help is often the hardest step. Once a problem is acknowledged, neighbours, friends and professionals can all help in different ways.

Preventing or helping with post-natal depression

What you can do

- Ask your LMC, post-natal midwife, Well Child or Plunket nurse, GP or practice nurse about support services in your area, and about other mothers with new babies.
- Join a new mothers' support group in your area or online. Go out and visit any friends, relations or neighbours who are at home, even if you don't know them very well.
- Get some exercise.
- Try to eat regularly and well; have bigger portions of any healthy food (see pp.20 and 134).
- Avoid alcohol and recreational drugs.
- Use music, yoga or meditation to help you relax.
- If no one offers, ask a friend or relation to give you some 'time out' from the baby. A couple of hours a week can make all the difference.
- If you really have to go back to work within the first three months, make sure you have good, reliable childcare and housekeeping arrangements in place. If you can't afford them, is it worth going back this early?
- Tell your LMC, post-natal midwife, Well Child nurse, GP or practice nurse if you feel tearful or sad much of the time.

How partners can help

- Listen – don't dismiss your partner's feelings as trivial or unimportant.
- Find out what your partner needs most – is it time alone? Time out with a friend? Or do you need to get someone else to look after the baby while the two of you go out together?
- Try not to offer just 'quick fixes' – doing the shopping once is not going to be enough. But do help out where you can, and be alert to things not coming right.
- Seek further help if you are concerned. You may need to persuade your partner that this is the right thing to do.

5. Cot death, or sudden infant death syndrome (SIDS)

Occasionally, small babies who are apparently well can suddenly die in their sleep for no obvious reason. Sudden infant death syndrome (SIDS) or sudden unexplained death in infancy (SUDI), as cot death is now called, is not new, and is one of the commonest causes of death in babies under one year in most developed countries – including, until recently, New Zealand.

In the early 1990s, when this country's death rate from SIDS was especially high, local research revealed that SIDS occurred much more often in:

- babies who slept on their tummies
- babies of mothers who smoked, especially if they also shared a bed
- babies who were not breastfed.[19]

Since then, these findings have been widely publicised, and the death rate from SIDS in New Zealand has continued to drop, reaching an all-time low in 2004.[20] Other countries have achieved similar results. The improvement is largely attributed to changes in recommended sleeping positions, with most parents now putting their babies to sleep on their back or side.

Despite the progress of the last few years, the underlying causes of SIDS are still not clear; this is why it is also becoming known as sudden unexplained death in infancy (SUDI). Many studies have tried to explain why the prone sleeping position is more likely to cause SIDS. Some suggest that babies can easily become overheated on their tummies; some speculate that their airways can become blocked more easily; and others indicate that they might rebreathe their own exhaled air. More recent research in the US has found that some babies who died of cot death had abnormalities in their brain stem that prevented their bodies realising they did not have enough oxygen.[21]

There are many other questions still to be answered. While the overall death rate from SIDS in New Zealand has dropped dramatically, the same drop has not yet been seen among Māori, for reasons that remain unclear.

However, previous studies have produced some important findings:

- Twins, and babies who are small at birth (less than 2.5kg) or premature are at greater risk.
- The most common age for SIDS is between two and six months. It becomes much less common as babies get older, and is very unusual in babies older than one year.
- Babies are at greater risk if they have had a previous episode where they stopped breathing but recovered (known as apnoea). If your baby seems to stop breathing, or becomes blue, limp or floppy, but then recovers when picked up or rubbed vigorously, he should be thoroughly checked as soon as possible. This is most easily done with both of you in hospital for close observation for some hours, or even a day.
- Babies who have already had to be resuscitated are also at greater risk.

Reducing the risk of cot death[22]

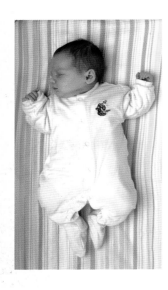

- *Always put your baby to sleep on his back.* This is the safest position, as babies who are put to sleep on their sides can sometimes roll forward onto their tummies.
- *Use a firm sleeping surface.* Soft materials or objects such as pillows, quilts or sheepskins should not be placed under the baby. A firm, correctly fitting bassinet or cot mattress, covered by a sheet, is best.
- *Keep soft objects and loose bedding out of the bassinet or cot altogether.* Soft objects such as pillows, quilts, comforters, sheepskins and toys should be kept out of the baby's bed.
- *Don't smoke during pregnancy or during the first year of your baby's life.* Nor should other people be allowed to smoke in the same room as your baby. It is also important that the house in which the baby lives, and the car in which he is transported, are smoke-free. If you are still smoking, you should not share a bed with your baby (although giving up smoking is the best option).
- *Breastfeed your baby fully until he is six months old.* Ideally, continue to breastfeed while you introduce other foods.
- *Never put a baby to sleep in a room on his own or without a responsible adult checking on him frequently.* The risk of SIDS has been shown to be less when babies under six months old sleep in the same room as their mother, but in their own separate bed.

Baby monitors

There are two main types of baby monitor. The more common are generally one-way intercom systems that allow you to hear a crying baby when out of direct earshot. However, these monitors are *not* designed to detect that a baby has stopped breathing. The Consumer NZ website has details of products available (see Appendix).

If your baby has a higher than normal risk of SIDS, and especially if you have already suffered the trauma of cot death with a previous baby, it may be advisable to use a more specialised type of monitor. An apnoea monitor is a small portable alarm that is attached to your baby, and makes a noise and flashes a light if he stops breathing. Then you or whoever is at hand must help your baby to start breathing again – the monitor cannot do this for you. The flashing light and loud alarm may sometimes be enough to stimulate the baby to take another breath, but this can never be relied on.

Picking your baby up and rubbing him vigorously may be sufficient to revive him. But if not, you should know how to do mouth-to-mouth rescue breathing, otherwise known as cardio-pulmonary resuscitation (CPR). It is not difficult to learn (see box on pp.384–385), but it helps if someone experienced in the technique can show you exactly what to do.

Having a baby on an apnoea monitor is a big responsibility, and the decision to use one cannot be taken lightly. You must be prepared to learn exactly how to manage the machine – how to change the batteries, how to attach it to the baby, and how to deal with false alarms. You also have to know exactly what to do if your baby has in fact stopped breathing. This obviously

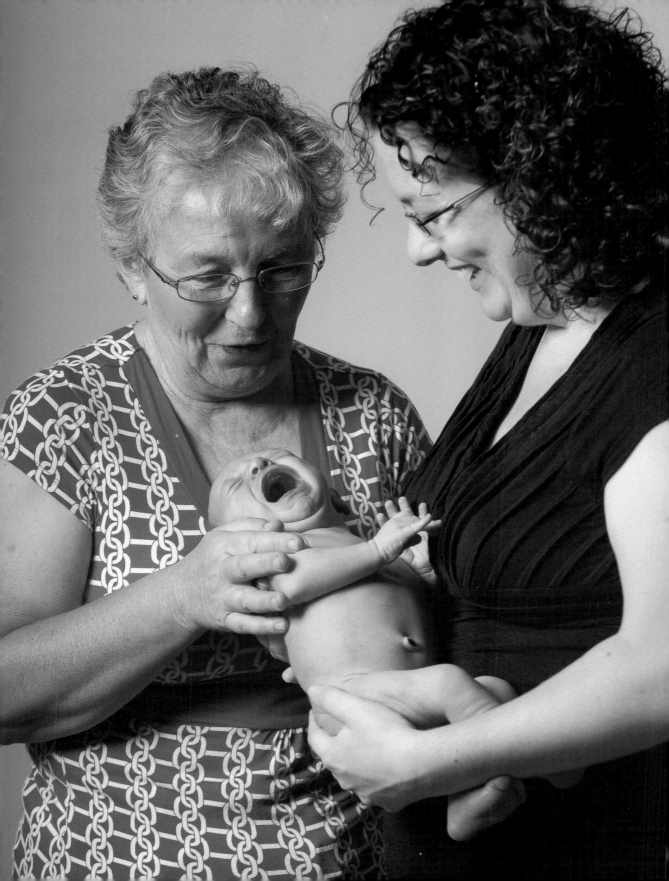

limits who can babysit for you in the early months, and may make you feel very tied down.

All the drawbacks of an apnoea monitor may be worth it, of course, if it means having a live, healthy baby and sane parents. But they are best reserved for special circumstances, rather than routine use.[23]

Apnoea monitors are available through your local hospital, and SIDS New Zealand has excellent information available on how to use them. (See Appendix: SIDS.) In some areas there is a special nurse available to assist with any problems; otherwise your Well Child nurse can help.

Cardio-pulmonary resuscitation (CPR)

Sometimes, babies with none of the risk factors stop breathing without any warning. That's why everyone who looks after a baby should know how to do mouth-to-mouth rescue breathing (CPR).

CPR can be used whenever a baby stops breathing for any reason. It could be because of SIDS, but CPR may also be required to help a baby who has choked, suffocated, breathed in water or smoke, had an electric shock or had a serious injury.

If you can, enrol on a first-aid course: you will be shown how to do CPR and have the chance to practise on a model. Good courses are available through organisations such as the New Zealand Resuscitation Council, the Red Cross, St John, and Surf Life Saving associations. (See Appendix: CPR.) But even if you have not done a course, you can still do CPR, and you may save a baby's life by doing so (see box below).

The basic steps of CPR[24]

If you find your baby blue and limp, follow the five basic CPR steps: Ensure safety, Check responsiveness, Open the airway, Breathing, and Circulation.

Ensure safety

- Check your own and the baby's safety (e.g. remove him from the water, check for live electricity, etc.).

Check responsiveness

- Pick him up and rub him vigorously. NEVER shake a baby.

- If he responds: carry him with you to the phone, dial 111 and ask for an ambulance. Say 'Baby not breathing', and give the address and phone number. Speak as slowly and as clearly as you can.

- If he does not respond: call out loudly for help – ask someone to phone 111 and request an ambulance. If you are by yourself, continue as below before phoning 111.

Open the airway

- Place the baby on his back on a firm surface.

- Open his airway by tilting his head back slightly over your arm, and lifting the chin up with your other hand. Hold the bony part of the chin, not the soft part.   *Continued on next page*

Breathing

Keeping his airway open, check if he is breathing:

- Watch to see if his chest rises and falls.
- Listen for the sound of breathing.
- Feel for air on your hand or cheek.

If he is now breathing:

- Keep him positioned so that his airway stays open.
- Phone 111. Take the baby with you, but make sure you keep his airway open.

If he does not start breathing:

- Keep his airway open with his head tilted slightly back and chin lifted.
- Remove any visible objects from his mouth with your fingers.
- Seal your mouth over his nose and mouth, or just his nose.
- Give five small puffs, looking to see if his chest is rising and falling each time.
- If his chest is not rising and falling, it means the airway is not open or is blocked for some reason. Reposition his head, and check inside his mouth to see whether the tongue has rolled backwards. (If it has, use your finger to flick it forward.)
- Look for any signs of life and check the heartbeat: feel for a pulse on his neck or on the inside of his arm (between shoulder and elbow).
- If there are signs of life (e.g. a pulse) but no breathing, continue giving one puff about every 3–6 seconds (10–20 per minute).

Circulation

If there are no signs of life or you cannot feel a pulse, start chest compressions, as follows:

- Imagine a line between the baby's nipples.
- Place two fingers below this line, where it crosses the breastbone.
- Press down firmly with both fingers (1–2cm), then release.
- Repeat about twice a second, or 100 times a minute.
- Do 30 compressions, then pause to give two puffs.
- Continue this pattern of 30 compressions to two puffs.
- Check for the return of his breathing and pulse every three minutes.

If you are alone, continue CPR for a full minute. Then take the baby to the phone with you, dial 111 and ask for an ambulance. Say 'Baby not breathing', and give the address and phone number. Speak as slowly and as clearly as you can.

- If signs of life return but there is still no breathing, keep the airway open and continue with the puffs only.
- If there are no signs of life, continue with both the puffs and the compressions.
- Carry on with CPR until help arrives.
- If you don't get the ratio of breaths to compressions quite right, it doesn't matter. As long as you have the airway open, it's better to have a go, even if you can't remember the technique exactly.

Resuscitation

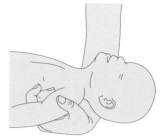

Tilt his head over your arm to open airway.

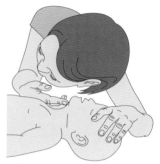

Seal your mouth over his nose and mouth. Give 3 slow puffs, checking that his chest rises and falls.

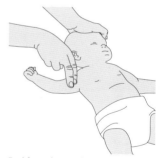

Feel for pulse on the inside of his arm between shoulder and elbow.

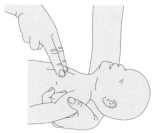

Press down firmly with both fingers 1–2cm, then release.

Charlotte's story: Cot death

This contribution has been retained from the earlier edition, published at a time when cot deaths were tragically much more common than they are now. Since the widespread adoption of a back sleeping position for babies, the incidence of SIDS in New Zealand has fallen to less than half what it was a decade ago. However, cot deaths do still occur, and the feelings of loss and subsequent healing expressed in this story are as relevant today as when it was written.

When I woke on 27 December I was certain that this was the first day of the rest of my life. Our two little boys were twittering on the end of our bed, clearly recovered from the virus that felled both of them on Christmas Day, and the younger one for the whole of Boxing Day too. Sun was filtering through the curtains after the oppressive iron skies of the previous day. The run-up to Christmas, 17 days of pleasure with no free evenings among them, was behind us. Only leisure lay ahead. I made two cups of tea and came back to the bedroom with them, intending to get the baby up and complete the five-on-the-bed family scene.

The clever girl had just slept through the night for the fourth night running and she wasn't four months old yet. I stepped smiling into her bedroom, an enclosed veranda that opened directly off ours. When I felt how chilly it was, and looked along to her cot where she lay face down, I felt so sickeningly certain that I was the only living creature in the room that I stepped back out into our room, softly, and took one last deep breath of the happiness that might not be mine again for months. Then I went to her.

Cold, stiff and clammy, like an underground cave, my precious Charlotte had been dead for hours. There was no question of applying rescue breathing to that squashed blue face, in which I could dimly make out her peaceful sleeping features. I called out for Richard.

Horror brings disorder with it, and my memories from here on are vivid but confused. Grief and guilt descended with equal speed and equal force. Holding her, waiting for the doctor, I heard someone shrieking her name aloud, and realised it was me. Later I stalked the most amiable of the three policemen, asking, 'What if she suffocated, what if she did?', and he parried me tenderly (just as the dandruffy, brown-toothed funeral director did, on another day) with 'Oh no, suffocation shows, on the face, completely differently from cot death.' I saw that the absence of struggle in Charlotte's face might comfort me later, but for the time being I felt as though I'd killed her.

I didn't dress her myself when the doctor took her from the house for the post-mortem, although I wrapped her in a shawl. As I said goodbye to her I knew that there would be more goodbyes. We took the boys to visit her twice before the funeral and kept the lid off her coffin until the last moment at the service. Then, as Richard carried her coffin to the waiting car, I realised how unfinished my goodbyes would be if I sent her coffin to the crematorium without accompanying it. So I asked friends who were staying with us to drive me there, behind the hearse. We ran out of petrol and Charlotte's car drove on without us. Eventually they stopped for us to catch up, and we all arrived together. The minister said a few words, and after a pause I asked if the cremation was over yet. No, they normally waited till the family had departed. 'But I can't say goodbye till she's really gone,' I mumbled. A few hurried words between the funeral director and the man inside the building, and it was done. I could say goodbye again.

Weeks later we went for a healing holiday to the Mahia Peninsula. Until then, I couldn't leave the house for more than an hour or two without feeling that I was leaving her at home on her own. Richard brought her ashes home on the Friday before we left, and suggested we scatter them on the sea at Mahia. I couldn't face having Charlotte's remains in the glove box, let alone trying to decide, when we stopped over-night en route, whether to leave them there or take them inside. Indecision pointed the way. We drove to Owhiro Bay and buried her ashes at the meeting of the sand and the incoming tide. We took photos of our little boys digging their hollows beside the water's edge. To this day we still call out, 'Hello Charlotte', as we ride past.

At Mahia we swam in the ocean and thought of the continuous body of water that connected us to Charlotte's last resting place and to the rest of the world. The sea isn't a universal symbol of life for nothing.

During the ensuing months, grief, guilt and longing pursued me equally. I'd said to Richard, on the that first morning, after the doctor and Charlotte and the police had gone, 'We're not going to be helpful to each other in this, you know, because our ways of handling pain are opposite. You cope with unhappiness by suppressing it, by battening down the hatches on it, and trusting that next time it pushes up the hatches and forces itself on you, it won't hurt as much. But I have to express everything that upsets me. Keeping it inside would destroy me in the end. So I'll be riding tractors across your wounds if I deal with my grief my way. And you'll be harming me with your inattention and unreceptiveness if your cope with your grief in your own way.'

'It'll be all right,' he said bleakly. It wasn't, of course. Our ways of responding were as extreme, and as difficult, as I had feared. Nonetheless we were kind to each other, respectful of our differences, charitable about our reciprocal uselessness.

He never suggested I should pull myself together, or develop a sense of propor-tion. I didn't accuse him of being a cold fish. He didn't remind me that infant deaths were commonplace until this century. I didn't call him emotionally stunted.

He holed up for months with his computer, which I came to call 'Your Friend'. I dug in with my friends, who allowed me to talk and cry by the hour, and wouldn't agree when I admitted that I was repeating myself. Initially they let me comfort them, too, which satisfied my deep need to see Charlotte herself figure in people's thoughts.

I was grateful to everyone who tried to lift the burden of personal liability off me. All the same, I couldn't doubt that my smoking and trying to keep thin during the pregnancy, the dotty action-packed life Charlotte had led in the days leading up to her death, the cold bedroom, and the boys' streaming colds had all contributed to loosen her grip on life. Why couldn't I have slowed down, eaten properly, stopped smoking, prevented the boys from kissing her when they were sick? In comparison, my grief over the loss, although overwhelming, felt very pure.

I even became fond of the huge egg-shaped pain that ran along the inside of one arm, across my breasts, along my other arm, and then extended out in front of me, phantom-like, as though marking my embrace with a vast ghost baby. Aches that I felt in the air in front of me didn't seem odd. Agony was the only bodily condition with which I felt comfortable. The rare times I felt briefly happy made me guilty anyway. How could I have forgotten my darling for two minutes?

While I cried my heart out every day for six months, I came to see that I would recover only when I'd had the time to absorb the loss and forgive myself the guilt. As neither was going to disappear miraculously, it became a matter of making them loved, accepted aspects of my life. I began to say 'Losing a baby is like travelling to Mars and finding that you've been diverted to undesirable Neptune. There's no getting back on track for Mars, and Neptune takes longer, but you just have to adjust to Neptune as your destination.'

By the beginning of winter, I had stopped my momentary response to all telephone calls and footsteps on the veranda: 'Ah, it was all a terrible mistake, and they're bringing Charlotte back.' My pain, regret and guilt were beginning to behave like manageable old friends. Richard, who had lost the look of being a thousand years old he'd had at Mahia, was still being patient with me. The little boys had been constantly delightful and comforting from the beginning. Sorrow began to reshape as a difficulty in starting another baby.

Frantic love-making was producing no outcome, although we concentrated our efforts around ovulation and I always lay rigidly still in the bed afterwards, tilting my pelvis upwards in the hope that nothing precious would escape.

The middle of winter saw me at the bottom of a trough, obsessed with conceiving another baby, yet certain that this anxiety was acting as a forceful contraceptive. I needed to map out a strategy to get my mind off conceiving. Clearly, I had to remove myself altogether from Richard at ovulation time. Then I got myself booked into hospital, straight after my next predicted period, for an operation on my piles. Not that I minded gushing blood daily from the anus. It suited my mental state and mirrored the accompanying neglect of my body. Still, an operation on my 'grandfather haemorrhoids' might remove me from the 'making babies' arena for two ovulations and bring about the defeat of my obsession.

When we made love on day seven of my cycle, the night before I went into hospital, I sat on the loo at quarter to one in the morning, contentedly watching those sperm drip into oblivion. For the first time in eight months I had freely sat up and risked being vertical after sex. The strategy was working. Conception could wait.

Recovery from the operation was painful, of course. There were times in hospital when I cried out for Charlotte and bawled so uncontrollably that the dear old soul in the next bed asked if I was okay through the curtain.

Still, I recovered. Mother came to look after us during my convalescence, and one glorious spring day I felt the astonishing, almost physical, sensation of a metal roof rolling back like a horizontal garage door, leaving my head exposed to the sun and the breeze and the smell of bustling life around me. 'Ma,' I said, 'in ten days, or ten months or ten years, I'll name this day as the day I recovered, healed from Charlotte's death.' It was as though I were pedalling away from my physical pain, only to discover that I'd left my grief behind too. Mother and I giggled about recommending unpleasant surgery to people as a method of easing bereavement. I told her how I could hold Charlotte in my mind's eye, all without misery or regret. Mother gazed at me with relief. After ten months the grief was behind me, and my baby daughter was mine to cherish in my memory.

A postscript. A month later, still floating on air and in love with life, I went to see the surgeon to be checked out. I was recovering well, but I asked him whether surgery in that part of a woman's body tended to delay her period. No, it didn't. Within 24 hours I had my answer. I was seven weeks pregnant. Thanks to our relaxed love-making the night before I went into hospital, Charlotte's sibling was on the way.

6. Continuing health care

Home or clinic visits

In most areas, a Well Child nurse who is specially trained in child development and baby care will contact you during the first four to six weeks after your baby is born. She will arrange either to visit you at home, or to see you at her local clinic.

In some areas, there may seem to be a gap between your LMC or post-natal midwife care finishing at about four to six weeks and your Well Child nurse contacting you. If you have any problems during this 'hand-over' time, phone or go to your local GP or practice nurse. After initial contact has been made with your Well Child nurse, you can continue to visit her regularly at the local clinic so that she can monitor your child's health and development.

Well Child care is offered to everyone, free of charge, and you may wonder why. A child's growth and development, particularly in the first two years of life, set the scene for his future mental and physical health. The sooner any delay or problem is detected, the sooner action can be taken to correct or minimise it. As a parent, you are in a very good position to notice delays or problems in your child, since you spend more time with him than anyone else. But Well Child care acts as a good back-up. A Well Child nurse also has the advantage of seeing lots of children of a similar age, so she has a good picture of the wide range of normal development.

Well Child nurses and provider organisations[25]

'Well Child care' is a term used to describe the government-funded screening, surveillance, education and support service offered to all New Zealand children from birth to five years and their family or whānau.

- A Well Child nurse is a fully trained nurse who has undertaken further accredited training to provide Well Child care.
- A Well Child nurse is usually employed by a Well Child provider to provide care for children up to five years of age.
- Often they will be trained and employed by the Plunket Society, and known as a Plunket nurse, Karitane or Kaiāwhina. (See Appendix: Plunket.)
- A number of other organisations (e.g. the Whare Mauri Ora Trust, HealthStar Pacific Trust and Ora Toa Well Child/Tamariki Ora services) also provide Well Child services via their fully trained Well Child nurses.
- Primary care providers such as GP teams and Well Child provider teams also provide Well Child services, including vaccination.
- The Well Child/Tamariki Ora website has more information about the range of Well Child providers. (See Appendix: Well Child/Tamariki Ora.)

'We had real trouble in the first couple of months getting her into a regular sleeping and feeding routine. She'd go to sleep a little while, and then wake up hungry again — it seemed like she was constantly on my breast. But it was because we didn't know enough about baby routines of feeding and sleeping. So she was just in a constant cycle of being overtired. During one visit, the Plunket nurse asked me how the sleeping was going and I just broke down. I felt so incredibly tired. She made an appointment for me, and I went to the Plunket centre. They told me about feeding and sleeping routines, and showed me a video on the "tired signs". It was such a revelation because her behaviour finally made sense. From then on, it worked like magic!'

> **Home and clinic visits – useful things to know**
>
> - Your Well Child nurse will usually contact you within two to six weeks of the birth.
> - If she visits you at home, she will want to wash her hands before handling your baby, so be prepared to show her the bathroom.
> - She will chat with you about how you're getting on – not to be nosy, but to try to help you if you have any worries.
> - She will usually want you to undress your baby to weigh him, so have a warm place available to do this.
> - At home, she will often weigh the baby by placing him in a clean cloth nappy, pinning the four corners together, and lifting him up on a spring-scale. Have a nappy or wrap and a nappy pin ready. At the clinic, she will have a set of more accurate baby-scales.
> - She may look at the baby's cord, and check his eyes, vision, ears, hearing, head movements, responses, etc. (depending on his age).
> - She will want to write important information about your baby in his *Well Child/Tamariki Ora* health book, so have it ready.
> - You will need to dress your baby again while she does this, so have a clean nappy etc. ready.
> - Be ready to ask about anything you're not sure of – your nurse is there to help you. Make a list so you can remember the questions you want to ask.
> - The whole visit usually lasts 15–30 minutes, or a bit less at the clinic.
> - If you're concerned about something, you can phone your nurse for advice or ask her for extra visits. Find out when and where you can contact her, and let her know if you're going to be out at a time when she might visit.

Your six-week check

The final phase of your post-natal care is a thorough check-up for both you and your baby, about six weeks after the birth. It is usually done by your LMC, although sometimes your GP may do it for you.

It may seem odd to still be having maternity care after you've had your baby. But this is an important health check to ensure that your body has recovered from pregnancy and childbirth, so that you may in time have more children should you choose to do so. And because you're now part of your own unique mother-baby unit, it's a good opportunity to check your baby's progress, too. Take your *Well Child/Tamariki Ora* health book with you.

Your LMC will usually allow at least half an hour for your six-week check, so make the most of it and ask all the questions you want. This visit is free, as it is still part of your maternity care, although it will be included in the charge if your LMC is a private specialist obstetrician (see p.97).

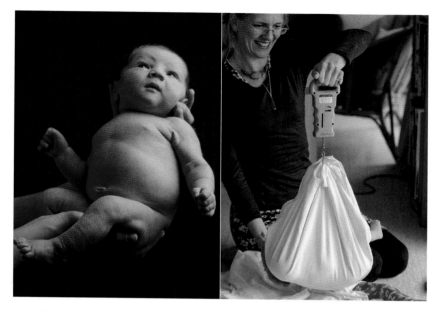

Questions your LMC or GP may ask you:

- The name, sex and birth weight of your baby. These will have been recorded at the birth, but your LMC may not have written them in their own notes.

- How you are feeding your baby – breast or formula, or both.

- How your breasts feel. Report any lumps or bumps, pain or discomfort, or any suspected mastitis (see p.344).

- How your bowels and bladder are. If you are having any problem at all, even if it seems trivial, say so. Your LMC or GP will then know to do an especially thorough examination.

- How intercourse is for you. If you haven't had intercourse yet, or if it has been painful, say so; the examination may need to be especially gentle.

- What you want to do about contraception (see p.395).

- How you feel in yourself. If you're down in the dumps, or feeling good but tired, say so. Your LMC or GP will be very aware of post-natal depression and distress, but are less likely to be alerted to it if you say everything is just fine.

- How you feel your baby's doing. If he's a gorgeous, settled baby, say so. But also say if he seems unsettled or fussy, if he cries for three hours in the evenings, or if you think he's not doing what he should.

- Is your baby smiling? Does he startle at a sudden loud noise out of sight? Has he had a routine hearing test (see p.330)? Does he turn towards a window or light? Does he follow a moving light with his eyes? Answer honestly – these are all early indications of normal vision and hearing. If you have any concerns, say so.

Examining you

Your LMC or GP will usually examine you first; someone else may be available to hold your baby while this is done.

- *Blood pressure and weight.* Your blood pressure should be back to normal, even if it was high during pregnancy or labour. Your weight may not be back to its pre-pregnancy level, but it should be less than it was after the birth.
- *Urine check.* This is not routine, but if there is any suspicion of urinary infection, a specimen will need to be taken.
- *Abdomen.* All your internal organs should be back in their usual places and your abdominal muscles should be starting to firm up. Your LMC or GP will check your liver, kidneys and intestines. If you had a Caesarean, the scar and surrounding area will be checked for pain and tenderness.
- *Breasts.* If you are not breastfeeding, your breasts should be quite soft and back to their normal size by now. If you are breastfeeding, they should be comfortable and free from lumps, although they may be larger than their pre-pregnancy size. The nipples should be comfortable and 'toughened up' by now, too. A quick check for lumps and bumps and a nipple inspection will usually be done.
- *Vaginal examination.* First the perineum and the area around the vaginal opening will be inspected. All should be well healed. A speculum may then be gently inserted so that the walls of the vagina and the cervix can be seen. Again, all should be well healed and the cervix tightly closed.

Swabs may be taken if there has been any infection during or after pregnancy. A cervical smear is not usually done at this time, because the results are often hard to interpret so soon after childbirth. If needed, it can be done later.

If you have decided to have an IUCD for contraception (see pp.37 and 395), this can now be inserted, although sometimes it may be advisable to wait another few weeks.

You may be asked to 'bear down' as if pushing in the second stage of labour (see p.363). This helps to check how firm the pelvic floor muscles are.

Finally, your LMC or GP may check the uterus by placing one hand on your abdomen and two gloved fingers in the vagina. The uterus should be back to its normal size. The tubes and ovaries will also be checked. If you have decided to have a diaphragm for contraception (see pp.36 and 395), this is a good time to fit it.

Examining your baby

You will need to undress your baby at least down to his singlet, and loosen his nappy. He may be weighed, unless this was done recently by your Well Child nurse.

- *Chest.* Your LMC or GP will watch your baby breathe, and listen to his chest (back and front) for breathing noises in the lungs. They will also listen carefully to his heart.

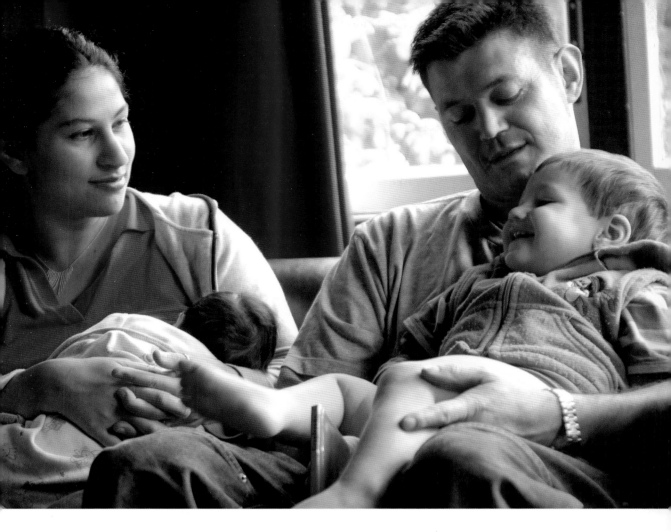

- *Abdomen*. The position of the liver, spleen, kidneys and intestines will all be checked. The umbilicus (tummy button) will be inspected – the cord should have dropped off by now, and the area be completely healed.
- *Genitals*. In a boy, the penis and scrotum will be inspected. The testes will be felt for in the scrotum to check that both are present. The foreskin will not be retracted, but left alone. If the baby has been circumcised, the scar will be checked. In a girl, the vaginal opening will be inspected – any discharge present at birth should be quite gone. The anal area will also be looked at, and any spots, marks or rashes noted and treated as necessary.
- *Back and limbs*. The back will be checked to make sure the vertebrae are straight and symmetrical, and any skin blemishes or marks noted. Many babies have an irregular, faintly bluish mark on their lower back (sometimes known as a Mongolian spot). This is normally harmless, and will fade with time. The limbs will be checked for straightness and firmness, and for symmetrical movements. In particular, the hip joints will be checked.

- *Head.* The head circumference may be measured, although this is usually not necessary if it has been done by your Well Child nurse, and the chart in your *Well Child/Tamariki Ora* health book has been filled in recently.

The fontanelles (the naturally occurring gaps between the skull bones which allow growth) will also be checked. The small one at the back of the head will be nearly closed by now, but the larger one in front will still be the size of a 50-cent piece.

The eyes, ears and mouth will be inspected. Any concerns will need to be followed up with more specific tests.

If this check is being done by your GP, your baby may be able to receive his six-week vaccination now from the practice nurse (see p.396); otherwise, you will need to make a separate appointment.

The lactational amenorrhoea method (LAM)

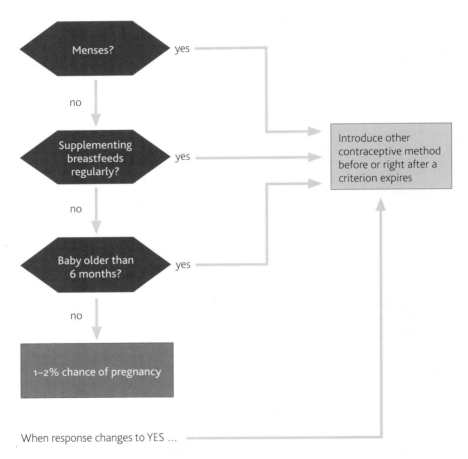

Adapted from M. Labbok, K. Cooney and S. Coly, *Guidelines: Breastfeeding, Family Planning, and the Lactational Amenorrhea Method – LAM*, Institute for Reproductive Health, Washington, DC, 1994.

Contraception after childbirth

After childbirth, you need to consider using some form of contraception to minimise the risk of becoming pregnant again before you are ready – unless of course you want another child very soon.

It is possible for normal fertility to return within a month or two of giving birth, particularly if you are not breastfeeding every two to three hours over a 24-hour period. Since ovulation occurs before the first menstrual period, you should start using contraception before your periods resume.

Contraception is usually discussed at your six-week check, but it's advisable to use a condom even before then if you want to be fully protected. If you are exclusively breastfeeding every two to three hours over a 24-hour period, you are in fact very unlikely to ovulate for some months – but as time goes on you should not rely on this for contraception.[26]

Not all forms of contraception are suitable at this time (see also pp.36–40).

- *Condoms.* Suitable. Vaginal dryness may be made worse unless you use some lubricant as well. Use a water-based product and avoid Vaseline, as it may damage the condom. Can be used soon after birth.

- *Diaphragms.* Suitable. You will need to be fitted about six weeks after birth to get the right size, even if you have worn a diaphragm before.

- *Cervical cap.* Suitable. Again, you will need to be refitted. The cervix tends to be softer than usual until 8–12 weeks after birth, so it may be more difficult to fit the cap properly.

- *Natural family planning (the lactational amenorrhoea method, or LAM).* Natural Fertility New Zealand offers specific advice and training on this method of contraception for women who are exclusively breastfeeding. LAM relies on the lack of ovulation and menstruation that most women experience while exclusively breastfeeding; nevertheless, there is still about a 2 per cent risk of pregnancy. Knowing about LAM can be a very helpful guide as to when to start using another method of contraception, because the combination of LAM and either condoms, a diaphragm or the mini-pill will greatly improve effectiveness (see diagram opposite).[27]

- *Intra-uterine contraceptive device (IUCD).* May be very suitable if you have no previous history of pelvic infection and no current infection (either a sexually transmitted disease or post-partum infection). Can be inserted four to eight weeks after birth with very little discomfort. Before this time, there is a higher risk of complications.

- *Standard (combined or ordinary) pill.* Generally unsuitable in the early weeks if breastfeeding, as it may interfere with milk production. Very suitable for women who are not breastfeeding. However, the combined pill should not be taken until at least four weeks after delivery, because the risk of blood clots remains heightened until this time.

- *Mini-pill (progestagen-only pill).* Suitable. Does not affect milk production and progestagen passes through breast milk only in minute amounts. Can be started within three weeks of birth, but very regular pill-taking is necessary, which may not be easy with a new baby. Will be a little less reliable once you stop breastfeeding, so a change of method may well be needed when you are weaning your baby.

- *Depo-Provera (contraceptive injection).* Suitable. Does not affect milk production or pass through breast milk in significant amounts. May make it harder to lose extra weight after childbirth. Best given about six weeks after birth, as bleeding problems may occur if given before this time.

- *Sterilisation.* It is possible to do a tubal ligation within a few days of childbirth or at the time of a Caesarean, but this is generally not recommended as there is a slightly higher risk of failure if the operation is done then. There may also be more complications with recovery. Many people feel that the period surrounding birth is not a good time to make decisions about permanent sterilisation (whether tubal ligation or vasectomy), and that it is wise to wait until the baby is at least a year old.

The most common forms of contraception after childbirth tend to be LAM and/or condoms initially, followed by the mini-pill, an IUCD or a diaphragm. But you and your partner both need to consider your own particular needs, and your previous experiences with contraception.

Vaccination programme

In New Zealand, all children are offered protection from a number of serious illnesses through a free vaccination programme. Vaccination is strongly recommended, but is not compulsory. Worldwide, vaccination programmes have greatly reduced the numbers of children dying or suffering permanent disability from potentially fatal diseases. The numbers can be further reduced if most children are immunised.

The benefits of immunisation far outweigh the risks for most children, but the risks do need to be considered carefully. There are a few children who have good reason not to be immunised. They will still be afforded some protection if most other children are immunised, because the disease is less likely to be present in their community.

When considering having your baby vaccinated, ask for current information about the New Zealand vaccination programme. Also check the Immunisation Advisory Centre's website (see Appendix: Vaccination) and/or the Ministry of Health's *Immunisation handbook* for reliable evidence-based information.[28]

A National Immunisation Register (NIR) has now been established; all newborn babies are put on it unless their parents decide to opt off (in which case you will need to fill in an 'opt off' form – available from your LMC, Well Child nurse or GP – and have it sent to the local NIR administrator). This register is designed to ensure that your baby gets recalled when particular immunisations are due and that, regardless of where you live in New Zealand, your child's immunisations will always be up to date.

If you decide not to immunise your baby, it should be a fully informed, active decision, and you need to inform your primary care provider as well as the NIR.

From 2008, the recommended immunisation schedule for all children includes free vaccination for the following serious diseases: diphtheria, tetanus, whooping cough (pertussis), polio, measles, mumps, rubella, hepatitis B, haemophilus influenzae type b (Hib), and pneumococcal disease.

Cases when vaccination is not recommended

Vaccination may not be recommended for a child who:

- is significantly unwell with an acute illness and a fever (vaccination should be postponed until he is better)

- has had a previous severe reaction to a vaccination

- has an ongoing serious illness such as HIV or cancer

If you have older children, they may not be immunised against Hib or pneumococcal disease, as these vaccinations have been added to the pro-gramme only recently. In special circumstances other vaccines, such as those for tuberculosis and meningitis type B, are available. (The meningitis type B (MeNZB) vaccination was widely and freely available to children and young adults from 2005 to 2008, as part of a campaign to deal with an epidemic.)

For easier administration and for your baby's comfort, combination vac-cines are given wherever possible. Some combinations also make each of the vaccines more effective than if they were given on their own. Combinations as of June 2008 are as follows (current brand names are shown):

- *Hexavalent vaccine (Infanrix-Hexa):* diphtheria, tetanus, whooping cough (pertussis), polio, Hib, hepatitis B
- *MMR (MMR-II):* measles, mumps, rubella
- *Quadrivalent vaccine (Infanrix-IPV):* diphtheria, tetanus, whooping cough, polio
- *Trivalent vaccine (Boostrix):* diphtheria, tetanus, whooping cough
- *Single vaccine:* pneumococcal disease (Prevenar).

Vaccination can be done by an authorised vaccinator, who is nearly always a nurse or a doctor. All vaccinations are now given by injection.

Immunisation schedule from June 2008

At six weeks (two injections)

- Infanrix-Hexa (diphtheria, tetanus, whooping cough, polio, Hib, hepatitis B)
- Prevenar (pneumococcal disease).

At three months (two injections)

- Infanrix-Hexa (diphtheria, tetanus, whooping cough, polio, Hib, hepatitis B)
- Prevenar (pneumococcal disease).

At five months (two injections)

- Infanrix-Hexa (diphtheria, tetanus, whooping cough, polio, Hib, hepatitis B)
- Prevenar (pneumococcal disease).

At 15 months (three injections)

- MMR-II (measles, mumps, rubella)
- Prevenar (pneumococcal disease)
- Hiberix (Hib).

At four years (two injections)

- MMR-II (measles, mumps, rubella)
- Infanrix-IPV (diphtheria, tetanus, whooping cough, polio).

At 11 years (one injection)

- Boostrix (diphtheria, tetanus, whooping cough).
- (The HPV vaccine, to protect against cervical cancer, is being introduced, and is to be given to girls aged 12–18 years.)

Adverse reactions

A small number of children have an adverse reaction to vaccines, the most common being:

- redness around the vaccination site
- a rash, either around the vaccination site or all over
- child grumpy or unsettled for a day or so
- a slight temperature
- with the MMR vaccine, there may be a mild delayed reaction seven to ten days later.

All of these will generally settle by themselves, although you should tell your GP or practice nurse about any reaction at your next visit.

Very rarely, a child can have a significant allergic (anaphylactic) reaction to the vaccine. These more serious reactions nearly always occur within a short time of having the injection, which is why vaccinators will ask you to wait in the clinic area for a minimum of 20 minutes afterwards.

If, after having a vaccination, your baby develops swelling around the mouth and eyes, or a severe red lumpy rash, or has difficulty breathing, take him *straight* back to the clinic or an after-hours medical centre. Authorised vaccinators are trained to manage and treat this type of reaction effectively. Very occasionally, observation in hospital will also be necessary.

Having a regular primary care provider

If this is your first baby, or if you have recently moved, you may not be enrolled yet with a primary care general practice service in your area. This is especially likely if your LMC was located some distance from where you live, or was not attached to a particular primary care provider. Once you have children, it is usually much more convenient to be enrolled with a provider close by, as you will probably be making many more visits to your practice or primary care nurse, GP and possibly other health professionals than you did before. If you have not done so already, you should enrol with a local primary care provider that offers comprehensive health care from GPs, practice nurses and other health professionals. Sometimes your chosen practice will be very busy and not taking new patients, particularly if you are new to the area. If so, you should see what other options there are nearby or, if necessary, apply again at a slightly later date. If you still have trouble getting enrolled, phone your local primary health organisation (PHO) directly (their number will be in the phone book) and ask for advice. (See Appendix: Primary health organisation.)

In general, the PHO system of funding (see p.27) means you can visit the primary health service at which you are enrolled at low or no cost. The government heavily subsidises visits for children under six years; at many practices, child visits during working hours are free (although a charge may apply for long or complicated visits, home visits and visits after hours). Whatever the arrangement, you will find it very helpful to get to know the nurses and doctors at the health service, well before you need them in an emergency.

Practice nurses at most health services can also provide excellent, personalised advice over the phone, which is helpful if you're unsure whether you need to bring your baby in. Primary care providers will also remind you (as an enrolled person) when vaccinations and other checks are due.

Good-quality free health advice (including Well Child and parenting advice) is also available by phone from Healthline (0800 611 116) 24 hours a day, seven days a week, 365 days a year. Plunket Line (0800 933 922) offers specific advice on children under five years, and is available from 7 a.m. to midnight seven days a week.

Getting the best from your primary care provider

- Enrol before you need an urgent visit.
- Keep the phone number of the health service and the after-hours number (if different) in a prominent position.
- If your child is unwell, ring earlier rather than later.
- If you're not sure whether you need to see a doctor, ask to speak to a practice nurse first.
- Explain clearly who you are, who is sick, how old they are, what the problem is, and how long it's been going on for.
- If you are ringing for advice, say so. If you want to be seen anyway, make this quite clear.
- When you talk to the practice nurse or see the doctor, explain what has happened, and what you are worried about.
- Make sure you understand what they think is wrong, and what treatment they think is necessary. Ask when you should expect to see an improvement. If no improvement has occurred, take your child back to the same doctor or nurse. If this is not possible, explain that you have already spoken to or seen Nurse X or Dr Y, and when that was.
- If you need to change or cancel an appointment, phone the service and say so. Don't just 'not go'; someone else may well be grateful for your appointment time.
- Respond to routine reminders about vaccinations or other health checks. While these are recommended, none is compulsory; if you really don't want to participate after being fully informed, you can ask to be taken off the recall system.

After-hours services

All primary care providers must have arrangements in place for their enrolled patients to be seen outside normal hours. Although many primary care practices are now open into the evening and at times over the weekend, very few are open 24 hours a day.

In urban and suburban areas, acute care is usually available outside normal hours from an after-hours clinic. In some places, all the GPs in the area work rotating shifts in the local after-hours clinic; in other areas, after-hours services are provided by commercial companies employing full-time permanent medical and nursing staff. Some clinics close between 11 p.m. and 7 or 8 a.m., and redirect patients to the local hospital emergency department during those times.

After-hours clinics are not ideal for routine or non-urgent medical care, because you have little choice as to which nurse or doctor you will see, you cannot usually follow up with the same staff, and your health records are often not accessible. In an acute situation, however, after-hours services can provide the prompt attention you need.

In rural areas, acute care outside normal hours is more often provided directly by local nurses and GPs, who take turns to provide an after-hours service. Because of the wide geographic area they cover, you may have to travel some distance to see them. When you have young children, it makes sense to have a reliable vehicle or other means of transport readily available for use in an emergency.

Registering the birth

The law in New Zealand requires that all births be recorded with the Registrar of Births, Deaths and Marriages as soon as possible, as this is the first official step that confirms your child is a New Zealand citizen. As a parent, you are responsible for completing the form provided with your baby's *Well Child/ Tamariki Ora health book*. Alternatively, you can get a form from regional offices of Births, Deaths and Marriages. The form should be posted to the Births, Deaths and Marriages Office in Lower Hutt, using the envelope enclosed with it. Registration is free, but you will have to pay for a birth certificate.

The registration form requires the full name, date of birth, ethnicity, place of birth and usual occupation or job of both natural parents (if known), and the full name, date of birth, sex, ethnicity and place of birth of the child. It requires the signature of at least one of the parents. If the parents are not married to each other and the father's details are to be included, both must sign the form.

If the birth is not registered, your child will not be able (among other things) to get a birth certificate or a passport, enrol in childcare or pre-school, or receive any benefits he may be entitled to.

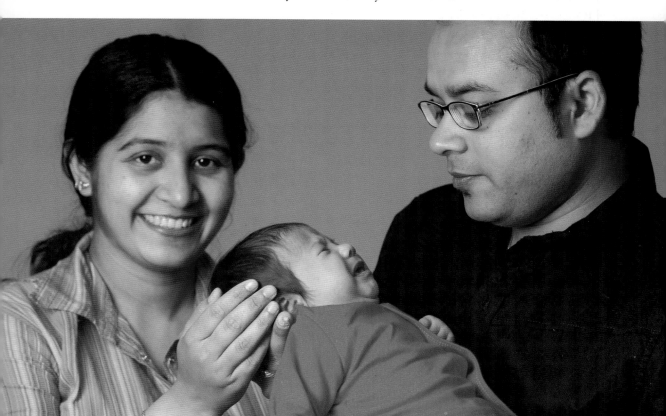

7. Life with a baby

Looking after yourself

Exercise

How are you getting on with the post-natal exercises you started in the first few days after the birth? Are your abdominal muscles nice and firm, your pelvic floor muscles strong, and your weight back to its pre-pregnancy level? If not, don't despair – most women find it quite hard to exercise regularly with a new baby.

But exercise does help, even if you do only a little bit. It's never too late to start, even though it may now be many weeks since the birth. The exercises described in Chapter 7 (pp.323–326) are still well worth starting and carrying on with. It's wise to begin slowly and build up gradually, but by about six weeks you can do as much moderate exercise as you can manage.

As you regain your pre-pregnancy fitness, go to the next level in strengthening your abdominal, back and leg muscles. Swiss ball exercises, Pilates-type exercises and swimming will all help to achieve this, and regular exercise regimes and classes can be resumed or started. If you find it difficult to get out with a young baby, look for good exercise DVDs you can play at home. Walking is a great way to exercise at a pace you are comfortable with, as well as getting you out and about again.

Be careful about lifting heavy or awkward objects until your back and abdominal muscles are back to full strength. The suggestions for lifting (see box on p.402) may be useful even if you haven't had a Caesarean.

When is it safe to start exercising more vigorously again?

You will probably be eager to get back into shape. As long as you return to your pre-pregnancy exercise routines gradually, following the advice given above, you can safely resume exercise and feel the better for it.

But be aware of the extra fatigue levels that result from childbirth and caring for a small baby. Some women who start too vigorously find they have to reduce the amount and intensity of exercise, and build up more gradually. Make sure you don't do any high-impact exercise until you know that your pelvic floor and abdominal muscles have recovered their strength. Because it takes a while for your hormonal levels to return to normal, especially if you are fully breastfeeding, it can take at least three months, and sometimes longer, for everything to return to normal – although between six and 12 weeks you should be aware of a steady improvement. If this is not the case, or if you feel things are taking much longer than you expected, discuss this with your health care provider and/or physiotherapist.

What about exercise and breastfeeding?

Moderate-intensity exercise during lactation does not negatively affect the quantity or composition of breast milk. Really high-intensity exercise may affect milk production in some women, so keeping exercise at moderate levels is best.[29] Even when doing light exercise, make sure your bra fits well and provides good support for your larger-than-normal breasts, especially in the first months (see p.168).

'One of the things I enjoyed most with my first baby was long walks with the pushchair (and before that the pram). I'd think nothing of a two-hour walk most afternoons, and she came to expect it…of course, it's much harder to do with two children, but now we tend to go the park or the beach instead.'

Exercising after a Caesarean

It's important to take things very easily in the first three weeks following a Caesarean. Have someone to help you for at least part of the day, and have a rest as soon as you feel tired – not later.

After any pregnancy, the abdominal muscles take time to regain their firmness and strength, and need protecting for at least six weeks after delivery. With a Caesarean, these muscles have suffered the additional trauma of being separated and then sewn together again. It takes longer for them to heal well, and they need extra protection for about 12 weeks. Wear clothes that give your tummy good support, such as bike pants or sports pants.

Remember that you are not exempt from doing pelvic floor exercises just because you have had a Caesarean birth! Have another look at the section on pelvic floor exercises and tummy tucks (see pp.126–133). Start with the pelvic floor exercises and see if you can manage a tummy tuck within a few days. To begin with, it will be easier to do these exercises lying on your side, and then progress to sitting or standing while doing them.

Lifting after a Caesarean

- Don't lift anything heavier than your baby for the first six weeks.
- Use a trolley for carrying the washing, or split the load into several smaller, lighter ones.
- Lift small loads from bench height if possible.
- If you do have to lift from the ground, do so with your knees bent and your back straight.
- Get someone else to carry the shopping and empty the baby's bath.
- Drive only very short distances in the first four weeks, and get help with lifting car seats or prams in and out of the car.
- From about six weeks, gradually build up your exercise and activity levels. You can expect to be back at your normal levels about three months after a Caesarean.

Weight loss

Many women worry about losing weight in the months after birth. Weight gain during pregnancy is normal, and some of the gain is extra fat laid down to meet the extra nutritional needs of pregnancy and breastfeeding. Originally, this was to help women get through times of critical food shortage. These days, serious food shortages are unlikely to occur in New Zealand, so the extra weight must be gradually lost after pregnancy. For most women, this takes several months.

Exercise and breastfeeding will help this process, although some women find that they get very hungry when breastfeeding so it's not easy to lose weight. Even though it's tempting, try to avoid snacking on sweets, cakes and biscuits when you're hungry, and get the extra energy you require from larger portions of fruit and vegetables, breads and cereals. Breastfeeding is an energy-intensive process, so strict weight-loss diets are inappropriate. Instead, it's best to aim for healthy eating habits that can be maintained long term (see pp.20 and 134).

Above all, try not to put unrealistic expectations on yourself. As a new mother, you have a responsible full-time job with lots of unpredictable demands, and this can be stressful. New babies tend to become unsettled if their mother is tense or worried, which in turn can create more stress and unhappiness. Additional worries about your weight are not going to help anyone, so you may need to accept being a larger size – for the time being at least.

Clothes for you

Suddenly, with the birth of your child, your body has changed dramatically and your clothing needs are completely different. Often it's not just a matter of stepping neatly into your pre-pregnancy clothes. You may be breastfeeding, you may be several sizes bigger – but you still want to look attractive.

Most women take some months to return to their pre-pregnancy size, so tracksuits, knit-fabric tops, loose shirts, and stretchy skirts and trousers are popular choices in the meantime.

Clothes to make you feel good

After months of being pregnant, most women enjoy getting back into 'normal' clothes. You may find that buying something new gives you a much-needed lift. If you can, get someone to look after your baby for an hour or two, go into town, and treat yourself to an attractive top or maybe just a new scarf. If you take your baby with you, most shop assistants will be more than happy to hold him while you try something on, as long as you choose a quiet time (such as mid-morning on a weekday).

It's perfectly possible to buy attractive but practical clothes that don't cost a fortune – and looking good may spur you on to continue those tummy-flattening exercises! Internet shopping is also a good way to find great new clothes that have been designed especially for breastfeeding women. (See Appendix: Breastfeeding.)

> **Clothes suitable for breastfeeding**
>
> When breastfeeding, remember that suitable clothes:
>
> - can be fashionable and flattering
> - should be roomy but not baggy around the bust area, as you will probably have larger breasts for a while
> - should either open up easily down the front, or be able to be lifted up with little fuss. A row of small buttons down the front may look pretty, but will be hard to undo with one hand while you're holding your hungry baby in the other. T-shirts and sweatshirts offer a much simpler alternative, and new styles enable you to breastfeed discreetly. Breastfeeding singlets, with an opening over each breast, can be a good option, worn under a shirt
> - should be tough enough to withstand the firm grip of your baby's hands (more than one favourite necklace has come adrift in this way)
> - should be easy to wash and care for – there won't be a lot of time in your day for fiddly ironing
> - should be able to cope with milk stains, although you can minimise this by using disposable nursing pads or a folded hankie or small cloth inside your bra.

'For me the key is to not be too idealistic. So many people have this ideal of how everything should be. But babies don't do that – they just do what they want to do, when they want to do it.'

'Dinnertime's one of the best times. She sits up in the high chair with the boys on either side of her. We all discuss our day and what was the best thing that happened. She just sits there and stares at the boys and watches them eating; they talk to her and it's so nice…And because my husband works shifts, he's often here with the kids during the day – he's not just seeing them when they're tired at night.'

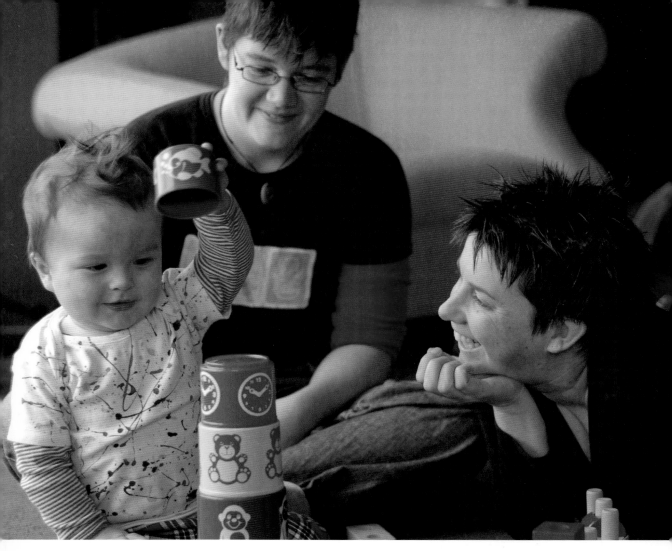

Enjoying your baby

So, in the end, has it all been worth it? Is life with a new baby rewarding – or perhaps not quite as you'd imagined…?

You might have the feeling, if you've read this far, that having a baby is a daunting prospect, full of pitfalls for the unwary. To some extent this is true, but most of the time becoming a parent is tremendously rewarding, and many people have been amazed at how much joy their baby has brought them.

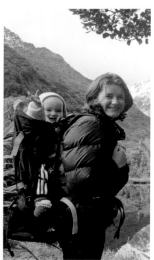

Anna's story: Three small children

Even though Margot is my third baby, I've still had the chance to have a bit of that 'bubble time' with her – that wonderful time after you've had a baby when there are no expectations on you. You can just hang out with the baby; people send you gifts and flowers, and pop around with a meal or baking. Even though people's lives seem so frantic, there's still this wonder about a child being born, especially a first baby. As a mother, you know that this bubble of time isn't going to last forever, and I think for each baby, it's smaller.

The first week at home is amazing – despair, wonder, the works. After our first baby Nadya was born, we stayed one night in hospital and it was all fine. So we brought her home, thinking to ourselves: oh, this is easy. And then she just screamed all night. Both of us were at a complete loss – what is this thing we've brought home? What do we do now? Breastfeeding was no good because my milk hadn't come in. My body was just going 'oh-oh' after the incredible adrenalin rush of giving birth, and poor Jeremy was sleepless too … Fortunately, both my mother and aunt were staying and in the end my aunt just took Nadya away and walked her round for an hour, rubbing her back.

But then there are all the wonderful times with a new baby. When they're asleep, and they turn into china dolls, the most perfect little creatures you've ever seen. And when you go out and see people, or you're in the supermarket and someone leans over and goes, 'Oh, that's a really new baby'. You're so proud! Even though all you did was pop them out, you're amazingly proud of how beautiful they are. And walking in the howling wind and rain with the baby all wrapped up in a front pack, snug and warm. When they smile for the first time and for the next 20,000 times. It never ceases to be amazing that there's this person who loves you so absolutely and unconditionally.

Before you have a baby, no one tells you how many hours you're going to spend sitting on a couch breastfeeding, with a peg on your bra to help you remember which side you're up to! No book prepares you for that, and all the mountains of washing you have to do, and for the wonder of it all. With all the babies, I've felt how lucky I am to have that time with them. You can't do anything else when you're breastfeeding: you just sit there, and look at them and love them.

It's really special to have that time with Margot right now. When the other kids have gone to bed at night, it's just her and me and Jeremy. She gets to be the only baby for a while, which is lovely for her and for us. But I try to have a bit of time with each of them on their own every day so they all feel equally important. Even if it's just a chore, like going to the shops, you can turn it into a really nice time together.

Sometimes you get overwhelmed. In amongst all the wonderful times, there are some really hard times too. When there are three kids screaming in the car, you just think – how did it come to this? It always seems to be when you want to do something nice for them, like taking them to the pool or the library. You expect them to be thrilled that you're going out of your way to do this special thing for them. Then when you get there, the kids are grumpy, nothing's working, they get hungry, you pack them back in the car and everyone screams all the way home. Usually, it's because you've tried to do too much with them – it's really hard not to fall into the trap of thinking they need all these activities. And, like everyone who tries to juggle paid work with babies, there are times when I'm really busy or stressed out and I'm not very nice with the kids.

When things have been hard, I've tended to turn to other women for support. The Plunket nurse was great at weighing and measuring and saying the babies were growing as they should, but I've mostly relied on my mother and other women I met through antenatal classes or already knew. Because I've been working as well, I never felt like I had to go to these groups just to meet people – I was always interacting with people through work. But it was still really good to be part of those groups where mums meet other mums.

After your baby is born, I think it takes quite a long time to feel like you're still an individual and not only a mother. It can take a while before you even want to be a separate person – I think Nadya was about two before I ever spent a night away from her. And the whole time, I was thinking: what's she doing, what's she thinking, is she OK without me? For quite a while, you just want to be part of that other little person.

It can also be a challenge to see yourselves as a couple, as well as parents. For Jeremy and me, it's so alien now to imagine not having little children around who need you all the time – what on earth did we do before we had them? And it's a struggle sometimes to tell yourself: I'm not just this scruffy person who sits around breastfeeding all day, I can still be attractive to someone else! It does happen eventually, though.

Physically, I've learnt to really listen to my body in the first three months. All these very well-meaning people come to see you – one day, there were about ten lots of people through the house. Even if they bring food, you still end up making them a cup of tea and then doing dishes and making the next person a cup of tea and then someone else arrives … You end up drinking all this tea, but you never have a proper meal! Now if anyone I know has a baby, I always take them food and just leave it on the doorstep until they're ready for visitors. It's also important to make a fuss over the older children – perhaps with a present – before turning your attention to the new arrival. Just after Nadya was born, I was rushing around and so excited about showing her to everyone. But almost straight away, I got mastitis and then the same thing happened about three weeks later. My body was just saying: don't do too much, just hang out at home and let people come to you. So now I know the signs and recognise when I need to slow down. Sometimes, the thing you need to do most is to sleep when the baby's asleep, but that's hard to do in practice. I think it feels quite strange to go to bed in the middle of the day, especially when it's the only time you have for yourself all day. But really, sometimes I know I should just lie down and cuddle up with the baby and sleep rather than clean the house or make phone calls.

With each baby, I've recovered from the birth itself much more quickly. I think my body's worked it out in some way. But as far as getting my figure back, well it's the other way. After Nadya it was really easy, after William it was okay but with Margot – well, I'm not worried about it, but I can see that it's not going to happen as quickly.

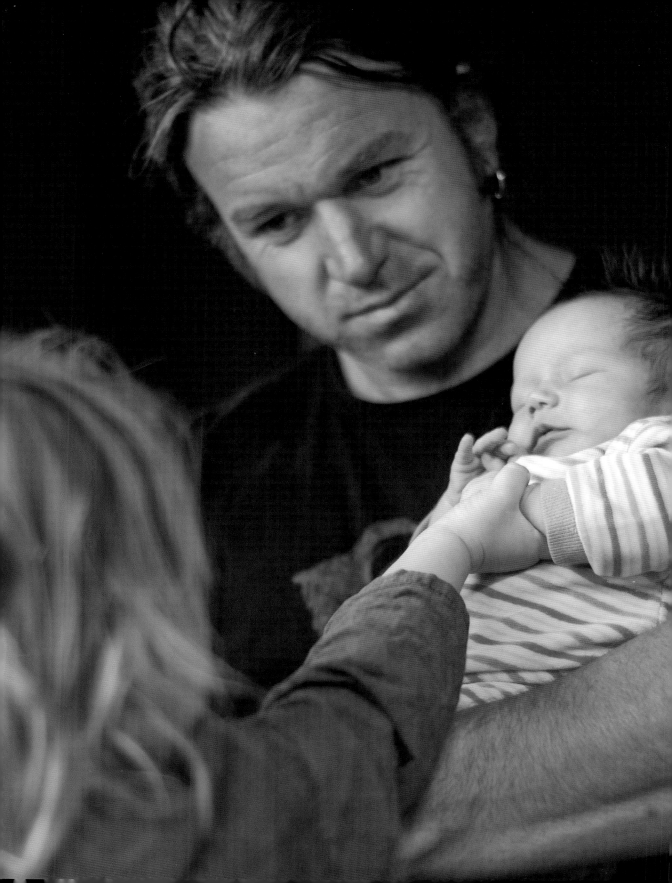

APPENDIX: USEFUL WEBSITES AND ORGANISATIONS

Adoption

Adoption Services is part of Child, Youth and Family (CYF, a service of the Ministry of Social Development), and provides advice and services relating to adoption both within New Zealand and from other countries. There are CYF Adoption Services offices throughout the country; all can be contacted by calling the freephone number.

www.cyf.govt.nz/adoptions.htm

Freephone: 0508 FAMILY
(0508 326 459)

Alcohol

For information and resources about alcohol use in pregnancy, see the website of the Alcohol Advisory Council of New Zealand (ALAC):

www.alac.org.nz/Pregnancy

The Alcohol Drug Helpline is a confidential information, referral and intervention service funded by the Alcohol Advisory Council and the Ministry of Health.

www.adanz.org.nz/Helpline

Freephone: 0800 787 797
(10 a.m. to 10 p.m. daily)

Antenatal care – see LMCs; Midwives; Doctors

Antenatal classes – see Pregnancy and parenting classes

Breastfeeding

La Leche League New Zealand is part of an international organisation that helps mothers to breastfeed by providing mother-to-mother support, education, information and advocacy. There are La Leche League support groups throughout New Zealand. For contact details, see:

www.lalecheleague.org.nz

The website of the NZ Lactation Consultants Association provides contact details of certificated lactation consultants throughout New Zealand:

www.nzlca.org.nz

Information and advice (including online antenatal education) is available from:

www.breast-feeding.co.nz

Clothes suitable for breastfeeding can be purchased online from several retailers, including:

www.mummymatters.co.nz/new_stocks.htm

Car seats

Information on buying, installing and using child restraints is available from Safe2Go, a programme funded by ACC and Land Transport New Zealand. There are Safe2Go technicians throughout New Zealand who can help fit a child restraint suitable for your vehicle and child. For details, see:

www.safe2go.co.nz

Tel: 09 827 6182

Car Seat Rentals – see Plunket; Well Child/Tamariki Ora

Cervical smears/testing

The National Cervical Screening Programme aims to reduce the incidence and effect of and deaths from cancer of the cervix by detecting pre-cancerous cervical changes, thus enabling appropriate and effective treatment. The programme is delivered by a large number of health providers. The various aspects of the programme are coordinated by the National Screening Unit:

www.nsu.govt.nz

Child, Youth and Family (CYF)

CYF is a service of the Ministry of Social Development. It works to ensure the well-being and safety of children, and supports positive parenting.

www.cyf.govt.nz

Freephone: 0508 FAMILY
(0508 326 459)

Citizens Advice Bureau – see Financial support/advice for families

Consumer NZ

An independent, non-profit organisation that tests and researches a wide range of consumer products, including baby equipment. Its monthly *Consumer* magazine is available by subscription and from public libraries.

www.consumer.org.nz

CPR (cardio-pulmonary resuscitation)

The following organisations provide CPR information and training:

New Zealand Resuscitation Council:
www.nzrc.org.nz

Red Cross:
www.redcross.org.nz

St John Ambulance:
www.stjohn.org.nz

Surf Lifesaving Associations:
www.slsnz.org.nz

Well Child/Tamariki Ora:
www.wellchild.org.nz

Disability

Parent to Parent (Matua ki te Matua) New Zealand is a support and information network for parents of children with special needs. Voluntary support is provided by trained parents who have a child with the same or similar needs.

www.parent2parent.org.nz

National Office: 07 853 8491 or freephone 0508 236 236

District Health Boards (DHBs)

DHBs are funded by the Ministry of Health to provide primary, secondary and tertiary health services to the population in their (geographically defined) area. The websites for all DHBs can be found at:

www.dhbnz.org.nz

www.moh.govt.nz

Doctors

The Medical Council of New Zealand registers doctors; oversees their practice standards, conduct and competence; and promotes professional education and training. Its website has an online register enabling people to check a doctor's registration; it also provides information about the patient/doctor relationship, the standards that doctors must meet, and how to make a complaint about a doctor.

www.mcnz.org.nz

Freephone: 0800 286 801

The Royal Australian and New Zealand College of Obstetricians and Gynaecologists (RANZCOG) trains and accredits obstetricians and gynaecologists in both countries. It also supports research into women's health and acts as an advocate for women's health care. Its website lists obstetricians, gynaecologists and GP obstetricians by area.

>www.ranzcog.edu.au
>Tel: 04 472 4608
>(Executive Officer, New Zealand Regional Committee)

The Royal New Zealand College of General Practitioners (RNZCGP) trains and accredits general practitioners (GPs). It supports research on and promotes many aspects of general practice and primary health care.

>www.rnzcgp.org.nz

Doulas

A 'doula' is a trained laywoman paid to support mothers and families during the birth and postnatal period. For more information and contact details, see:

>www.kiwifamilies.co.nz/Topics/ Pregnancy/Doula
>www.organicbaby.co.nz/articles/ pregnancy/doula

Equipment and clothing – see Car seats; Consumer NZ; Monitors; Nappies

Family doctors – see Doctors; General practitioners; Primary health organisations

Family planning/sexual health – see also Sexual health

Family Planning (the Family Planning Association) is a non-profit charitable organisation providing sexual and reproductive health information, clinical services, education, training and research.

>www.fpanz.org.nz
>Helpline: 0800 FPA LINE
>(0800 372 5463)

Fertility awareness

Natural Fertility NZ Inc. is a non-profit organisation that provides information and teaching about natural family planning and fertility awareness. Fertility educators are based throughout New Zealand; for contact details, see website:

>www.naturalfertility.co.nz
>Freephone: 0800 178 637
>Email: info@naturalfertility.co.nz

Financial support/advice for families

Citizens Advice Bureau is an independent community organisation providing information, advice, advocacy and support to individuals. There are bureaux in 90 locations in New Zealand, and also a freephone service.

>www.cab.org.nz
>Freephone: 0800 FOR CAB
>(0800 367 222)

Work and Income is part of the Ministry of Social Development, and administers benefits and a range of other services (such as childcare subsidies).

>www.workandincome.govt.nz
>Freephone: 0800 559 009

Working for Families is a tax credit scheme provided by Work and Income and the Inland Revenue Department.

>www.workingforfamilies.govt.nz
>Freephone: 0800 227 773

General practitioners (GPs) – see also Doctors; Primary health organisations

For local GPs and other doctors, see the front section of your White Pages telephone book, under 'Registered Medical Practitioners and Medical Centres'.

Health and Disability Commissioner

This independent agency was established under the Health and Disability Commissioner Act 1994 to promote and protect the rights of consumers of health and disability services, and to help resolve problems between consumers and providers. The Commissioner enforces the Code of Health and Disability Services Consumers' Rights.

>www.hdc.org.nz
>Freephone: 0800 11 22 33

Health professionals' education & qualifications – see Doctors; Midwives

Healthline

A free 24-hour health advice telephone service staffed by registered nurses and funded by the Ministry of Health. It includes the Well Child telephone advice service.

>Freephone: 0800 611 116

Hearing Testing Programme for all Newborns

This countrywide programme for newborn babies is delivered by the National Screening Unit (a unit of the Ministry of Health).

>www.nsu.govt.nz

Home Birth Aotearoa

This national organisation represents local home birth associations throughout New Zealand. The website provides the contact details of those associations, and of midwives offering a home birth service.

>www.homebirth.org.nz

Homeopathy

For information about homeopathy and homeopathic practitioners in New Zealand:

>www.homeopathy.co.nz

For information on Bach flower remedies (which include Rescue Remedy) used by some women in pregnancy and labour:

>www.bachcentre.com

Human Rights Commission

For information about your rights during pregnancy, especially in relation to employment, see:

>www.hrc.co.nz

Infertility

The New Zealand Infertility Society (also known as Fertility New Zealand) is a non-profit, consumer-based organisation which offers support, networking services, information and advocacy to anyone with an interest in fertility issues.

>www.fertilitynz.org.nz
>Freephone: 0800 333 306

Fertility Associates is a private provider of fertility diagnosis, support and treatment, with three treatment clinics and peripheral consultation clinics throughout the North Island.

>www.fertilityassociates.co.nz
>Tel: 09 520 9520 (Auckland clinic)

Lactation consultants – see Breastfeeding

LMCs (lead maternity carers) – see also Doctors; Midwives

Details of LMCs in your area are available through the maternity consumer phone line run by the Ministry of Health.

>Freephone: 0800 MUM 2 BE
>(0800 686 223)

Māori health providers

Māori health providers deliver health and disability services predominantly (but not exclusively) to Māori clients, using a distinctively Māori kaupapa and delivery framework. A directory of providers is available from the Ministry of Health:

>www.maorihealth.govt.nz/moh.nsf/ menuma/Maori+Health+Providers

Medicines

Medsafe is the independent monitoring agency responsible for the safety of prescription drugs and medical devices in New Zealand. It is a business unit of the Ministry of Health, and its website has useful information on medicines and medical devices.

> www.medsafe.govt.nz

Mental health – see also District Health Boards (DHBs); Mothers Online; Post-traumatic stress disorder

District Health Boards provide services for women in their region who have mental health needs related to pregnancy, childbirth and parenting. See, for example, the Auckland District Health Board website:

> www.adhb.govt.nz/NWHealthInfo/
> MaternityServices/mental_health.htm

Midwives – see also LMCs (lead maternity carers)

The Midwifery Council of New Zealand oversees midwifery training, qualifications and practice. It publishes an online register of midwives, listing the name, location and practising status of every registered midwife in New Zealand. It also provides information about the standards that midwives must meet, and how to make a complaint about a midwife.

> www.midwiferycouncil.org.nz
> Tel: 04 499 7979

Miscarriage

Miscarriage Support Auckland Inc. is an independent group of volunteers who have themselves experienced miscarriage. They provide support and information for women and their families during and after miscarriage, and during subsequent pregnancies. Their website has helpful resources and contact details of miscarriage support groups throughout the country; they also provide support by phone and email, and run an Internet bulletin board.

> www.miscarriage.org.nz
> Supportline: 09 378 4060
> Bulletin board: www2.everybody.co.nz/
> bulletinboard.html

Monitors

For information about baby monitors:

> www.consumer.org.nz

For information about apnoea monitors:

> www.sids.org.nz

Mothers Online

This website offers a chat-room, discussion groups, articles, expert advice, and directories of products and services. It covers a wide range of subjects associated with pregnancy, birth, parenting and women's health, including confidence, self-esteem, relationships and depression.

> www.mothersonline.co.nz

Multiple Birth Association

This national body supports parents who are expecting or raising 'multiples'. Its website provides contact details of local clubs throughout the country.

> www.nzmba.info
> Freephone: 0800 4 TWINS ETC
> (0800 489 467)

Nappies

Online suppliers of new reusable nappies include:

> 100% NZ suppliers:
> www.econappies.co.nz
> www.yoyonappy.com

> Other popular suppliers:
> www.snazzipants.co.nz
> www.honeychild.co.nz
> www.fuzzibunz.co.nz

> Sew-your-own patterns:
> www.greenbeans.co.nz

> Washing products:
> www.ecover.com/au/en/Products/

> Local councils offering cash-back or hire schemes for cloth nappies include the Kaikoura District Council (www.kaikoura.govt.nz) and Waitakere City Council (www.waitakere.govt.nz).

National Screening Unit

A unit set up by the Ministry of Health to oversee current national screening programmes (e.g. cervical screening, newborn hearing programme, newborn metabolic testing, HIV testing in pregnancy) and to investigate possible new programmes.

> www.nsu.govt.nz

Parental leave

The Department of Labour website provides basic information about the rights and obligations of employees, employers and self-employed people. An online calculator allows you to work out your own parental leave entitlement.

> www.ers.dol.govt.nz/parentalleave
> Freephone: 0800 20 90 20

Parents Centre

A nationwide volunteer-based organisation with 52 centres offering wide-ranging support and education on all aspects of parenting, from pre-birth to school age. It is the largest provider of childbirth education and antenatal support in New Zealand, and has more than 120 qualified childbirth educators. The website provides contact details of all Parents Centres in the country.

> www.parentscentre.org.nz
> Tel: 04 233 2022 (National Support Team)

Physiotherapy

The website of the New Zealand Society of Physiotherapists Inc. lists qualified physiotherapists by region, and provides information on how physiotherapy can help you to manage pregnancy and childbirth.

> www.physiotherapy.org.nz

Plagiocephaly (flat head syndrome)

Helpful information is available from the UK Institute of Child Health:

> www.ich.ucl.ac.uk/factsheets/families/
> F040171/index.html

Plunket

Plunket (the Royal New Zealand Plunket Society) is New Zealand's largest provider of support services for the development, health and well-being of children under the age of five. It is a non-profit organisation with clinical staff and a volunteer network providing services to help families throughout New Zealand. Those services include **Plunketline**, a free telephone helpline for parents and caregivers (7 a.m. to midnight, seven days a week).

> www.plunket.org.nz
> Plunketline: 0800 933 922

Post-traumatic stress disorder (PTSD)

TABS (Trauma and Birth Stress) is a charitable trust supporting mothers who have experienced stressful or traumatic pregnancies or births.

> www.tabs.org.nz
> P O Box 18002, Glen Innes, Auckland

Pregnancy and parenting classes – see Home Birth Aotearoa; Multiple Birth Association; Parents Centre; Plunket

Wide-ranging antenatal advice is also available via Internet courses, email, CDs and booklets from:

> www.breast-feeding.co.nz

Primary Health Organisations (PHOs)

The Ministry of Health publishes a list of Primary Health Organisations throughout New Zealand, listed by District Health Board.

> www.moh.govt.nz/moh.nsf/indexmh/contact-us-pho
>
> Freephone: 0800 HLTH 4 U
> (0800 252 464)
> to check if you are enrolled in a PHO.

Quitline

This free telephone service offers support, resources and low-cost nicotine patches or gum to New Zealanders wanting to stop smoking. More resources and tools are available on the website.

> www.quit.org.nz
>
> Quitline: 0800 778 778

Reproductive technologies

For information on new developments and research, see the websites of the Ethics Committee on Assisted Reproductive Technology (ECART) and the Advisory Committee on Assisted Reproductive Technology (ACART):

> www.ecart.health.govt.nz
>
> www.acart.health.govt.nz

Section 88

The Ministry of Health's requirements for maternity services are set out in Section 88 of the Public Health and Disability Act 2000. For more information, see:

> www.moh.govt.nz/moh.nsf/indexmh/section88-maternity-notice-2007-feb07

Sexual health

The Ministry of Health website provides information and useful links on a wide range of sexual health matters, including sexually transmitted infections:

> www.moh.govt.nz/sexualhealth

Sexually transmitted infections (STIs)

The New Zealand Herpes Foundation provides support and education for people affected by genital herpes:

> www.herpes.org.nz
>
> Freephone: 0508 11 12 13

The New Zealand HPV Project provides support and education for people affected by the human papilloma virus (genital warts and/or HPV):

> www.hpv.org.nz
>
> Freephone: 0508 11 12 13

SIDS (sudden infant death syndrome, or cot death)

SIDS New Zealand Inc. is a national organisation of parents, families and friends of children who have died suddenly and/or unexpectedly of any cause, including SIDS. It provides services and support for families and communities.

> www.sids.org.nz
>
> Freephone: 0800 164 455

Smoking cessation – see Quitline

Special needs – see Disability

Stillbirth and neonatal deaths

The Stillbirth and Neonatal Death Support Association (SANDS) is a voluntary organisation set up and run by parents to support other parents and families who have experienced the death of a baby. For details of SANDS support groups and contact people throughout the country, see the website:

> www.sands.org.nz

Termination of pregnancy (abortion) – see also Family planning/sexual health

Women intending to have a termination can find information on New Zealand's abortion law, abortion counselling, available methods of abortion, and how to access abortion services in different regions of New Zealand at this website:

> www.abortion.gen.nz

Unplanned pregnancy

For information on available options, see:

> www.fpanz.org.nz/OurClinics/NeedHelpNow/UnplannedPregnancy/tabid/338/Default.aspx

Vaccination

The Immunisation Advisory Centre, based at the University of Auckland, offers independent, factual information on immunisation and vaccine-preventable disease. All information is based on international and New Zealand medical research and is supported by a large network of health professionals.

> www.immune.org.nz
>
> Freephone: 0800 IMMUNE
> (0800 466 863)

Well Child/Tamariki Ora

Under the government's Well Child/Tamariki Ora Framework, screening, education and support services are available to all New Zealand children (aged 0–5) and their families/whānau. The services help families to improve and protect their children's health, and are provided by registered nurses and community health workers with specific training in child health.

> www.wellchild.org.nz
>
> www.plunket.org.nz

Women's Refuge

This independent community organisation provides services for women and children facing violence, including 24-hour access to emergency accommodation. Their website has resources for people who are thinking about leaving a violent relationship, people who already have left, and those wanting to help others stay safe. It also provides contact details of local Refuges.

> www.womensrefuge.org.nz

Work and Income – see Financial support/advice for families

Working for Families – see Financial support/advice for families

GLOSSARY AND ABBREVIATIONS

A

Abdomen Region of body between chest and pelvis; tummy.

Acne Skin condition characterised by pimples and blackheads, common in teenagers.

Acupuncture/acupressure Chinese method of clinical treatment which usually involves pressure over, or placement of small needles at, identified acupuncture points in the body.

Afoetal sac A fluid-filled sac that persists after a foetus dies very early in pregnancy.

Afterbirth See Placenta.

AIDS Acquired immunodeficiency syndrome. An infectious, eventually fatal disease, resulting from infection by the human immunodeficiency virus (see HIV).

Alpha fetoprotein A substance found in the mother's blood which is abnormally high if the foetus has one of certain types of spina bifida or related conditions.

Alveoli Tiny grape-like structures within the breast where milk is made and collected. (There are also alveoli in the lungs, which have a somewhat similar structure.)

Amniocentesis A method of collecting a sample of amniotic fluid from a pregnant woman.

Amniotic fluid The fluid surrounding the foetus, and contained by the membranes. Also known as 'waters'.

Anaemia Condition where the number of healthy red cells in the blood is too low. This may be due to a lack of iron, but there are many other possible causes.

Anaesthetic Can be either a general anaesthetic (GA), where consciousness is reduced so that all sensation is absent, or a local anaesthetic, where sensation is reduced in part of the body.

Anaesthetist A doctor with postgraduate training and qualifications in anaesthetics.

Anencephaly A type of neural tube defect. A fault of early development of the brain. See also NTD.

Anorexia nervosa An eating disorder, which can have serious consequences. Sufferers often have poor self-esteem and a distorted body perception, which results in extreme weight loss.

Antacid A type of medication which helps neutralise the acid in the stomach and eases heartburn.

Antenatal Before birth.

Antepartum haemorrhage See APH.

Anterior To the front.

Anterior lip (of the cervix) Last area of the cervix to retract out of the baby's way during the transition phase of labour.

Anteverted uterus A uterus in its normal position, tipped forward within the pelvis.

Antibiotics Class of drugs which combat bacterial infection.

Anti-D Substance administered to Rhesus-negative women to prevent Rhesus disease.

Antihistamines Class of drugs used to treat allergies. Can also be used as a sedative and to prevent travel sickness.

Anus Posterior opening of the bowel. Back passage.

APH Antepartum haemorrhage. Bleeding from the uterus during pregnancy.

Areola Dark area surrounding the nipple.

ARM Artificial rupture of the membranes that contain the fluid ('waters') surrounding the foetus.

ART Assisted reproduction technologies. The range of artificial techniques available to assist people to achieve a pregnancy. Includes donor insemination (DI) IVF, GIFT and surrogacy.

Atherosclerosis Hardening of the arteries. A disease process where material is laid down within the arteries, making them narrower than normal, and more prone to blockages which can reduce or stop blood flow to vital organs.

B

Bacterial vaginosis (BV) An imbalance in the normal bacteria of the vagina, which may cause a vaginal discharge. Has been associated with miscarriage and premature birth.

BCG Vaccine used to prevent tuberculosis.

Bicornuate uterus Uterus partially divided in two as a result of its development at the embryo stage.

Bilirubin Substance normally produced by the liver, and passed into the intestine. If too much is produced, or its normal passage is blocked, it accumulates in the blood and causes jaundice.

Blastocyst Collection of cells which forms once a human egg is fertilised. It becomes two groups of cells, and some fluid. One of the groups of cells becomes the embryo, and the other group becomes the future placenta.

Blood pressure Pressure of the blood within the circulatory system.

BMI Body mass index. Weight in kilograms divided by height in metres squared. A method of estimating whether a person's weight for height is ideal, too low (underweight) or too high (overweight). An approximate measure only, as it does not properly account for muscle mass, body type or ethnic variation.

Braxton-Hicks contractions Mild contractions of the uterus which occur later in pregnancy.

Breech Position of foetus lying within the uterus with its bottom towards the cervix and its head toward the fundus (top of the uterus). See also Extended breech, Flexed breech.

Bronchitis Inflammation of the bronchial tubes within the lungs. Can cause coughing and difficulty with breathing. Chronic bronchitis is common in smokers, and is sometimes known as COPD.

Bulimia Self-induced vomiting associated with poor self-esteem. Often part of a cycle of binge eating and vomiting. An eating disorder, related to anorexia nervosa.

C

Caesarean section Operation in which a baby is delivered through a surgical incision in the mother's abdomen.

Cancer A disease process whereby a group of cells replicates in a disordered manner and can spread to distant parts of the body. If left unchecked, many cancers will eventually be fatal.

Cannula Small hollow tube, usually made of flexible plastic.

Cardio-pulmonary resuscitation See CPR.

Cardiotocograph See CTG.

Carpal tunnel syndrome Tingling and numbness in the thumb and index finger of the hand, caused by pressure on the nerve that runs through the narrow carpal tunnel at the wrist.

CBC Complete blood count. See FBC.

Catheter (urinary) Flexible, hollow plastic tube inserted into the bladder to keep it empty by continuously draining away the urine.

CDH Congenital dislocation of the hip. Condition in which the hip joint in a baby is unstable because of lax ligaments and an unusually shallow cup in the hip bone into which the head of the femur (thigh bone) sits.

Cephalic presentation Position of the foetus lying within the uterus with its head presenting at the cervix. Normal presentation.

Cervical os Opening in the cervix.

Cervix Entrance to the uterus, situated at the top of the vagina.

Chlamydia A common sexually transmitted infection (STI) which may cause infertility, or be passed on to a baby during birth.

CHD Congenital heart disease. Malformations within the heart which have occurred in the embryo phase of development.

Chorionic villus biopsy Procedure in which a sample is taken from the placental tissue in early pregnancy.

Chromosome Structure within the nucleus of every living cell which carries the genetic code for that cell. In humans, there are normally 46 chromosomes in every cell.

Circumcision Removal of the foreskin from the penis.

Cleft palate Malformation of the roof of the mouth, often associated with a malformation of the upper lip.

CMV Cytomegalovirus. A virus which is sometimes responsible for miscarriage.

COC Combined oral contraceptive pill. Contains two hormones, oestrogen and progestagen.

Colic Term used to describe spasmodic abdominal pain.

Colicky Term often used to describe an unsettled, crying baby who possibly has tummy pain.

Colostrum Rich yellow breast milk, containing immunoglobulins. Produced within the breast from as early as 16 weeks of pregnancy, increasing in late pregnancy and immediately after birth.

Combined oral contraceptive pill See COC.

Combined spinal-epidural See CSE.

Computerised tomography See CT.

Congenital dislocation of the hips See CDH.

Congenital heart disease See CHD.

Conjunctivitis Inflammation of the thin clear tissue that lines the eyelids and the eyeball.

Constipation Condition in which faeces are hard, making it difficult to empty the bowel.

Contraception Method of preventing conception (pregnancy).

Contractions (of the uterus) Coordinated tightening of the muscles within the uterus wall during labour in order to bring about the birth of a baby.

Cord (umbilical) Structure that connects the foetus to the placenta within the uterus.

Corpus luteum Fluid-filled sac left behind in the ovary after an egg is released at ovulation.

CPR Cardio-pulmonary resuscitation, or 'rescue breathing'. A method of restarting breathing and circulation in someone who has stopped breathing.

Cranial stenosis A condition where the bones of the skull fuse together too early in an infant or small child, restricting normal brain growth and development.

CSE Combined spinal-epidural. Used during labour to alleviate pain. An anaesthetic drug is inserted both into and around the spinal cord to decrease sensation in the lower half of the body. See also Epidural (anaesthetic).

CT Computerised tomography. A type of x-ray using multiple computer images.

CTG Cardiotocograph. A graphic recording of the foetal heartbeat and the mother's uterine contractions during pregnancy and/or labour.

Curette See D&C.

CVS Chorionic villus sampling. A technique for sampling the tissue of part of the placenta (the chorion) during pregnancy.

CYF The Child Youth and Family service, part of the Ministry of Social Development.

Cytogeneticist Genetics specialist. Doctor with postgraduate training and qualifications in genetics and genetic disorders.

Cytomegalovirus See CMV.

D

D&C Dilatation and curettage. A procedure done under general anaesthetic in which the cervix is dilated and the contents of the uterus are scraped out.

Depo-Provera Long-acting progestagen-only contraceptive, given by injection.

Deep vein thrombosis See DVT.

Depression State of mind characterised by persistent feelings of deep sadness, and sometimes by dulling of the senses, altered sleep patterns and altered appetite. Associated with biochemical changes in the brain.

DI Donor insemination. Artificial placing at the cervix of semen from a donor. An assisted reproduction technology treatment for infertility. Also used when intercourse is not appropriate and/or acceptable.

Diabetes (diabetes mellitus or 'sugar diabetes') Condition in which there is a lack of (or resistance of the tissue to) insulin in the body, and sugar cannot be removed normally from the blood.

Diagnostic test A test done to make a specific diagnosis for an individual as accurately as possible. In relation to prenatal testing, to check whether a baby is developing normally, this may be a test such as amniocentesis, which is accurate but carries a small risk for the baby. See also Prenatal testing or prenatal diagnosis, Screening test.

Diarrhoea Loose, frequent, watery bowel motions.

Diastasis Separation. Often referring to separation of the abdominal muscles.

Dilation (of the cervix) The opening up of the cervix in labour.

Diphtheria Infectious disease affecting the respiratory system, which can be fatal in children.

Diuresis Change in kidney function which produces an increased amount of urine.

Donor insemination See DI.

DOSA Day of surgery area.

Down syndrome (Trisomy 21) A condition caused by a defect on the 21st chromosome during early development, resulting in characteristic facial features, and varying degrees of intellectual, cardiac and other disabilities.

DPB Domestic purposes benefit.

Drip See IV line.

DVT Deep vein thrombosis. A blood clot that develops in the deep veins, usually in the leg. See also Pulmonary embolus.

E

EC Emergency contraception. Also known as the 'morning-after pill'. Pills taken after unprotected intercourse to prevent pregnancy.

Eclampsia, pre-eclampsia Disease of pregnancy in which there is high blood pressure, oedema, protein in the urine, and an adverse effect on placental function. In its severe form, pre-eclampsia becomes eclampsia, threatening the life of the baby and/or the mother.

Ectopic (pregnancy) Early pregnancy sac which implants outside the uterus, usually in the fallopian tube.

ECV External cephalic version. A method of turning a breech baby into a head-down position prior to birth.

EDB Estimated date of birth (same as EDD).

EDD Estimated date of delivery (same as EDB).

Effacement Shortening of the cervix in early labour, prior to dilation.

Egg (human) or ovum Sex cell of a woman, released from her ovary during the reproductive cycle.

Embryo Developing baby within the uterus, from implantation to the end of the eighth week of development.

Emergency contraception See EC.

Endometriosis Condition in which fragments of uterine lining (endometrium) are found within the pelvis, outside the uterus, causing pain.

Engagement (of foetal head) Positioning of the head of the foetus in the mother's bony pelvic ring.

Entonox Mixture of air and nitrous oxide, used to dull sensation and lower the level of consciousness. Sometimes used towards the end of labour.

Epidural (anaesthetic) An anaesthetic used during labour to alleviate pain. An anaesthetic drug is inserted around, but not into, the spinal cord to decrease sensation in the lower half of the body. See also CSE.

Episiotomy Cut made in the perineum immediately prior to birth to prevent tearing of the tissue as the baby is born.

Exchange transfusion Replacement of a baby's blood with donated, antibody-free blood. Only a few millilitres of blood can be changed at a time, so a series of small exchanges are done, and this can take 2–3 hours. Part of the treatment for Rhesus disease.

Extended breech Position of the foetus lying in the uterus with its bottom towards the cervix and with straight, extended legs.

External cephalic version See ECV.

F

Faeces Waste material formed in the bowel and expelled from the body through the anus.

Fallopian tube (oviduct) Structure that carries a human egg from the ovary to the uterus.

FASD Foetal alcohol syndrome disorder.

FBC Full blood count. Measure of types and amounts of red and white blood cells in a blood sample. Also called CBC (complete blood count).

Femur The long bone in the upper leg.

Fertility awareness A method of contraception that relies on accurate detection of ovulation and avoidance of sexual intercourse during the fertile time in a woman's menstrual cycle. Knowledge of this technique can also be used to promote conception.

FGR Foetal growth restriction. Also known as IUGR. Slower growth than usual of a foetus within the uterus.

FISH Foetal in-situ hybridisation. A technique for rapidly analysing the results from an amniocentesis.

Flexed breech Position of foetus lying in the uterus with its bottom towards the cervix and with crossed or bent legs.

Foetal growth restriction See FGR.

Foetus Unborn baby within the uterus, from the ninth week of development until birth.

Folic acid A vitamin essential for health. A woman's requirement is increased before and during pregnancy, in order to complete the proper development of the baby's brain and spinal cord.

Follicle Fluid-filled sac within the ovary, containing an egg.

Follicle stimulating hormone See FSH.

Fontanelles Naturally occurring gaps in a baby's skull bones, present at birth and for some months afterwards.

Forceps (obstetric) Thin metal blades, like slim hands, used to assist the baby to move down and out of the birth canal during the second stage of labour.

Foreskin Cover of thin skin around the tip of the penis.

FSH Follicle stimulating hormone. Hormone produced by the pituitary gland, which acts on the ovaries.

Full blood count See FBC.

Fundal height Distance from the symphysis pubis to the top of the uterus in pregnancy.

Fundus (of uterus) Top portion of the uterus.

G

GA General anaesthetic. In which consciousness is reduced so that all sensation is absent.

Gene A genetic message within a chromosome. There are many genes on each chromosome.

General anaesthetic See GA.

General practitioner See GP.

Genetics specialist See Cytogeneticist.

Genital tract (female) The vagina, cervix, uterus and fallopian tubes.

Gestation The duration of pregnancy.

Gestational diabetes Diabetes that becomes apparent only during pregnancy.

GIFT Gamete intra-fallopian transfer. An assisted reproduction technology treatment for infertility, in which an egg and sperm are artificially placed in the fallopian tube for fertilisation to take place in the normal way.

GP General practitioner or family doctor. Doctor with postgraduate training and qualifications in primary health care and family medicine.

GP obstetrician A GP who may also be an LMC, with experience and postgraduate qualifications in obstetrics.

Gullet See Oesophagus.

Gynaecologist Doctor with postgraduate training and qualifications in gynaecology.

Gynaecology The science and medicine of disorders particular to women. Usually studied in conjunction with obstetrics.

H

Haemophilia Condition in which the blood fails to clot, caused by a lack of one or more clotting factors.

Haemorrhage Heavy bleeding.

Haemorrhoids Piles. Swellings around the anus caused by pressure on the veins in that area.

HCG Human chorionic gonadotrophin. A hormone produced in pregnancy which acts on the ovaries to stimulate production of oestrogen and progesterone. This is the hormone measured in pregnancy tests.

HDC Health and Disability Commissioner.

Heart attack Myocardial infarction. Blockage in the blood supply to the heart (see Atherosclerosis), causing the death of a portion of heart muscle. Usually heralded by severe chest pain.

Heartburn Condition in which acid from the stomach is regurgitated into the oesophagus, causing pain in the chest.

Hepatitis Infection of the liver. Can be severe. There are several types: hepatitis A (infectious hepatitis) and hepatitis B (serum hepatitis) are the most common.

Herpes (herpes simplex) Viral infection which can occur in the genital area. Usually sexually transmitted. Can be recurrent.

Hib Haemophilus influenzae type b. A common bacteria which can cause ear, throat and chest infections and some types of meningitis.

HIV Human immunodeficiency virus. A virus which eventually leads to AIDS (Acquired immunodeficiency syndrome). With modern treatment, this may not happen for many years. Most often sexually transmitted, but can be transmitted via blood products, or passed from mother to baby during pregnancy, labour or breastfeeding.

Homeopathy Treatment of disease by homeopathic drugs (usually in minute doses) which in healthy people would produce symptoms like those of the disease.

HPL Human placental lactogen. Hormone produced in pregnancy to prepare the breasts for lactation.

HPV Human papilloma virus. A common virus group, some of which may cause cervical abnormalities (detected by cervical smears) or genital warts.

Human Assisted Reproduction Technologies (HART) Act An Act of Parliament setting out provisions for the use of assisted reproduction technologies in New Zealand. See also ART.

Human chorionic gonadotrophin See HCG.

Human placental lactogen See HPL.

Human papilloma virus See HPV.

Hydrocephalus Condition in which the circulation of cerebrospinal fluid around the brain is obstructed, causing swelling within the skull which restricts brain growth and development.

Hyperemesis (gravidarum) Severe vomiting in pregnancy.

Hypertension High blood pressure.

Hypertension of pregnancy See Pre-eclampsia.

Hypothyroidism Condition in which hormone production from the thyroid gland is deficient. In infants, it can cause permanent mental retardation.

I

Immune Resistant (to a particular disease).

Immunoglobulins Complex protein molecules in the body which help it to develop resistance to infection.

Incontinence (urinary) Involuntary leaking of urine from the bladder via the urethra.

Insulin Substance produced by the pancreas which removes sugar from the blood to the cells of the body. Absent or deficient in diabetes.

Intercourse (sexual) Coitus. Insertion of the penis into the vagina during sexual arousal.

Intestine Coiled, tube-like structure within the abdomen where nutrients are absorbed from food.

In vitro fertilisation See IVF.

Intubation Insertion of a tube into the trachea (windpipe) to assist breathing.

Intra-uterine contraceptive device See IUCD.

Intra-uterine growth restriction See IUGR.

Intravenous line See IV line.

IRD Inland Revenue Department.

Ischium One of the bones in the pelvic ring.

IUCD (or IUD) Intra-uterine contraceptive device. A small plastic device introduced into the uterus to prevent pregnancy.

IUGR Intra-uterine growth restriction. Slower than usual growth of a foetus within the uterus.

IV line Intravenous line. Sometimes known as a drip. Plastic tube inserted into a vein to provide a continuous supply of fluid.

IVF In vitro fertilisation. An advanced treatment for infertility, in which a human egg is fertilised outside the body and then implanted into the uterus.

J

Jaundice A yellow hue of the skin, found in people with high levels of bilirubin in their blood. Common in infants.

K

Kidneys Paired organs in the loin where toxic substances are removed from the blood, and urine is made to enable these substances to be passed out of the body via the ureters, bladder and urethra.

Konakion Vitamin K.

L

Lacrimal (duct) Channel which drains tears from the eye into the nasal passages.

Lactation Process of producing milk within the breast.

Lactation consultant A midwife, nurse, doctor or other person who has training and qualifications in the art and science of lactation and breastfeeding (IBCLC – International Board Certified Lactation Consultant).

LAM Lactational amenorrhoea method. A method of contraception suitable for use when women are fully breastfeeding.

Lead maternity carer See LMC.

LH Luteinising hormone. One of the hormones produced from the pituitary gland which acts on the ovary.

Lie (of a foetus) Way in which the foetus is lying within the uterus, e.g. transverse.

Ligaments Bundles of tissue which hold bones together.

Listeriosis Uncommon disease, caused by a bacterial infection, which may result in miscarriage, premature birth or still birth.

Liver Large organ in the upper right region of the abdomen where potentially harmful substances are broken down into other less harmful substances which can then be excreted from the body.

LMC (lead maternity carer) The health professional (most often a midwife, but occasionally a doctor) who is responsible for the overall health care of a woman during pregnancy, labour, birth, and after the birth.

LMP First day of the last menstrual period. Pregnancy is usually regarded as starting on this date.

LOA Left occipito anterior. One of the positions a baby's head may assume within the pelvis before birth.

LOP Left occipito posterior. One of the positions a baby's head may assume within the pelvis before birth.

LSCS Lower segment Caesarean section. See Caesarean.

Luteinising hormone See LH.

M

Mammography A soft-tissue X-ray of the breast tissue, used to screen women for possible breast cancer. Can also be used to detect other breast conditions.

Mastitis Inflammation of lactating breast tissue.

Measles (English) Childhood infection characterised by a rash, lethargy, runny nose and sore eyes. Can lead to pneumonia and, rarely, death.

Meconium Sticky black substance within the bowel of a foetus. Passed during or soon after birth.

Membranes Bag of tissue containing the amniotic fluid which surrounds a foetus.

Menarche A young woman's first menstrual period.

Meningitis A serious, rapidly progressive infection of the coverings of the brain (meninges) and sometimes also the blood (septicaemia). Often fatal without immediate treatment.

Menopause A woman's last menstrual period. Has also come to mean the time around the last menstrual period, and may be associated with hot flushes, sleep disturbances and mood swings.

Menstruation Menstrual period. The monthly blood loss from the vagina during the female reproductive cycle, where the lining of the uterus is shed if the egg (ovum) has not been fertilised.

Metabolism The normal body function. Often used to mean specifically the processing and changing of food and other substances (e.g. food, drugs, poisons) within the body.

Mid-stream urine See MSU.

Midwife Health professional with training and qualifications in maternity care who has specialised in the care of women during pregnancy, labour and birth, and the post-natal period.

Miscarriage Spontaneous abortion. The spontaneous loss of a pregnancy, usually within the first 3–4 months.

MMR Measles, mumps and rubella vaccine.

MRI Magnetic resonance imaging. A detailed imaging technique for viewing many internal organs.

MSS Maternal serum screening. A prenatal screening test, using a blood sample from the mother to assess the risk of some foetal abnormalities.

MSU Mid-stream urine. The type of urine sample required to check for infection in the urine.

Mucous Thick fluid secreted in various parts of the body.

Multipara Woman who is giving (or has given) birth to her second or subsequent child.

N

Narcotic Class of drugs which affect the senses and are used principally to relieve pain.

Nasogastric tube Tube passed through the nose, down the oesophagus and into the stomach.

Nausea Feeling of wanting to vomit.

Neonate Newborn baby up to one month old. If premature, the baby will be a neonate for the number of weeks premature plus one month.

Neural tube defect See NTD.

NIR National Immunisation Register.

NTD Neural tube defect. A fault in the early development of the tissue that becomes the brain and spinal cord in an embryo. Anencephaly and spina bifida are different types of neural tube defect.

NTS Nuchal translucency scan. An ultrasound scan done at 11-13 weeks to measure the neck (nuchal) thickness. When combined with other information, this is a prenatal screening test for Down syndrome and other chromosomal abnormalities. See also Prenatal testing or prenatal diagnosis, Screening test.

Nullipara Woman who has never borne a child.

NVD Normal vaginal delivery

O

Obstetrician Doctor with postgraduate training and qualifications in obstetrics.

Obstetrics The science and medicine of pregnancy and childbirth.

Occiput Area of the head on the opposite side to the face.

Oedema Swelling of the body tissues, usually with excess fluid.

Oesophagus Gullet. Tube-like structure connecting the mouth with the stomach.

Oestriol A type of oestrogen.

Oestrogen A hormone produced cyclically by the ovaries throughout a woman's reproductive years.

Oligohydramnios Condition in which there is less amniotic fluid than usual within the pregnancy sac.

Orthopaedic surgeon Doctor with postgraduate training and qualifications in orthopaedics.

Orthopaedics The science and medicine of the limbs, principally the bones, muscles, joints, tendons and ligaments.

OSFA One size fits all (in relation to nappy sizes).

Ovaries Paired organs within a woman's pelvis which contain eggs (ova). Also responsible for the production of oestrogen and progesterone.

Ovulation Process of releasing a human egg from the ovary.

Oxytocin Hormone which allows milk to be released from the breast and encourages the uterus to contract after childbirth.

P

Paediatrician Doctor with postgraduate training and qualifications in paediatrics.

Paediatrics The science and medicine of children's diseases.

Palpation (of the abdomen) Examination of the abdominal area, using one or two hands.

Pancreas Organ at the back of the abdominal cavity, where insulin is produced.

Paracetamol Panadol. A pain-relieving drug, often given to children in liquid form.

Parturition Birth.

Pathologist Doctor with postgraduate training and qualifications in pathology.

Pathology The study of human tissue, including blood, and bacteria found within the body.

PD Peak day. Time in a woman's reproductive cycle when fertility is at its peak.

Pelvic inlet Space formed by the top of the pelvic ring.

Pelvic outlet Space formed by the bottom of the pelvic ring.

Pelvimetry Measurement of the spaces within the pelvic ring. Can now be done by CT-scan.

Penis The male sex organ.

Perinatal Around the time of birth.

Perineum Area of skin and tissue between the vaginal opening and the anal opening.

Peritonitis Inflammation of the covering of the bowel.

Pertussis Whooping cough. An infectious disease of childhood, characterised by a peculiar cough.

Pessaries Tablets made to be inserted into the vagina.

Pethidine Narcotic drug, used to relieve pain.

Phenylketonuria See PKU.

PHO Primary Health Organisation.

Phototherapy Exposure of an infant to the blue spectrum of light to reduce the amount of bilirubin in the blood when the level is too high.

Physiology The study of body function.

Pituitary gland Small gland at the base of the brain which produces hormones.

PKU Phenylketonuria. A condition where the lack of a particular enzyme in the body results in failure to process some proteins. Can lead to severe mental retardation.

Placenta Afterbirth. Whenua. Organ within a pregnant uterus which is responsible for obtaining oxygen and nutrients from the mother's bloodstream for the growing foetus.

Plagiocephaly Flat head. A condition where a baby's head becomes slightly misshapen due to persistent pressure on one part of the head, often from sleeping in only one position.

Pneumonia Severe infection of a section of the lungs.

Polio (poliomyelitis) Infectious disease causing inflammation of part of the spinal cord. Can cause partial or complete paralysis.

Polyhydramnios Condition in which there is a larger amount of amniotic fluid than usual.

POP Progestagen-only pill. A type of contraceptive pill.

Posterior To the back.

Post-mortem Medical examination of the body of someone who has died, in order to establish the cause of death.

Post-natal After birth.

Post-natal depression See Depression.

Post-natal midwife A fully trained midwife who specialises in looking after women in the post-natal period, often in conjunction with one or more LMCs.

Post-partum After birth.

PPH Post-partum haemorrhage. Heavy bleeding after birth from the uterus, cervix or vagina.

Practice nurse Nurse who works in primary care, often as a member of a general practice health care team.

Pre-eclampsia Disease of pregnancy in which there is high blood pressure, oedema, protein in the urine, and an adverse effect on placental function. In its severe form, pre-eclampsia becomes eclampsia, threatening the life of the baby and/or the mother.

Premature (baby) Baby born before 37 weeks' gestation.

Prenatal testing or prenatal diagnosis Tests that can be done to check whether a baby is developing normally in the uterus. Some are initial screening tests, which estimate the risk of the baby having a problem. Others are diagnostic tests, which are much more accurate in detecting a developmental problem. See also Diagnostic test, Screening test.

Primipara Woman who is giving (or has given) birth to her first child.

Progestagen Synthetic analogue of progesterone.

Progesterone Hormone produced by the ovaries.

Prolapse (of the uterus) Abnormally low position of the uterus within the pelvis, caused by lax ligaments and muscles at the base of the pelvis.

Prostaglandins Group of hormones produced within the body. One type of prostaglandins makes the uterus contract.

PT Pregnancy test.

PTSD Post-traumatic stress disorder.

Puerperal sepsis (puerperal fever) Infection within the genital tract after childbirth. Can be fatal without antibiotic treatment.

Pulmonary embolus Clot of blood, usually formed in the leg, which moves into the lungs and severely affects breathing. May be fatal.

PV Per vaginum. A vaginal examination (also known as VE).

Pyelonephritis Infection within the kidney.

Pyridoxine Vitamin B6.

R

Rectum Area of the bowel immediately before the anus.

Renal colic Pain caused by a kidney stone moving down the ureter.

Retroverted (uterus) Uterus which is tipped backwards within the pelvis.

Rh Rhesus factor. Name given to a series of blood groups. Lack of the Rhesus factor in a mother (Rh-negative) may result in Rhesus disease if her baby is Rh-positive.

Ripening (of the cervix) Softening and shortening of the cervix in preparation for labour.

RM Ruptured membranes.

ROA Right occipito anterior. One of the positions a baby's head may assume in the pelvis before birth.

Rooting reflex Instinctive turning of a newborn baby's head when the cheek is touched.

ROP Right occipito posterior. One of the positions a baby's head may assume in the pelvis before birth.

Rubella German measles. An infectious disease which may severely affect a foetus if the mother contracts it during pregnancy.

S

Sac (pregnancy) Bag containing amniotic fluid and the foetus, formed by the membranes within the uterus in pregnancy.

Schizophrenia Disorder of the mind, possibly caused by biochemical changes. Characterised by periods of hallucination.

Screening test A test that is available to screen everyone in an apparently well population for a particular condition. In relation to prenatal testing, to check whether a baby is developing normally, this may be a maternal serum test (MSS) or a nuchal transluceny scan (NTS), which is safe for the baby but only estimates the risk of having a certain condition. See also Diagnostic test, Prenatal testing or prenatal diagnosis.

Scrotum Bag of tissue containing the testes in a male.

Semen Fluid produced from a man's penis during ejaculation. It normally contains sperm.

Septicaemia Infection of the blood, causing severe illness.

SIDS Sudden infant death syndrome. Cot death. See also SUDI.

Sign (of illness) Something that is apparent to another person, e.g. a rash.

SPD Symphysis pubis dysfunction. Softening of the ligaments, causing pain at the symphysis pubis during pregnancy.

Speculum An instrument used to clinically examine the vagina and cervix.

Sperm Male sex cells produced within the testes.

Spermicide Substance that kills sperm if in direct contact.

Spina bifida A type of neural tube defect. A fault in the early development of the spinal cord and/or its coverings. See also NTD.

SRM Spontaneous rupture of the membranes.

Stethoscope Instrument used to listen to sounds within the body, principally in the heart and lungs.

STI Sexually transmitted infection.

Stroke Blockage in the blood supply to a portion of the brain, resulting in death of an area of tissue and consequent lack of function, often in an arm or a leg, or affecting speech.

Sudden infant death syndrome See SIDS.

SUDI Sudden unexplained death in infancy. Term sometimes used instead of SIDS or cot death.

Sutures Stitches used to hold tissue on either side of a wound together so that it may heal.

Swab Sample of material taken from the body in order to identify bacteria which may be causing infection.

Symphysis pubis Place where the pelvic bones join in the midline at the front.

Symptom (of illness) Something a person has noticed themselves which may indicate disease, but is not necessarily apparent to anyone else, e.g. tiredness.

T

TENS Transcutaneous electrical nerve stimulation. A method of relieving pain in labour.

Testes Paired male organs in the scrotum where sperm are made. Commonly known as 'balls'.

Tetanus Infection caused by bacteria which live in the soil. Can be fatal in severe cases.

Thrombosis Clot which forms in a blood vessel. See also DVT.

Thrush (infection) Yeast infection which may occur in the vagina as well as in other places. May cause an itchy vaginal discharge.

Thyroid A gland at the front of the neck which controls the metabolic rate of the body functions. If under-active, causes hypothyroidism; if over-active, causes hyperthyroidism.

Toxaemia See Eclampsia, Pre-eclampsia.

Toxoplasmosis Infection often carried by domestic cats which in rare cases can cause miscarriage in humans.

Trachea Windpipe. Structure connecting the mouth and nose to the lungs.

Transverse lie Position of foetus lying across the uterus with its back or shoulder towards the cervix). See also Lie (of a foetus).

Trimester Three-month period of pregnancy.

Tuberculosis Disease caused by the tubercle bacteria which can affect the whole body but commonly affects the lungs. Can be fatal if left untreated.

Tummy tuck An exercise recommended during lifting, and for strengthening the abdominal muscles during and after pregnancy.

U

Ultrasound scan A method of visualising soft-tissue structures within the body. Used during pregnancy to check the growing foetus and uterus.

Umbilicus Tummy button. Place on the abdomen where the umbilical cord was attached before birth.

Ureter Tube which carries urine from the kidney to the bladder.

Urethra Tube which carries urine from the bladder to outside the body.

Urine Fluid produced by the kidneys to carry waste products out of the body.

Uterus Womb. Organ at the top of the vagina. Has a lining which is normally shed monthly unless pregnancy occurs. During pregnancy, the uterus greatly enlarges, containing the growing foetus within the pregnancy sac.

V

Vagina Passage from the outside of a woman's body to the uterus, in which a man's penis is placed during sexual intercourse. Forms part of the birth canal during childbirth.

Vas deferens Tube which carries sperm from the testes to the urethra in a man.

VBAC Vaginal birth after a Caesarean. Having a baby by vaginal delivery after a Caesarean delivery in an earlier pregnancy.

VE Vaginal examination, also known as PV.

Ventouse (vacuum) A suction device used to assist the birth of a baby during the second stage of labour.

Vernix White, cheesy material which covers a foetus within the uterus.

Vitamin K Substance required in tiny amounts for the clotting of blood.

W

Waters See amniotic fluid.

Whenua See placenta.

Whooping cough See Pertussis.

LIST OF ILLUSTRATIONS

This list includes captioned photographs, drawings and diagrams.

REFERENCES

Introduction

1 Statistics New Zealand, *Births and deaths; March 2008 quarter*, p.4, www.stats.govt.nz/NR/rdonlyres/98E7CDCE-888B-4068-8A00-A14D7E5CE24C/0/birthsanddeathsmaro8qtrhotp.pdf (accessed 29 June 2008).

Chapter 1: Planning for pregnancy

1 P. Bateson, D. Barker & T. Clutton-Brock, 'Developmental plasticity and human health', *Nature*, Vol.430, 2004, pp.419–21.

2 Ministry of Health, *Food and nutrition guidelines for healthy pregnant and breastfeeding women*, Wellington, 2006.

Ministry of Health, *Food and nutrition guidelines for healthy adults: A background paper*, Wellington, 2003.

3 Ministry of Health, *Food and nutrition guidelines for healthy pregnant and breastfeeding women*, Wellington, 2006.

4 Hillary Commission, *Movement = health*, Wellington, 2001.

5 Cancer Society of New Zealand, *The quit book*, revised edn, Ministry of Health, Wellington, 2004.

6 Alcohol Advisory Council of New Zealand, 'Pregnancy', www.alac.org.nz/Pregnancy (accessed 12 February 2008).

7 B. Sood, V. Delaney-Black, C. Covington, et al., 'Prenatal alcohol exposure and childhood behaviour at 6 to 7 years', *Pediatrics*, Vol.108, August 2001, p.E34.

8 Alcohol Advisory Council of New Zealand, 'Pregnancy', www.alac.org.nz/Pregnancy (accessed 12 February 2008).

9 Ministry of Health, Chapter 13: 'Cervical cancer', in *Cancer in New Zealand: Trends and projections*, Wellington, 2002.

10 Ministry of Health, *HPV Immunisation Programme overview*, www.moh.govt.nz/moh.nsf/indexmh/immunisation-diseasesandvaccines-hpv-programme#overview (accessed 8 July 2008).

Helen Clark, 2 May 2008, *Announcement of the HPV Vaccine Programme*, www.beehive.govt.nz/speech/announcement+hpv+vaccine+programme (accessed 8 July 2008)

11 National Cervical Screening Programme, *Cervical screening: A guide for women in New Zealand*, Ministry of Health, Wellington, 2005.

12 E. Davey, A. Barrett, L. Irwig, et al., 'Effect of study design and quality on unsatisfactory rates, cytology classifications, and accuracy in liquid-based versus conventional cervical cytology: A systematic review', *The Lancet*, Vol.367, 2006, pp.122–32.

13 Ministry of Health, *Sexual and reproductive health: A resource book for New Zealand health care organisations*, Wellington, 2003.

14 Ministry of Health, *Sexual and reproductive health: A resource book for New Zealand health care organisations*, Wellington, 2003.

15 S. McAlister, AIDS Epidemiology Group, 'HIV and AIDS in New Zealand 2006', *AIDS – New Zealand*, Vol.59, 2007.

16 Ministry of Health, Chapter 12: 'Breast cancer', in *Cancer in New Zealand: Trends and projections*, Wellington, 2002.

17 National Screening Unit, *Breastscreen Aotearoa: National policy and quality standards*, Ministry of Health, Wellington, 2004.

National Screening Unit, *A literature review to inform a decision on the most appropriate breast screening interval for women aged 45–49 years in New Zealand*, Ministry of Health, Wellington, 2004.

18 J. Guillebaud, *Contraception: Your questions answered*, 4th edn, Churchill Livingstone, Edinburgh, 2004.

19 D. Scholes, A.Z. LaCroix, L.E. Ichikawa, W.E. Barlow & S.M. Ott, 'Change in bone mineral density among adolescent women using and discontinuing depot medroxyprogesterone acetate contraception', *Archives of Pediatric and Adolescent Medicine*, Vol.159, 2005, pp.139–44.

20 L. Cheng, A. Gülmezoglu & C. Van Oel, 'Interventions for emergency contraception', *Cochrane Database of Systematic Reviews*, Issue 3, 2004.

21 C. Paul, 'Contraceptive practice in New Zealand', *New Zealand Medical Journal*, Vol.101, 1988, pp.809–13.

22 Auckland District Health Board, 'National Women's Newborn Services Clinical Guideline – Down syndrome', www.adhb.govt.nz/newborn/guidelines/anomalies/downsyndrome.htm (accessed 12 February 2008).

23 Statistics New Zealand, *Births and deaths; March 2008 quarter*, p.4, www.stats.govt.nz/NR/rdonlyres/98E7CDCE-888B-4068-8A00-A14D7E5CE24C/0/birthsanddeathsmaro8qtrhotp.pdf (accessed 29 June 2008).

24 MRC Vitamin Study Group, 'Prevention of neural tube defects: Results of a Medical Research Council vitamin study', *The Lancet*, Vol.338, 1991, pp.131–7.

25 J. Dixon, 'Folic acid and neural tube defects in New Zealand: A cautionary tale?', *New Zealand Medical Journal*, Vol.120, No.1254, 2007.

26 Ministry of Health, *Food and nutrition guidelines for healthy pregnant and breastfeeding women*, Wellington, 2006.

27 Ministry of Health, *Immunisation handbook 2006*, Wellington, 2006.

28 Ministry of Health, *Smoking cessation guidelines*, Wellington, 2007.

29 L. Craig, L. Miller & A. Criniti, 'Rapid resumption of ovulation and menstruation following continuous use of the combination oral contraceptive', *Fertility and Sterility*, Vol.83, 2005, p.S16.

A. Farrow, M. Hull, K. Northstone, H. Taylor, W. Ford & J. Golding, 'Prolonged use of oral contraception before a planned pregnancy is associated with a decreased risk of delayed conception', *Human Reproduction*, Vol.17, 2002, pp.2754–61.

30 M. Zinaman, E. Clegg, C. Brown, et al., 'Estimates of human fertility and pregnancy loss', *Fertility and Sterility*, Vol.65, 1996, p.503.

31 W. Kuohung & R. Barbieri, 'Overview of female fertility', in B. Rose (ed.), *UpToDate*, UptoDate, Waltham, MA, 2007.

32 Advisory Committee on Assisted Reproductive Technology, *Annual report 2005–2006*, Wellington, 2007.

33 Advisory Committee on Assisted Reproductive Technology, *Annual report 2005–2006*, Wellington, 2007.

34 C. Gnoth, E. Godehardt, P. Frank-Hermann, K. Friol, J. Tigges & G. Freundl, 'Definition and prevalence of sub-fertility and infertility', *Human Reproduction*, Vol.20, 2005, pp.1144–7.

Chapter 2: Suspecting and confirming pregnancy

1 Family Planning Association, *Pregnancy testing*, www.fpanz.org.nz/OurClinics/NeedHelpNow/PregnancyTesting (accessed 12 February 2008).

2 Health and Disability Commissioner, *The Code of Health and Disability Services Consumers' Rights*, www.hdc.org.nz/theact/theact-thecode (accessed 12 February 2008).

3 Abortion Services in New Zealand, *Abortion procedures*, www.abortion.gen.nz/procedures/index.html (accessed 12 February 2008).

4 K. McRae & L. Nikora, 'Whāngai: Remembering, understanding and experiencing'. MAI Review, Intern Research Report 7, University of Waikato, Hamilton, 2006, p.1.

Chapter 3: The first three months

1 E.D. Albrecht & G.J. Pepe, 'Estrogen maintains pregnancy, triggers fetal maturation', in *ScienceDaily*, 1997, www.sciencedaily.com/releases/1997/03/970321141042.htm

2 Statistics New Zealand, *Demographic trends 2006*, Wellington, 2007.

3 New Zealand Food Safety Authority, *Food safety in pregnancy*, Wellington, 2004.

4 M. Verberg, D. Gillott, N. Al-Fardan & J. Grudzinskas, 'Hyperemesis gravidarum: A literature review', *Human Reproduction Update*, Vol.11, 2005, pp.527–39.

5 E. Furneaux, A. Langley-Evans & S. Langley-Evans, 'Nausea and vomiting of pregnancy: Endocrine basis and contribution to pregnancy outcome', *Obstetrical and Gynecological Survey*, Vol.56, 2001, pp.775–82.

P. Lagiou, R. Tamimi, L. Mucci, D. Trichopoulos, H. Adami & C. Hsieh, 'Nausea and vomiting in pregnancy in relation to prolactin, estrogens, and progesterone: A prospective study', *Obstetrics and Gynecology*, Vol.101, 2003, pp.639–44.

6 E. Werntoft & A. Dykes, 'Effect of acupressure on nausea and vomiting during pregnancy: A randomized, placebo-controlled, pilot study', *Journal of Reproductive Medicine*, Vol.46, 2001, pp.835–9.

7 P. Aikins Murphy, 'Alternative therapies for nausea and vomiting of pregnancy', *Obstetrics and Gynecology*, Vol.91, 1998, pp.149–55.

K. Willetts, A. Ekangaki & J. Eden, 'Effect of a ginger extract on pregnancy-induced nausea: A randomised controlled trial', *Australian and New Zealand Journal of Obstetrics and Gynaecology*, Vol.43, 2003, pp.139–44.

Ministry of Health, *Food and nutrition guidelines for healthy adults: A background paper*, Wellington, 2003.

8 D. Tiran, *Nausea and vomiting in pregnancy: An integrated approach to care*, Churchill Livingston, London, 2004.

9 As at 2008, such products include 'Inner Health Plus'.

10 As at 2008, such products include 'KiwiCrush', available from most supermarkets.

11 S. Bryan, 'Current challenges in the assessment and management of patients with bleeding in early pregnancy', *Emergency Medicine Australasia*, Vol.15, 2003, pp.219–22.

12 Miscarriage Support, *Understanding miscarriage*, Pamphlet, Miscarriage Support Auckland Inc.

13 E. Jauniaux, R. Farquharson, O. Christiansen & N. Exalto, 'Evidence-based guidelines for the investigation and medical treatment of recurrent miscarriage', *Human Reproduction*, Vol.21, 2006, pp.2216–22.

14 Midwifery Council of New Zealand, www.midwiferycouncil.org.nz

15 Royal Australian and New Zealand College of Obstetricians and Gynaecologists, 'Membership/fellowship elevation', www.ranzcog.edu.au/about/pdfs/Constitution.pdf (accessed 3 November 2007).

Medical Council of New Zealand, www.mcnz.org.nz

16 Ministry of Health, *Your pregnancy: Tō hapūtanga*, Wellington, 2004.

17 Ministry of Health, *Your pregnancy: Tō hapūtanga*, Wellington, 2004.

18 J. Sherwood, *Chlamydia screening in New Zealand: Report for the National Screening Unit*, Ministry of Health, Wellington, 2006.

19 Ministry of Health, *Immunisation handbook 2006*, Wellington, 2006.

20 National Health and Medical Research Council, *Australian immunization handbook*, 2003, www9.health.gov.au/immhandbook

21 National Screening Unit, Ministry of Health, 'Antenatal HIV screening', www.nsu.govt.nz/current-nsu-programmes (accessed 12 February 2008).

22 Antenatal Down Syndrome Advisory Group, *Antenatal Down syndrome screening in New Zealand 2007*, Ministry of Health, Wellington, 2007.

23 J. Dixon, *Prenatal diagnosis information sheet*, New Zealand Genetic Services, Wellington, 2005.

24 Z. Alfirevic, K. Sundberg & S. Brigham, 'Amniocentesis and chorionic villus sampling for prenatal diagnosis', *Cochrane Database of Systematic Reviews*, Issue 3, 2003.

Chapter 4: The second three months

1 D. Betts, *The essential guide to acupuncture in pregnancy and childbirth*, The Journal of Chinese Medicine, Hove, 2006.

2 M. Sutton, 'Planning for a healthy pregnancy and traveling while pregnant', in *CDC Health Information for International Travel Yellow Book*, Centers for Disease Control and Prevention, Atlanta, GA, 2008.

3 The Travel Doctor, 'New Zealand clinics', www.traveldoctor.co.nz/NZclinics/NZclinics.php (accessed 12 February 2008).

4 D. Carroll & A. Van Gompel, 'The pregnant wilderness traveler', *Travel Medicine and Infectious Disease*, Vol.3, 2005, pp.225–38.

5 G. Davies, L. Wolfe, M. Mottola & C. MacKinnon, 'Exercise in pregnancy and the postpartum period', SOGC/CSEP Joint Clinical Practice Guideline 129, *Journal of Obstetrics and Gynaecology Canada*, Vol.25, 2003, pp.516–22.

6 M. Kramer & S. McDonald, 'Aerobic exercise for women during pregnancy', *Cochrane Database of Systematic Reviews*, Issue 3, 2006.

7 E. Lumbers, 'Exercise in pregnancy: Physiological basis of exercise prescription for the pregnant woman', *Journal of Science and Medicine in Sport*, Vol.5, 2002, pp.20–31.

8   G. Davies, L. Wolfe, M. Mottola & C. MacKinnon, 'Exercise in pregnancy and the postpartum period', SOGC/CSEP Joint Clinical Practice Guideline 129, *Journal of Obstetrics and Gynaecology Canada*, Vol.25, 2003, pp.516–22.

D. Araujo, 'Expecting questions about exercise and pregnancy?', *The Physician and Sports Medicine*, Vol.25, 1997, pp.85–93.

9   G. Davies, L. Wolfe, M. Mottola & C. MacKinnon, 'Exercise in pregnancy and the postpartum period', SOGC/CSEP Joint Clinical Practice Guideline 129, *Journal of Obstetrics and Gynaecology Canada*, Vol.25, 2003, pp.516–22.

10 Continence Foundation of Australia, *Pelvic floor muscle training for women*, Information leaflet, Parkville, 2006.

Continence Foundation of Australia, *Pelvic floor muscles: A consumer education resource for health professionals*, Parkville, 2006.

11 K. Bo, B. Berghmans, S. Morkved & M. Van Kampen, *Evidence-based physical therapy for the pelvic floor: Bridging science and clinical practice*, Elsevier, Amsterdam, 2007.

12 R. Sapsford, J. Bullock-Saxton & S. Markswell, *Women's health: A text book for physiotherapists*, Saunders, London, 1998.

13 T. Spitznagle, F. Leong & L. Van Dillen, 'Prevalence of diastasis recti abdominis in a urogynecological patient population', *International Urogynecology Journal*, Vol.18, 2007, pp.321–8.

14 Ministry of Health, *Food and nutrition guidelines for healthy pregnant and breastfeeding women*, Wellington, 2006.

15 T. Scholl, 'Iron status during pregnancy: Setting the stage for mother and infant', *American Journal of Clinical Nutrition*, 81 (Supplement), 2005, pp.1218–22.

16 A. Heath & S. Fairweather-Tait, 'Health implications of iron overload: The role of diet and genotype', *Nutrition Reviews*, Vol.61, 2003, pp.45–62.

17 A. Judkins & C. Eagleton, 'Vitamin D deficiency in pregnant New Zealand women', *New Zealand Medical Journal*, Vol.119, No.1241, 2006.

18 L. Magloire & E. Funai, 'Gestational hypertension', in B. Rose (ed.), *UpToDate*, UpToDate, Waltham, MA, 2007.

19 V. Barss & R. Blatman, 'Obstetrical management of pregnancy complicated by diabetes mellitus', in B. Rose (ed.), *UpToDate*, UpToDate, Waltham, MA, 2007.

20 L. Jovanovic, 'Screening and diagnosis of gestational diabetes mellitus', in B. Rose (ed.), *UpToDate*, UpToDate, Waltham, MA, 2007.

21 Y. Divon & A. Ferber, 'Fetal growth restriction: Etiology', in B. Rose (ed.), *UpToDate*, UpToDate, Waltham, MA, 2007.

22 J. Johnson & J. Iams, 'Cervical insufficiency', in B. Rose (ed.), *UpToDate*, UpToDate, Waltham, MA, 2008.

23 A. Cust, B.A. Darlow & D.A. Donoghue, on behalf of the Australian New Zealand Neonatal Network (ANZNN), 'Outcomes for high risk New Zealand newborn infants in 1998–1999: A population based, national study', *Archives of Disease in Childhood – Fetal and Neonatal Edition*, Vol.88, 2003, pp.F15–F22.

24 Z. Alfirevic, K. Sundberg & S. Brigham, 'Amniocentesis and chorionic villus sampling for prenatal diagnosis', *Cochrane Database of Systematic Reviews*, Issue 3, 2003.

25 M. Sangalli, F. Langdana & C. Thurlow, 'Pregnancy loss rate following routine genetic amniocentesis at Wellington Hospital', *New Zealand Medical Journal*, Vol.117, No.1191, 2004.

26 Royal Australian and New Zealand College of Obstetricians and Gynaecologists, 'Amniocentesis and chorionic villus sampling (CVS)', in *A guide on prenatal diagnostic procedures*, 3rd edn, Mi-tec Medical Publishing, Melbourne, 2006.

27 J. Ferguson, W. Hansen, K. Novak & M. Novak, 'Should we treat periodontal disease during gestation to improve pregnancy outcomes?', *Clinical Obstetrics and Gynaecology*, Vol.50, 2007, pp.454–67.

K. Boggess & B. Edelstein, 'Oral health in women during preconception and pregnancy: Implications for birth outcomes and infant oral health', *Maternal Child Health Journal*, Vol.10, 2006, pp.S169–74.

28 Ministry of Health, *Food and nutrition guidelines for healthy pregnant and breastfeeding women*, Wellington, 2006.

29 M. Bates, *Fluoridation of water supplies: An evaluation of the recent epidemiological evidence*, ESR for Ministry of Health, Wellington, 2000.

Public Health Commission, *Fluoride and oral health: The Public Health Commission's advice to the Minister of Health*, Wellington, 1995.

30 World Health Organization, *Environmental health criteria for fluorides (EHC227): International programme for chemical safety*, Geneva, 2002.

31 New Zealand Health Information Service, *Report on maternity: Maternal and newborn information 2004*, Ministry of Health, Wellington, 2007.

32 Statistics New Zealand, 'Births and deaths: September 2007 quarter', www.stats.govt.nz/products-and-services/hot-off-the-press/births-and-deaths/births-and-death-sep07qtr-hotp.htm (accessed 12 February 2008).

33 New Zealand Health Information Service, *Report on maternity: Maternal and newborn information 2004*, Ministry of Health, Wellington, 2007.

34 New Zealand Health Information Service, *Report on maternity: Maternal and newborn information 2004*, Ministry of Health, Wellington, 2007.

35 New Zealand Health Information Service, *Report on maternity: Maternal and newborn information 2004*, Ministry of Health, Wellington, 2007.

36 New Zealand Health Information Service, *Report on maternity: Maternal and newborn information 2004*, Ministry of Health, Wellington, 2007.

37 Ministry of Health, *Food and nutrition guidelines for healthy infants and toddlers (aged 0–2): A background paper*, Wellington, 2007.

38 Department of Labour, 'Parental leave', www.ers.dol.govt.nz/parentalleave (accessed 12 February 2008).

39 Department of Labour, 'Parental leave', www.ers.dol.govt.nz/parentalleave (accessed 12 February 2008).

40 Department of Labour, 'Forms and sample letters', www.ers.dol.govt.nz/parentalleave/forms (accessed 12 February 2008).

41 Statistics New Zealand, 'A profile of people not in the labour force', www.stats.govt.nz/products-and-services/articles (accessed 6 December 2007).

42 Ministry of Social Development, 'Domestic Purposes Benefit', www.workandincome.govt.nz (accessed 12 February 2008).

43 Kaikoura District Council, 'Cloth Nappy Cash Back Scheme', www.kaikoura.govt.nz/projects/cloth_nappy_schemeclo.htm?xhighlightwords=nappy (accessed 29 June 2008).

44 E. Mitchell, E. Robinson, P. Black, et al., 'Risk factors for asthma at 3.5 and 7 years of age', *Clinical and Experimental Allergy*, Vol.37, 2007, pp.1747–55.

45 Child Safety Foundation NZ, *Child restraints save lives*, Information leaflet, Land Transport NZ, Wellington, 2007.

46 Royal NZ Plunket Society, *Children, car seats and airbags*, Information leaflet, Wellington, 2004.

47 Consumer NZ, 'Baby buggies – checklist', www.consumer.org.nz (accessed 12 February 2008).

48 Consumer NZ, 'Baby buggies – safety issues', www.consumer.org.nz (accessed 12 February 2008).

Chapter 5: The last three months

1 G. Hofmeyr, 'Approach to breech presentation', in B. Rose (ed.), *UpToDate*, UpToDate, Waltham, MA, 2008.

2 G. Hofmeyr, 'Approach to breech presentation', in B. Rose (ed.), *UpToDate*, UpToDate, Waltham, MA, 2008.

3 W. Bowes, 'Management of the fetus in transverse lie', in B. Rose (ed.), *UpToDate*, UpToDate, Waltham, MA, 2008.

4 J. Lauwers & A. Swisher, *Counseling the nursing mother: A lactation consultant's guide*, Jones & Bartlett, Sudbury, MA, 2005.

5 C. Lockwood & K. Russo-Stieglitz, 'Clinical manifestations and diagnosis of placenta previa', in B. Rose (ed.), *UpToDate*, UpToDate, Waltham, MA, 2008.

6 D. Fry, 'Perinatal symphysis pubis dysfunction: A review of the literature', *Journal – Association of Chartered Physiotherapists in Women's Health*, Vol.85, 1999, pp.11–18.

7 Y. Ferguson, *Symphysis pubis joint in pregnancy*, Information leaflet, Nelson Marlborough District Health Board, Nelson, 2005.

8 G. Davies, L. Wolfe, M. Mottola & C. MacKinnon, 'Exercise in pregnancy and the postpartum period', SOGC/CSEP Joint Clinical Practice Guideline 129, *Journal of Obstetrics and Gynaecology Canada*, Vol.25, 2003, pp.516–22.

9 J. Robinson, 'Approach to episiotomy', in B. Rose (ed.), *UpToDate*, UpToDate, Waltham, MA, 2008.

10 M. Labreque, E. Eason, S. Marcoux, et al., 'Randomized controlled trial of prevention of perineal trauma by perineal massage during pregnancy', *American Journal of Obstetrics and Gynecology*, Vol.180, 1999, pp.593–600.

11 M. Pomeranz, 'Physiologic changes of the skin, hair, nails and mucous membranes during pregnancy', in B. Rose (ed.), *UpToDate*, UpToDate, Waltham, MA, 2008.

12 New Zealand Health Information Service, *Report on maternity: Maternal and newborn information 2004*, Ministry of Health, Wellington, 2007.

13 S. Chasen & F. Chervenak, 'Antepartum assessment of twin gestations', in B. Rose (ed.), *UpToDate*, UpToDate, Waltham, MA, 2008.

14 E. Norwitz & J. Park, 'Overview of etiology and evaluation of vaginal bleeding in pregnant women', in B. Rose (ed.), *UpToDate*, UpToDate, Waltham, MA, 2008.

15 C. Lockwood, 'Overview of prevention of venous thrombosis in pregnant and postpartum women', in B. Rose (ed.), *UpToDate*, UpToDate, Waltham, MA, 2008.

16 C. Lockwood, 'Overview of prevention of venous thrombosis in pregnant and postpartum women', in B. Rose (ed.), *UpToDate*, UpToDate, Waltham, MA, 2008.

17 K. Moise, 'Prevention of Rh (D) alloimmunization', in B. Rose (ed.), *UpToDate*, UpToDate, Waltham, MA, 2008.

18 Ministry of Health, 'RhoGAM data sheet', www.medsafe.govt.nz/profs/datasheet/r/rhogaminj.htm (accessed 30 January 2008).

19 J. Perloff, C. Waksmonski & M. Foley, 'Pregnancy in women with congenital heart disease', in B. Rose (ed.), *UpToDate*, UpToDate, Waltham, MA, 2008.

20 A. Cust, B.A. Darlow & D.A. Donoghue, on behalf of the Australian New Zealand Neonatal Network (ANZNN), 'Outcomes for high risk New Zealand newborn infants in 1998–1999: A population based, national study', *Archives of Disease in Childhood – Fetal and Neonatal Edition*, Vol.88, 2003, pp.F15–F22.

21 K. Puopolo, L. Madoff & C. Baker, 'Group B streptococcal infection in pregnant women', in B. Rose (ed.), *UpToDate*, UpToDate, Waltham, MA, 2008.

22 New Zealand Herpes Foundation, *Guidelines for the management of genital herpes in New Zealand*, Auckland, 2007.

23 C. Bree, 'Lesbian mothers: Queer families: The experience of planned pregnancy', MHSc thesis, Auckland University of Technology, 2003.

24 D. Mitchell & P. Chapman, *Dads: Part of the team or warming the bench?* Nelson Marlborough Institute of Technology, Nelson, 2002.

25 R. Sapsford, J. Bullock-Saxton & S. Markswell, *Women's health: A text book for physiotherapists*, Saunders, London, 1998.

26 R. Sapsford, J. Bullock-Saxton & S. Markswell, *Women's health: A text book for physiotherapists*, Saunders, London, 1998.

27 A. Frye, *Holistic midwifery. Vol. 1: Care during pregnancy*, Labrys Press, Portland, OR, 1998.

28 New Zealand Guidelines Group, 'Care of women with breech presentation or previous caesarean birth: Best practice evidence-based guideline', www.nzgg.org.nz/guidelines/0074/Caesarean_Full_Guide_(web).pdf#page=52 (accessed 20 April 2008).

M. Coyle, C. Smith & B. Peat, 'Cephalic version by moxibustion for breech presentation', *Cochrane Database of Systematic Reviews*, Issue 2, 2005.

29 A. Jacobs, 'Causes and treatment of postpartum haemorrhage', in B. Rose (ed.), *UpToDate*, UpToDate, Waltham, MA, 2008.

30 W. Prendiville, D. Elbourne & S. McDonald, 'Active versus expectant management in the third stage of labour', *Cochrane Database of Systematic Reviews*, Issue 3, 2000.

Chapter 6: Birth

1 A. Basbaum & H. Fields, 'Endogenous pain control systems: Brainstem spinal pathways and endorphin circuitry', *Annual Reviews of Neuroscience*, Vol.7, 1984, pp.309–38.

New Zealand Council of Midwives, *Labour pains? Making choices*, Christchurch, 2003.

2 S. Jordan, 'Infant feeding and analgesia in labour: The evidence is accumulating', *International Breastfeeding Journal*, Vol.1, 2006, p.25.

3 S. Simmons, A. Cyna, A. Dennis & D. Hughes, 'Combined spinal-epidural versus epidural analgesia in labour', *Cochrane Database of Systematic Reviews*, Issue 3, 2007.

4 D. Betts, *The essential guide to acupuncture in pregnancy and childbirth*, The Journal of Chinese Medicine, Hove, 2006.

5 S. Carlan, J. Lense, W. O'Brien & M. Parsons, 'Preterm premature rupture of membranes: A randomized study of home versus hospital management', *Obstetrics and Gynecology*, Vol.81, 1993, pp.61–4.

6 B. Mercer, 'Preterm premature rupture of membranes', *Obstetrics and Gynecology*, Vol.101, 2003, pp.178–93.

7 S. Kenyon, M. Boulvain & J. Neilson, 'Antibiotics for preterm rupture of membranes', *Cochrane Database of Systematic Reviews*, Issue 2, 2003.

8 H. Scheepers, P. de Jong, G. Essed, et al., 'Fetal and maternal energy metabolism during labor in relation to the available caloric substrate', *Journal of Perinatal Medicine*, Vol.29, 2001, pp.457–64.

9 M. Westgren, K. Kruger, S. Ek, et al., 'Lactate compared with pH analysis at fetal scalp blood sampling: A prospective randomised study', *British Journal of Obstetrics and Gynaecology*, Vol.105, 1998, pp.29–33.

   R. Mason & S. Paterson-Brown, 'Fetal distress and blood lactate monitoring', *British Journal of Midwifery*, Vol.9, 2001, pp.507–9.

10 G. Carroli & J. Belizan, 'Episiotomy for vaginal birth', *Cochrane Database of Systematic Reviews*, Issue 3, 1999.

11 J. Mercer, D. Erickson-Owens, B. Graves & M. Haley, 'Evidence-based practices for the fetal to newborn transition', *Journal of Midwifery and Women's Health*, Vol.52, No.3, 2007, pp.262–72.

12 New Zealand Resuscitation Council, *Newborn life support*, Wellington, 2006.

13 E.R. Cluett, V.C. Nikodem, R. McCandlish & E.E. Burns, 'Immersion in water in pregnancy, labour and birth', *Cochrane Database of Systematic Reviews*, Issue 2, 2002.

   D. Garland, *Waterbirth – an attitude to care*, Oxford Books for Midwives, Oxford, 2000.

14 A. Deans & P. Steer, 'Labour and birth in water: To breathe or not to breathe', *British Medical Journal*, Vol.311, 1995, pp.390–1.

15 T. Levy & I. Blickstein, 'Timing of cord clamping revisited', *Journal of Perinatal Medicine*, Vol.34, 2006, pp.293–7.

   P. Van Rheenen, L. de Moor, S. Eschbach, H. De Grooth & B. Brabin, 'Delayed cord clamping and haemoglobin levels in infancy: A randomised controlled trial in term babies', *Tropical Medicine and International Health*, Vol.12, 2007, pp.603–16.

   C. Chaparro, L. Neufeld, G. Alavex, R. Cedillo & K. Dewey, 'Effect of timing of umbilical cord clamping on iron status in Mexican infants: A randomised controlled trial', *The Lancet*, Vol.367, 2006, pp.1997–2004.

16 A. Kugelman, L. Borenstein-Levin, A. Riskin, et al., 'Immediate versus delayed umbilical cord clamping in premature neonates born <35 weeks: A prospective, randomized, controlled study', *American Journal of Perinatology*, Vol.24, 2007, pp.307–15.

17 W. Prendiville, D. Elbourne & S. McDonald, 'Active versus expectant management in the third stage of labour', *Cochrane Database of Systematic Reviews*, Issue 3, 2000.

18 A. Frye, *Holistic midwifery. Vol. 1: Care during pregnancy*, Labrys Press, Portland, OR, 1998.

19 New Zealand Guidelines Group, *Care of women with breech presentation or previous caesarean birth: Best practice evidence-based guideline*, Ministry of Health, Welington, 2004.

20 F. O'Mahony , G. Hofmeyr & V. Menon, 'Instruments for assisted vaginal delivery (protocol)', *Cochrane Database of Systematic Reviews*, Issue 3, 2005.

21 F. O'Mahony , G. Hofmeyr & V. Menon, 'Instruments for assisted vaginal delivery (protocol)', *Cochrane Database of Systematic Reviews*, Issue 3, 2005.

22 F. Silverman, 'Management of the third stage of labour', in B. Rose (ed.), *UpToDate*, UpToDate, Waltham, MA, 2008.

23 A. Jacobs, 'Causes and treatment of postpartum haemorrhage', in B. Rose (ed.), *UpToDate*, UpToDate, Waltham, MA, 2008.

24 A. Jacobs, 'Causes and treatment of postpartum haemorrhage', in B. Rose (ed.), *UpToDate*, UpToDate, Waltham, MA, 2008.

25 E. Norwitz, 'Patient choice Caesarean delivery', in B. Rose (ed.), *UpToDate*, UpToDate, Waltham, MA, 2008.

26 New Zealand Guidelines Group, *Care of women with breech presentation or previous caesarean birth: Best practice evidence-based guideline*, Ministry of Health, Wellington, 2004.

27 E. Capeless & D. Damron, 'Cesarean delivery', in B. Rose (ed.), *UpToDate*, UpToDate, Waltham, MA, 2008.

28 New Zealand Resuscitation Council, *Newborn life support*, Wellington, 2006.

   C. Fernandes, 'Neonatal resuscitation in the delivery room', in B. Rose (ed.), *UpToDate*, UpToDate, Waltham, MA, 2008.

29 Parent to Parent (Matua ki te Matua) New Zealand, 'Mission statement', www.parent2parent.org.nz/start.htm (accessed 26 January 2008).

Chapter 7: The week after birth

1 National Health and Medical Research Council (NHMRC), *Vitamin K for newborn babies: Information for parents*, Canberra, 2006.

2 National Health and Medical Research Council (NHMRC), *Vitamin K for newborn babies: Information for parents*, Canberra, 2006.

3 E. Moore, G. Anderson & N. Bergman, 'Early skin-to-skin contact for mothers and their healthy newborn infants', *Cochrane Database of Systematic Reviews*, Issue 3, 2007.

4 J. Kinlay, D. O'Connell & S. Kinlay, 'Risk factors for mastitis in breastfeeding women: Results of a prospective cohort study', *Australian and New Zealand Journal of Public Health*, Vol.25, 2001, pp.115–20.

5 S. Cox, *Breastfeeding with confidence: A do-it-yourself guide*, Finch, Sydney, 2004.

6 D. Betts, *The essential guide to acupuncture in pregnancy and childbirth*, The Journal of Chinese Medicine, Hove, 2006.

7 K. Roberts et al., 'A comparison of chilled and room temperature cabbage leaves in treating breast engorgement', *Journal of Human Lactation*, Vol.11, 1995, pp.191–4.

8 World Health Organisation, *HIV transmission through breastfeeding: A review of available evidence*, Geneva, 2004.

9 S. Benson, 'What is normal? A study of normal breastfeeding dyads during the first sixty hours of life', *Breastfeeding Review*, Vol.9, 2001, pp.27–32.

10 D. Stables & J. Rankin (eds), *Physiology in childbearing: With anatomy and related biosciences*, Elsevier, Edinburgh, 2005.

11 Ministry of Health, *Food and nutrition guidelines for healthy pregnant and breastfeeding women*, Wellington, 2004.

12 As at 2008, such products include 'KiwiCrush'.

13 D. Betts, *The essential guide to acupuncture in pregnancy and childbirth*, The Journal of Chinese Medicine, Hove, 2006.

14 P. Chiarelli, *Women's waterworks: Curing incontinence*, Khera Publications, Snohomish, WA, 2004.

15 C. Wilson, N. Kerruish, B. Wilcken, E. Wiltshire & D. Webster, 'The failure to diagnose inborn errors of metabolism in New Zealand: The case for expanded newborn screening', *New Zealand Medical Journal*, Vol.120, No.1262, 2007.

16 National Screening Unit, 'Universal Newborn Hearing Programme', www.nsu.govt.nz/Current-NSU-Programmes/568.asp (accessed 6 February 2008).

17 Ministry of Internal Affairs, 'Notice pursuant to Section 88 of the New Zealand Public Health and Disability Act 2000', *New Zealand Gazette*, Vol.41, 2007, pp.1025–111.

Chapter 8: The first three months with a baby

1 L. Thornley, A. Waa & J. Ball, *Comprehensive plan to inform the design of a national breastfeeding promotion campaign*, Quigley Watts Ltd, for the Ministry of Health, Wellington, 2007.

World Health Organization, *Global strategy for infant and young child feeding*, Geneva, 2003.

2 K. Basire, S. Pullon & D. McLeod, 'Babyfeeding: The thoughts behind the statistics', *New Zealand Medical Journal*, Vol.110, 1997, pp.184–7.

3 J. Kinlay, D. O'Connell & S. Kinlay, 'Risk factors for mastitis in breastfeeding women: Results of a prospective cohort study', *Australian and New Zealand Journal of Public Health*, Vol.25, 2001, pp.115–20.

4 S.H. Wakelin, H. Smith, I.R. White, R.J.G. Rycroft & J.P. McFadden, 'A retrospective analysis of contact allergy to lanolin', *British Journal of Dermatology*, Vol.145, 2001, pp.28–31.

5 L. Amir, D. Forster, H. McLachlan & J. Lumley, 'Incidence of breast abscess in lactating women: Report from an Australian cohort', BJOG: *An International Journal of Obstetrics and Gynaecology*, Vol.111, 2004, pp.1378–81.

6 Ministry of Health, *Food and nutrition guidelines for healthy pregnant and breastfeeding women*, Wellington, 2006.

7 C.M. Hall & L.T. Brody, *Therapeutic exercise: Moving toward function*, Lippincott Williams & Wilkins, Philadelphia, PA, 2004.

8 The Meningitis Trust, 'The glass test', www.meningitis-trust.org/signs-symptoms.html (accessed 4 February 2008).

9 H. Cooke, Child Development Services, *Plagiocephaly*, Information leaflet, Nelson Marlborough District Health Board, Nelson, 2007.

Great Ormond Street Hospital (GOSH), 'Positional plagiocephaly', www.ich.ucl.ac.uk/factsheets/families/F040171/index.html (accessed 4 February 2008).

10 H. Cooke, Child Development Services, *Tummy time*, Information leaflet, Nelson Marlborough District Health Board, Nelson, 2007.

11 New Zealand Health Information Service, *Fetal and infant deaths 2003 and 2004*, Ministry of Health, Wellington, 2007.

12 As at 2008, such products include Mother-Well 'Cap it off'.

13 S. Jones, *Crying babies, sleepless nights: Why your baby is crying and what you can do about it*, The Harvard Common Press, Boston, 1992.

14 M. Donohoe, 'Evidence-based medicine and shaken baby syndrome. Part I: Literature review, 1966–1998', *American Journal of Forensic Medicine and Pathology*, Vol.24, 2003, pp.239–42.

15 S. Lusskin & S. Misri, 'Postpartum blues and depression', in B. Rose (ed.), *UpToDate*, UpToDate, Waltham, MA, 2008.

16 J. Cox & J. Holden, *Perinatal mental health: A guide to the Edinburgh postnatal depression scale (EPDS)*, Gaskell, London, 2003.

Mental Health Foundation of New Zealand, *Postnatal depression: Getting the support you need*, Information leaflet, Auckland, 2007.

17 D. Bick, C. MacArthur, H. Knowles & H. Winter, *Postnatal care: Evidence and guidelines for management*, Churchill Livingstone, Edinburgh, 2002.

18 Mental Health Foundation of New Zealand, *Postnatal depression: Getting the support you need*, Information leaflet, Auckland, 2007.

19 R. Scragg, E. Mitchell, S. Tonkin & J. Nassall, 'Evaluation of the Cot Death Prevention Programme in South Auckland', *New Zealand Medical Journal*, Vol.106, 1993, pp.8–10.

20 New Zealand Health Information Service, *Fetal and infant deaths 2003 and 2004*, Ministry of Health, Wellington, 2007.

21 D. Paterson, F. Trachtenberg, E. Thompson, et al., 'Multiple serotonergic brainstem abnormalities in sudden infant death syndrome', *Journal of the American Medical Association*, Vol.296, 2006, pp.2124–32.

22 Task Force on Sudden Infant Death Syndrome, 'The changing concept of sudden infant death syndrome: Diagnostic coding shifts, controversies regarding the sleeping environment, and new variables to consider in reducing risk: Policy statement', *Pediatrics*, Vol.116, No.5, 2005, pp.1245–55.

23 Task Force on Sudden Infant Death Syndrome, 'The changing concept of sudden infant death syndrome: Diagnostic coding shifts, controversies regarding the sleeping environment, and new variables to consider in reducing risk: Policy statement', *Pediatrics*, Vol.116, No.5, 2005, pp.1245–55.

24 New Zealand Resuscitation Council, *Resuscitation level 7*, Wellington, 2007.

New Zealand Resuscitation Council, *DRS ABC infant or child collapse – level 2/3*, Wallet card, Wellington, 2007.

25 Ministry of Health, *Well Child – Tamariki Ora National Schedule Handbook*, Wellington, 2002.

26 J. Guillebaud, *Contraception: Your questions answered*, 4th edn, Churchill Livingstone, Edinburgh, 2004.

27 M. Labbok, K. Cooney & S. Coly, *Guidelines: Breastfeeding, family planning, and the lactational amenorrhea method – LAM*, Institute for Reproductive Health, Washington, DC, 1994.

28 Ministry of Health, *Immunisation handbook 2006*, Wellington, 2006.

29 G. Davies, L. Wolfe, M. Mottola & C. MacKinnon, 'Exercise in pregnancy and the postpartum period: SOGC/CSEP Joint Clinical Practice Guideline 129', *Journal of Obstetrics and Gynaecology Canada*, Vol.25, 2003, pp.516–22.

INDEX